Retroperitoneal Robotic and Laparoscopic Surgery

Jean V. Joseph • Hitendra R.H. Patel
(Editors)

Retroperitoneal Robotic and Laparoscopic Surgery

Springer

Editors
Jean V. Joseph, M.D., M.B.A.,
Head-Section of Urologic Laparoscopy and Robotic Surgery, Department of Urology
Wilmot Cancer Center, Center for Robotic Surgery and Innovation
University of Rochester Medical Center
Rochester, New York
USA

Hitendra R.H. Patel, Ph.D., FRCS,
Director of Minimal Access Surgery
Department of Surgery, Endocrine
Women's Health and Urology
University Hospital of North Norway
N-9038 Tromsø, Norway
www.hrhpatel.org

ISBN 978-0-85729-484-5 e-ISBN 978-0-85729-485-2
DOI 10.1007/978-0-85729-485-2
Springer Dordrecht Heidelberg London New York

British Library Cataloguing in Publication Data
A catalogue record for this book is available from the British Library

Library of Congress Control Number: 2011922533

Cover design: eStudioCalamar, Figueres/Berlin

Printed on acid-free paper

Springer is part of Springer Science+Business Media (www.springer.com)

Hitendra dedicates this book to all those wonderful people who support the wonderful world we live in by selfless living (www.mdcf.org)

To the contributors to this text, and to our many colleagues who continue to innovate, and to redefine what is accepted as gold standard, for the betterment of our patients.

Jean V. Joseph

Foreword I

Longevity allows for the witnessing of change and progress over an extended period of time. My personal focus incorporated a period of dramatic technologic advance. From a time when anticipated technology resided in the inventive mind of authors such as Jules Verne and cartoons such as Buck Rogers, the futurists' visions have been exceeded by reality. Medicine has shared in an extraordinary evolution.

Nowhere is this more apparent than in the realm of Urology. The introduction of the PSA determination has markedly improved the prognosis for a large population of men afflicted with the pervasive disorder of prostatic malignancy. The vistas for technologic innovation were opened by the introduction and rapid acceptance of minimally invasive surgical approaches to the removal of disease. The kidney, adrenal, and prostate presented as logical targets. Subsequently, robotic surgery was developed and advanced throughout the panorama of diverse surgical specialties. No specialty has had a more privileged position, in this regard, than Urology.

The editors along with the contributors of this thoroughly current text share their expertise, which is based on a broad personal experience and the critical encounters that they have been exposed to in their pioneering work. As such, their words and accompanying lucid illustrations provide for the readership a compendium that charts a course, which expedites performance, minimizes hazard, and maximizes success in dealing with technical adversity.

Seymour I. Schwartz
Distinguished Alumni Professor of Surgery
University of Rochester School of Medicine and Dentistry

Foreword II

I am honored that Doctors Joseph and Patel have asked me to write an introduction to their text, *Retroperitoneal Robotic and Laparoscopic Surgery.* They did so without knowledge of my experience with, or opinion of, robotic and minimally invasive surgery. With regard to the former, as an aging urologist, I have never performed a "minimally invasive procedure" and therefore can claim a neutral and unbiased stance concerning this technology. With regard to the latter, I can be counted among those in favor of the technology.

I have had the opportunity to watch many minimally invasive and robotic procedures as demonstrated in conferences featuring live surgery and at my home hospital where four urologic oncologists in the department perform these procedures. They are all of an age whereby they were trained extensively, and some exclusively with open surgery, but all, specifically with regard to robotic radical prostatectomy, prefer this, and would rue a return to the open approach. This sentiment is virtually universal among open surgeons who have embarked on a minimally invasive/robotic-controlled approach.

Minimally invasive surgery has brought all surgical procedures under a microscope demanding more precise recording of intra- and postoperative outcomes. In a relatively short period of time minimally invasive surgery has achieved results parallel to open surgery. I believe the promise for further improvement in outcomes is likely because, unlike open surgery, each step is clearly demonstrated and visualized by any number of viewers before the console, each step can be rigidly standardized, and the future of simulator surgery will provide greater opportunity for support of the adage "practice makes perfect." Practice will demand more than performance of an occasional procedure; practice will lead to more adept and therefore more successful "performance of surgery" with better outcomes and reduction of the traumatic insult.

The editors have brought together a timely piece of work, which will truly help current and future surgeons improve their patient outcomes, in the quest of delivering a minimally invasive procedure.

Paul F. Schellhammer
Professor of Urology
Eastern Virginia Medical School

Preface

Minimally invasive surgery has experienced significant growth over the past decades. When compared to other disciplines, the growth in the urology arena has been unrivaled. Procedures that were routinely done using an open approach have been quickly converted to a laparoscopic approach. Nearly every urological procedure has been performed laparoscopically. From the simple to the most complex, the common theme has been the development of a minimally invasive approach to lessen the collateral damage to adjacent structures. There is hardly a laparoscopic urologic procedure where safety and reproducibility have not been demonstrated.

Although laparoscopic urologic procedures are performed worldwide, the growth of minimally invasive urology took a different dimension with the arrival of robot assisted surgery over a decade ago. Many surgeons without laparoscopic skills have successfully made the transition from open to robotic surgery with the goal of providing their patients with an effective – yet minimally invasive – approach and decreasing the burden associated with surgical interventions.

Open abdominal urological procedures evolved from a transabdominal to a retroperitoneal route. Currently the standard open approach to the prostate, whether for benign disease or malignancy, is through the retroperitoneum. Similarly in most open kidney, adrenal, and ureteral cases, the standard approach has been by way of the loin to the retroperitoneal region. However, the vast majority of present day minimally invasive urology is performed transperitoneally.

Although these laparoscopic and robotic procedures were initially defined transperitoneally, extraperitoneal approaches have been thoroughly described, with several centers amassing large amount of experience with this technique. For many, the difficulty in adapting to the laparoscopic equipment is compounded by the unrecognizable anatomy of the retroperitoneal space, where the covering preperitoneal loose areolar or fatty tissue makes most structures similar.

Our objective is to produce a manual focused on the extraperitoneal space, which has long been the domain of the urologist. We have assembled a number of authors who are leaders in the areas they have covered. Detailed descriptions of the retroperitoneal anatomy, and a variety of procedures, with first hand experiences, or "how I do it" are reported, followed by key points at the end of the chapters, to help urologists at every stage make the transition to working in the extraperitoneal space, shortening their learning curve. Whether one is using a laparoscopic or robot assisted approach, the extraperitoneal technique remains an excellent method, to approach the target organ avoiding the abdominal cavity.

A number of individuals have contributed to bringing this manual to fruition. We are grateful to the contributing authors who have taken time from their busy lives as surgeons and teachers to share their talent and experience. It is our sincere hope that sharing their expertise will translate into many more of our urological colleagues learning the extraperitoneal technique for the laparoscopic and robot assisted procedures, as they did for open surgical cases.

We also wish to express our gratitude to Barbara Lopez-Lucio, Melissa Morton, Denise Roland, and the Springer staff for their tireless support and editorial work they contributed in the preparation of this book.

Jean V. Joseph
Hitendra R.H. Patel

Contents

Contributors

Claude C. Abbou, M.D., Ph.D. Department of Urology, CHU Mondor, Créteil, France

Satya B. Allaparthi, MRCS, M.D. Department of Urology, Caritas St. Elizabeth Hospital, Boston, MA, USA

Hany N. Atalah, M.D. Department of Robotic and Minimally Invasive Surgery and Department of Urology, University of Florida, Gainesville, FL, USA

Eric Barret, M.D. Department of Urology, Institut Montsouris, Paris, France

Xavier Cathelineau, M.D. Department of Urology, Institut Montsouris, Paris, France

Douglas M. Dahl, M.D. Department of Urology, Massachusetts General Hospital, Boston, MA, USA

Alexandre de la Taille, M.D., Ph.D. Department of Urology, CHU Mondor, Créteil, France

Minh Do, M.D., Ph.D. Department of Urology, University of Leipzig, Leipzig, Germany

Lori M. Dulabon, D.O. Department of Urology, New York University School of Medicine, New York, NY, USA

Marc Galiano, M.D. Department of Urology, Institut Montsouris, Paris, France

Roman Ganzer, M.D., Ph.D. Department of Urology, University of Regensburg, Regensburg, Germany

Matthew T. Gettman, M.D. Department of Urology, Mayo Clinic, Rochester, MN, USA

Ahmed E. Ghazi, M.D., FEBU Department of Urology, University of Rochester Medical Center, Rochester, NY, USA

Ty T. Higuchi, M.D., Ph.D. Department of Urology, Mayo Clinic, Rochester, MN, USA

Thomas T. Hoang, M.D. Department of Urology, Caritas St. Elizabeth's Medical Center, Tufts University School of Medicine, Houston, TX, USA

Andras Hoznek, M.D. Department of Urology, CHU Mondor, Créteil, France

Mitchell R. Humphreys, M.D. Department of Urology, Mayo Clinic, Phoenix, AZ, USA

Jean V. Joseph, M.D., M.B.A. Professor of Urology and Oncology, Head-Section of Urologic Laparoscopy and Robotic Surgery, Department of Urology, Wilmot Cancer Center, Center for Robotic Surgery and Innovation University of Rochester Medical Center, Rochester, New York NY, USA

Panagiotis Kallidonis, M.D. Department of Urology, University of Patras, Rion, Patras, Greece

Jihad H. Kaouk, M.D. Director, Robotic and Laparoscopic Surgery, Department of Urology, Cleveland Clinic Foundation, Cleveland, OH, USA

Edmund Y. Ko, M.D. Department of Urology, Mayo Clinic, Phoenix, AZ, USA

Iason Kyriazis, M.D. Department of Urology, University of Patras, Rion, Patras, Greece

Evangelos Liatsikos, M.D., Ph.D. Department of Urology, University of Patras, Rion, Patras, Greece

Alan McNeil, M.D., Ph.D. Department of Urology, Western General Hospital, Edinburgh, UK

Alireza Moinzadeh, M.D. Institute of Urology, Lahey Clinic Medical Center, Burlington, MA, USA

Sijo J. Parekattil, M.D. Department of Urology, University of Florida, Gainesville, FL, USA

Hitendra R.H. Patel, Ph.D., FRCS Director of Minimal Access Surgery, Department of Surgery, Endocrine, Women's Health and Urology University Hospital of North Norway, N-9038 Tromsø, Norway

Guillaume Ploussard, M.D. Department of Urology, CHU Mondor, Créteil, France

James R. Porter, M.D. Surgical Robotics, Department of Urology, Swedish Medical Center, Seattle, WA, USA

Sarah P. Psutka, M.D. Department of Urology, Massachusetts General Hospital, Boston, MA, USA

Francois Rozet, M.D. Department of Urology, Institut Montsouris, Paris, France

Laurent Salomon, M.D., Ph.D. Department of Urology, CHU Mondor, Créteil, France

Rafael E. Sanchez-Salas, M.D. Department of Urology, Institut Montsouris, Paris, France

Richard T. Schlinkert, M.D. Department of Surgery, Mayo Clinic, Phoenix, AZ, USA

Michael D. Stifelman, M.D. Department of Urology, NYU Langone Medical Center, New York University School of Medicine, New York, NY, USA

Jens-Uwe Stolzenburg, M.D., Ph.D. Department of Urology, University of Leipzig, Leipzig, Germany

Li-Ming Su, M.D. Department of Urology, University of Florida, Gainesville, FL, USA

Ingolf A. Tuerk, M.D., Ph.D. Department of Urology, St. Elizabeth's Medical Center, Boston, MA, USA

Guy Vallancien, M.D. Department of Urology, Institut Montsouris, Paris, France

Michael A. White, D.O. Center for Laparoscopic and Robotic Surgery, Cleveland Clinic, Glickman Urological and Kidney Institute, Cleveland, OH, USA

Anatomical Aspects of the Extra– and Retroperitoneal Space

1

Ahmed E. Ghazi and Jean V. Joseph

Abstract Laparoscopy has become the forefront of urologic surgery for the management of malignant and nonmalignant diseases. With this, an increasing number of urologists are performing routine and complex laparoscopic procedures with the aim of more minimal invasive approaches, which have the potential for significant reduction in patient morbidity. Understanding the anatomical landmarks and relationships of the urinary tract of these approaches is therefore vital to minimizing complications and maximizing success. Retroperitoneal laparoscopic surgery in urology is becoming relatively common and has led to great familiarity with the retroperitoneal anatomy. Knowledge of the complex anatomy of the entities lying between the posterior abdominal wall and peritoneum and recognition of common variations and their potential implications are crucial for successful surgery of retroperitoneal organs.

This chapter describes the important surface anatomy, relationship of the urinary tract to surrounding organs, and their clinical applications for a better understanding of the extraperitoneal approach to the kidney and pelvis.

Keywords Anatomy • Extraperitoneal space • Laparoscopy • Renal pedicle • Retroperitoneal space

Key Points

- Knowledge of key anatomical surface landmarks (12th rib, iliac crest, anterior superior iliac spine) is essential for optimum trocar placement.
- The psoas muscle is always first to be identified during retroperitoneal access and must always be kept in a horizontal plane.
- The orientation of the vascular pedicle during the retroperitoneal approach due to the lateral positioning of the patient and exposure of the posterior surface of the kidney, in contrast to the anterior surface visualized intraperitoneal.
- On the right, renal arterial pulsations can be easily appreciated and identified; therefore the renal artery is encountered first, followed by the right renal vein. On the other hand, the renal vein and artery are identified at the same time running parallel to one another on the left.
- In cases of selective identification of the adrenal vein (adrenalectomy); the right adrenal vein is often identified without dissection of the renal vein. In contrast, prior dissection of the renal pedicle is essential to secure the left adrenal vein.
- During dissection of the space of Retzius, the pubic symphysis serves as the main landmark for proper orientation.
- During dissection of the lateral peritoneal reflection, identification of the epigastric vessels is important to avoid their injury.

A.E. Ghazi (✉)
Department of Urology, University of Rochester Medical Center, 601 Elmwood Ave., Box 656,14642 Rochester, NY, USA
e-mail: ahmed_ghazimd@yahoo.com, ahmed_ghazi@urmc.rochester.edu

J.V. Joseph and H.R.H. Patel (eds.), *Retroperitoneal Robotic and Laparoscopic Surgery*,
DOI: 10.1007/978-0-85729-485-2_1, © Springer-Verlag London Limited 2011

1.1 Introduction

The breadth of urologic pathology that can be managed using a robot-assisted laparoscopic approach continues to expand as technology and surgeon's experience with this method improves. There is mounting evidence demonstrating that many urologic procedures can be performed efficiently and effectively using a robot-assisted laparoscopic approach, while significantly decreasing the pain and convalescence traditionally associated with ablative and reconstructive open urologic procedures.

One of the challenges of learning robot-assisted laparoscopic surgery remains the novel perspective on well-known anatomy. For many years, clinical anatomists and surgeons have admired and described anatomy from the outside in. Using direct vision, palpation and external perspective, the human body has been precisely characterized. Similarly, traditional medical education has focused on teaching and learning anatomy in this manner. Laparoscopic surgery, however, presents a novel perspective on a traditional science. In addition, the laparoscopic or robotic surgeon must work with limited or no tactile feedback. However, the technology used in laparoscopic surgery with or without robot assistance provides the surgeon with a view that may be considered superior to that of the traditional open surgical approach. The standard laparoscope provides the surgeon with a well-lit field and magnification 12 times greater than that afforded with the naked eye. The surgeon experiences a wealth of exquisite anatomic detail that cannot be appreciated without the laparoscope. The superior visualization of structures potentially allows compensation for the lack of tactile feedback. The laparoscopic surgeon relies on detail such as alteration in the weave of suture material to determine tension during laparoscopic suturing.

Although not intended to be an inclusive and complete description of urologic anatomy, this chapter will focus on assisting the urologic surgeon to learn key anatomical landmarks to facilitate performing laparoscopic procedures extraperitoneally.[1]

1.2 Body Surface Anatomy

Successful laparoscopic surgery or access relies on successful trocar placement. Unlike open surgery, where the incision can be extended to allow better visualization or exposure, the trocar sites cannot be extended during laparoscopic or robotic surgery. Appropriate planning and knowledge of the surgical anatomy are paramount in guiding the location of trocars. Thoughtful trocar placement incorporates parameters that include the surgical objectives, anatomic considerations, and body habitus. Although trocar templates are available for each procedure, trocar positioning must be individualized for each patient, location of the pathology, route of access, and surgeon preference. The key surface landmarks for urologic laparoscopic access are the umbilicus, the anterior superior iliac spine (ASIS), the costal margin, and the 12th rib. These important surface landmarks help the urologic surgeon choose appropriate trocar access sites and orient the operator to the underlying visceral anatomy. Another important structure is the rectus abdominis muscle, which may be difficult to appreciate by inspection and palpation, particularly in obese individuals. The location of the epigastric vessels coursing beneath the rectus muscles must be identified to avoid injury to these structures and subsequent bleeding.

1.2.1 Anatomical Landmarks

1.2.1.1 Umbilicus

The umbilicus is an optimal site for laparoscopic access. Because of its central location, it provides an intuitive perspective for laparoscopic visual orientation. Cosmetically, it is a superior site. Incisions in the periumbilical crease generally retract into the umbilicus and become nearly invisible when fully healed. When the patient is in the supine position the periumbilical area and not the umbilicus is an excellent site for primary access to the extraperitoneal space, because the preperitoneum is closest to the skin at the umbilicus on the abdominal wall. The preperitoneal layer of fatty tissue, which lies between the linea alba and the peritoneum, is thinnest at the level of the umbilicus. The latter is also an excellent extraction site for intact removal of the specimen. Only a single layer of suture is necessary to close the linea alba following specimen retrieval.

In establishing umbilical or periumbilical access, special consideration must be given to extremely obese or very thin body habitus. Hurd and colleagues evaluated the relationship of the umbilicus to the aortic bifurcation using magnetic resonance imaging (MRI) and computed tomography (CT). They assessed the effect of obesity on this relationship. In nonobese patients weighing <160 lb (73 kg), the umbilicus is at a mean distance 0.4 cm caudal to the aortic bifurcation, with a skin-to-peritoneum distance of 2 cm. In obese patients weighing more than 200 lb (91 kg), the umbilicus is located 2.9 cm caudal to the aortic bifurcation, with a skin-to-peritoneum distance of 12 cm.

1.2.1.2 Anterior Superior Iliac Spine

The ASIS is an excellent surface landmark that is easily discernible even in the most obese patient. Many urologic procedures are performed with the patient in the lateral decubitus position. Trocar placement at a site just cephalad and medial to the ASIS is useful because this is a common left-handed working site for laparoscopic procedures. The ASIS is a site of attachment for the internal oblique, external oblique, and transversalis fascial layers. Penetration of the abdominal wall is facilitated at this site by the tenting up of the abdominal wall by this bony prominence.

1.2.1.3 Twelfth Rib

Retroperitoneal access in the flank position is usually gained through an incision just caudal to the tip of the 12th rib. The 12th rib is usually discernible by palpation. In the very obese patient, the surgeon may estimate the location of the 12th rib. Digital palpation and dissection of the superficial fatty layers through a small incision will allow localization of the 12th rib in the minority of patients and will facilitate proper selection of the primary access site.

1.3 Body Habitus/Obesity

There are multiple physiologic and anatomic considerations that occur with obesity. Fat distribution will frequently alter the choice of access sites. Abdominal fat may be distributed primarily in the form of a pannus or the patient may have a more even barrel-like distribution of fat. The operating surgeon should assess fat distribution after the patient is properly positioned. When the patient is in the lateral decubitus position, a large pannus may frequently fall medially, allowing the surgeon to enter laterally through a relatively thinner abdominal wall. In these cases, the umbilicus is displaced to the contralateral side and should not be utilized as an access site. Medial access may be obtained at any site lateral to the margin of the rectus abdominis muscle; the location of this margin must frequently be estimated. In contrast, the more evenly distributed barrel-like body habitus may have little change in the position of the umbilicus relative to the midline.

When attempting a retroperitoneal approach, the location of the lateral peritoneal reflection is a crucial consideration. This reflection is dependent on the position of the patient. With the patient supine, the lateral peritoneal reflection is located at the posterior axillary line. With the patient placed in the flank (lateral) position, gravity-induced downward movement of the ipsilateral colon causes anterior displacement of the mesocolon and thus its peritoneal reflection. Chiu and co-workers[2] demonstrated that moving the patient from the supine to the lateral position increases the distance between the quadratus lumborum and colon by a mean of 23 mm (range, 8.7–27.3 mm on the left side and 4.6–18.1 mm on the right side). Capelouto and co-workers[3] showed that moving the patient from the supine to the flank position displaces the peritoneal reflection anteriorly, thereby increasing the anteroposterior dimension of the potential retroperitoneal space twofold.

1.4 Surgical Anatomy of the Posterior (Lumbar) Body Wall

The lumbar area of the posterior abdominal wall is bounded[4]:

- Superiorly: by the 12th rib
- Inferiorly: by the ASIS and iliac crest
- Posteriorly: by the erector spinae (sacrospinalis) muscles
- Anteriorly: by the posterior border of the external oblique muscle

In this area, the body wall is composed of the following layers of muscle and fascia:

1. Skin
2. Superficial fascia: two layers of fibrous tissue with an intervening layer of loose fatty areolar tissue
3. A superficial muscle layer composed of the latissimus dorsi muscle posterolaterally and the external oblique muscle anterolaterally
4. Thoracolumbar fascia containing three layers: posterior, middle, and anterior. The posterior and

middle layers envelop the sacrospinalis muscle and the middle anterior layer envelops the quadratus lumborum. Another characteristic of the middle layer of the thoracolumbar fascia is its lateral communication to the transversus abdominis aponeurosis by fusion of all three layers. Therefore, the transversus abdominis aponeurosis should be accepted as part of the thoracolumbar fascia.
5. A middle muscular layer of the sacrospinalis, internal oblique, serratus posterior inferior muscles
6. A deep muscular layer composed of the quadratus lumborum and psoas muscles
7. Transversalis fascia
8. Preperitoneal fat
9. Peritoneum

Within this area, two triangles may be described: the superior lumbar triangle (Grynfeltt's) and the inferior lumbar triangle (Petit's). The inferior lumbar triangle is of particular interest to urologist during retroperitonoscopy, as it is the area where access to the retroperitoneum is initiated. The base of the inferior lumbar triangle is the iliac crest. The anterior (abdominal) boundary is the posterior border of the external oblique muscle. The posterior (lumbar) boundary is the anterior border of the latissimus dorsi muscle. The floor of the triangle is formed by the internal oblique muscle with contributions from the transversus abdominis muscle and the posterior lamina of the thoracolumbar fascia. The triangle is covered by superficial fascia and skin.

1.5 Anatomical Considerations

Knowledge of anatomic landmarks is essential to orientation in the extraperitoneal space. The retroperitoneum can be divided into three spaces[5]:

- The retropubic space (space of Retzius) is the space between the pubic bone and the bladder.
- The space of Bogros is lateral and cephalad to the space of Retzius.
- The lumbar retroperitoneal space is the posterior continuation of the space of Bogros bounded by the vena cava and aorta medially, the psoas dorsally, the colon ventrally, and transversalis fascia laterally. This space contains the kidney, adrenal, and Gerota's fascia.

The Retzius space is located posterior to the abdominal rectus muscle and the pubic bone. Its lateral boundaries are the epigastric vessels and the spermatic cord. It contains loose fatty tissue and also denser condensations that form the pubovesical and puboprostatic ligaments in the male and the pubovesical ligaments in the female.

The space of Bogros is located lateral to the Retzius space. The psoas, iliacus, and transversus abdominis muscles form its posterior and lateral boundaries. The lumbar space is the cranial extension of the Bogros space. The medial boundaries are the vena cava, the aorta, and the vertebral column. The lateral boundaries are the transversus abdominis muscles. The floor of the lumbar space consists of the psoas and the quadratus lumborum muscles.

The lumbar retroperitoneal space is a potential space between the parietal peritoneum and posterior abdominal wall that is occupied by the retroperitoneal connective tissue. This tissue is composed of three layers called strata; the inner stratum lies immediately behind the peritoneum and covers the gastrointestinal viscera along with their blood supply. The intermediate stratum envelops the adrenals, kidneys, ureters, and great vessels. The outer stratum forms the fascia of the posterior abdominal wall. The boundaries of the retroperitoneum are the muscular diaphragm superiorly, the posterior parietal peritoneum anteriorly, the body wall both posteriorly and laterally, and the pelvic diaphragm inferiorly.

1.6 Clinical Applications

1.6.1 Upper Abdomen/Retroperitoneal Space

The anatomical perspective of the surgical field during the extraperitoneal approach to the upper urinary tract is somewhat different from the one visualized via an intraperitoneal approach. Although the anatomical relations of the kidney and related structures are similar, the position of the patient (more lateral than the transperitoneal approach) gives a different anatomical perspective. The surgeon must take this into consideration and realign the anatomical structures. There are certain anatomical landmarks that need to be identified to allow the surgeon to realign this anatomy and place a roadmap to readily define important structures. The psoas muscle is one of the first landmarks encountered in identifying the retroperitoneal anatomy. It should always be kept in a horizontal plane as a reference point (Fig. 1.1) while other structures are identified. Once the retroperitoneal space is created and the 30° laparoscope is inserted, the psoas muscle and one or more of the following structures can be visualized with the following frequency: Gerota's fascia (100%), peritoneal reflection (83%), ureter and/or gonadal vein (61%), pulsations of the fat-covered renal artery (56%), aortic pulsations (left side 90%), and the compressed, ribbon-like inferior vena cava (right side 25%). Following retraction of the kidney anterolaterally, a generous longitudinal incision in Gerota's fascia, parallel and close to the psoas muscle, allows access to the renal hilar area. A search for vascular pulsations is initiated. Although gentle, undulating pulsations are characteristic of the inferior vena cava, sharp, well-defined pulsations reveal the location of the fat-covered renal artery or, on the left side, the aorta.[6]

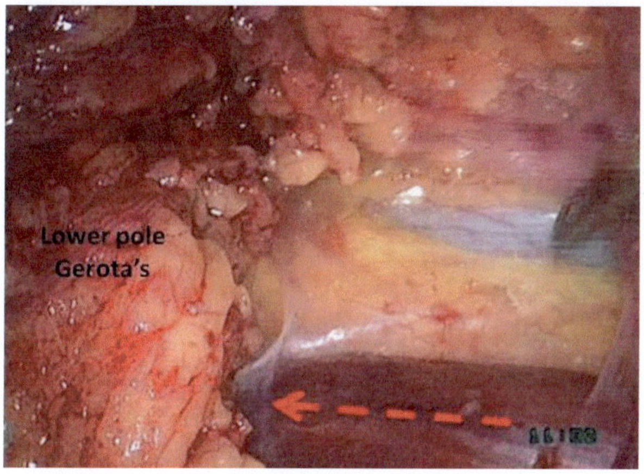

Fig. 1.1 Horizontal position of the Psoas muscle that facilitates orientation during retroperitoneal surgery.

As in the transperitoneal approach, the anatomical relations of the renal hilar structures differ from right to left. Figure 1.2 shows a schematic view of the vessels as seen during retroperitoneal surgery in an attempt to simplify these anatomical relations. On the left side, the aorta instead of the inferior vena cava is the first major vessel encountered, lying horizontally. Its sharp, horizontal pulsations are appreciated when the kidney is lifted anteriorly, away from the psoas muscle. During access of the right renal hilum, the renal arterial pulsations can be appreciated and easily identified. This poses no difficulty in control of the renal pedicle as the renal artery can be approached and controlled first, followed by the right renal vein (Fig. 1.3a). Similarly the approach to the right adrenal vein requires no dissection of the renal vein (as in the transperitoneal approach). It often courses approximately 0.5–1 cm anterior and parallel to the horizon of the anterior psoas muscle (Fig. 1.4).

On the other hand on the left side, the renal vein and artery can be seen at the same time running parallel to

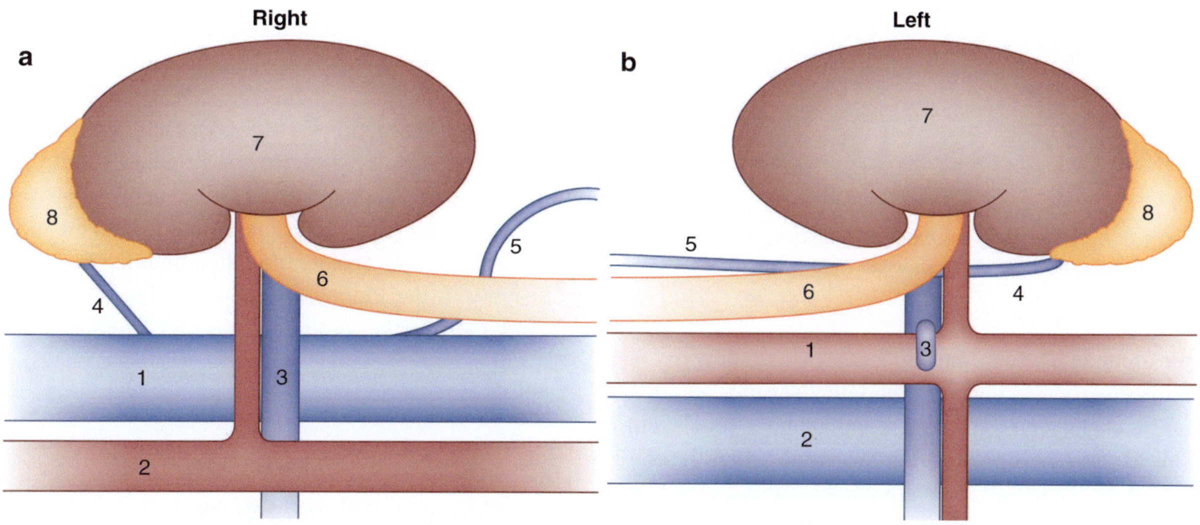

Fig. 1.2 Schematic view of the vessels as seen during retroperitoneal surgery; (**a**) *Right* side and. *1* inferior vena cava, *2* aorta, *3* renal pedicle, *4* adrenal vein, *5* gonadal vein, *6* pelvis and ureter, *7* kidney, *8* adrenal gland. (**b**) *left* side; *1* Aorta, *2* Inferior vena cava, *3*:Renal pedicle, *4*:Adrenal vein, *5*:Gonadal vein, *6*:Pelvis and ureter, *7*:Kidney, *8*:Adrenal gland, *9*:Lumbar vein.

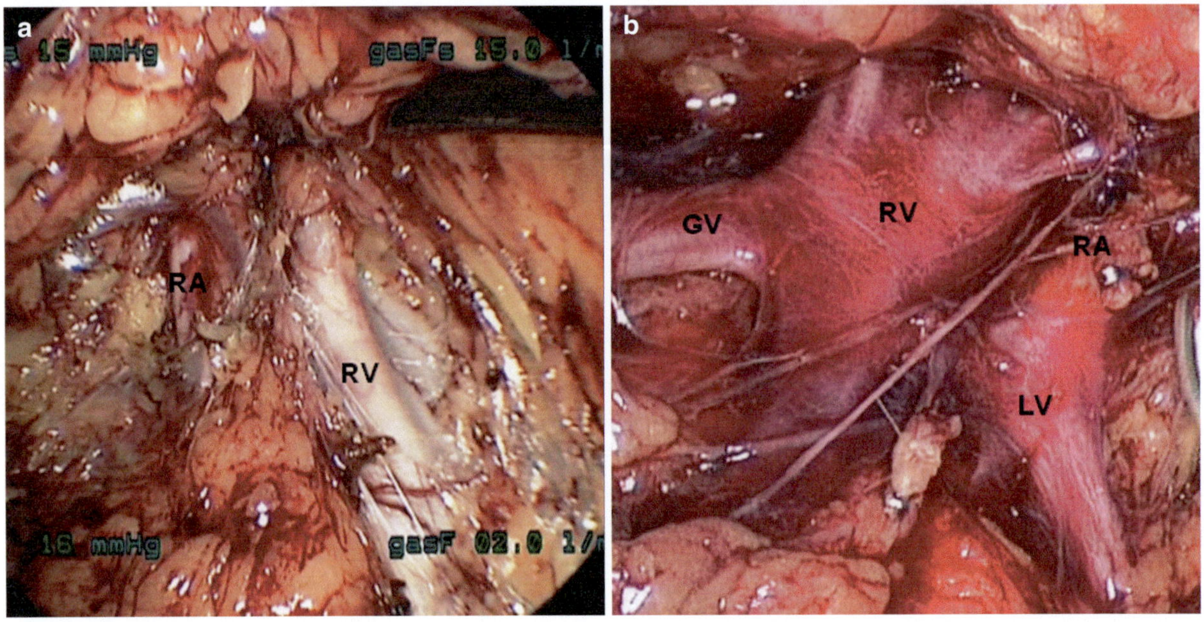

Fig. 1.3 (**a**) Operative view of the right renal pedicle. (**b**) Operative view of the left renal pedicle. *RA* Renal vein, *RV* Renal vein, *GV* Gonadal vein, *LV* Lumbar vein.

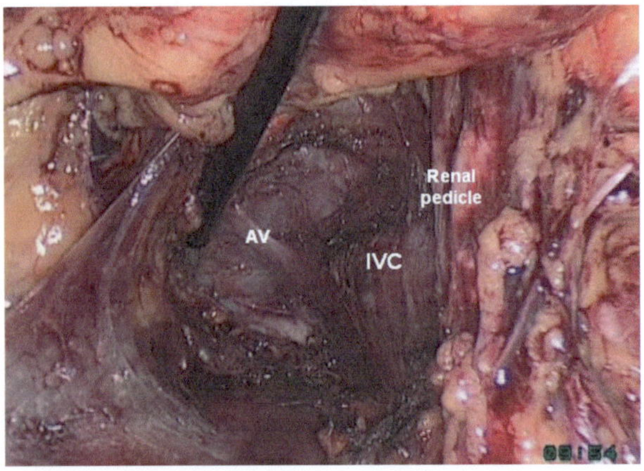

Fig. 1.4 Intraoperative view showing dissection of the right adrenal vein during retroperitoneal right adrenalectomy, *AV* Adrenal vein.

one another. The adrenal vein enters the renal vein cranially and the gonadal vein caudally. At times a lumbar vein can be seen entering the gonadal or renal vein. This should be ligated after the renal artery is controlled. When the lumbar vein is adequately controlled, the renal vein releases, facilitating further renal vein dissection. It may at times be necessary to control the lumbar vein to facilitate dissection of the renal artery. (Fig. 1.3b). Unlike a right adrenalectomy, during a left adrenalectomy the renal pedicle is dissected and displaced caudally to visualize where the adrenal vein enters the left renal vein (Fig. 1.5a). Alternatively, the renal artery and vein are dissected and separated to allow cranial displacement of the renal artery and to secure the left adrenal vein (Fig. 1.5b). The superior mesenteric artery runs anterior to the aorta and medial to the renal artery and vein. Dissection anterior to the aorta may lead to the identification of the superior mesenteric artery or celiac trunk. During a left-sided nephrectomy, these structures should not be confused for the main renal artery, which exits the aorta laterally coursing toward the kidney. Medial attachments of the kidney to the aorta or posterior peritoneum should be approached from an anterior and lateral approach (over the kidney rather than under the kidney). This enables the surgeon to appreciate the attachments that run exclusively to the kidney, thereby avoiding the superior mesenteric artery.[7]

1.6.2 Lower Abdomen/Pelvis/ Extraperitoneal Space

Similarly following development of the extraperitoneal space in the pelvis, there are certain landmarks that should be identified as the laparoscope is introduced.

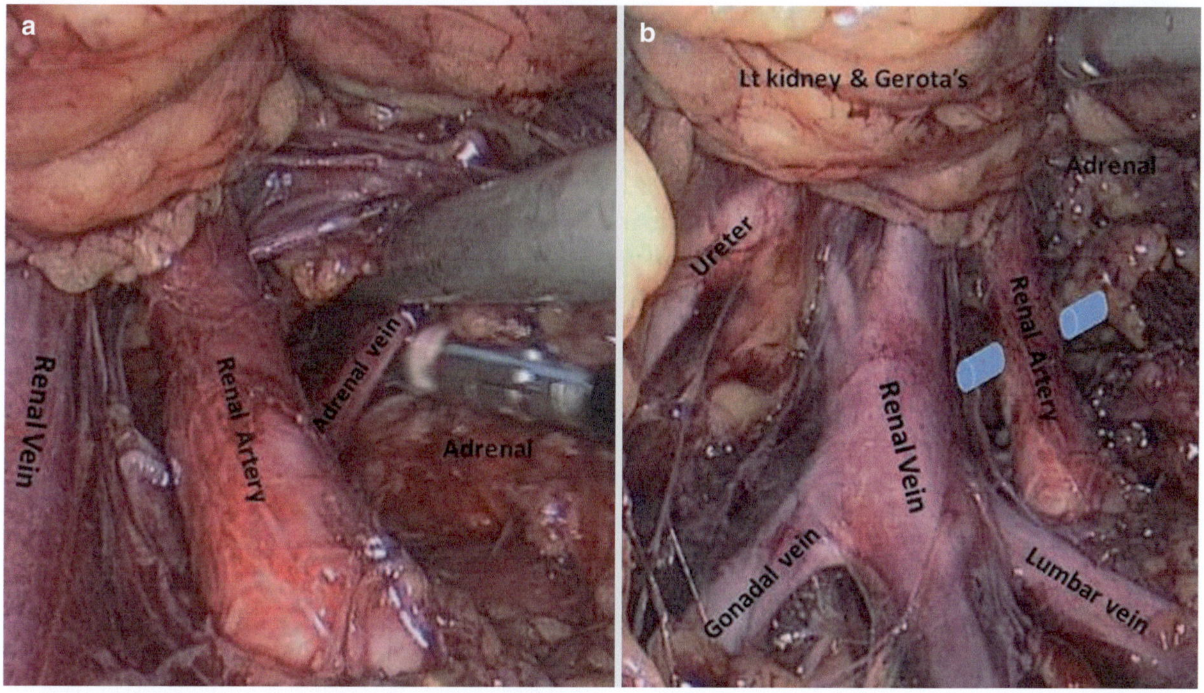

Fig. 1.5 Intraoperative view showing dissection of the left adrenal vein during retroperitoneal left adrenalectomy; (**a**) Pedicle is dissected and displaced caudally to view the left adrenal vein (**b**) After ligation of adrenal vein (blue vein shows position of left adrenal vein after renal artery and vein are dissected and separated.

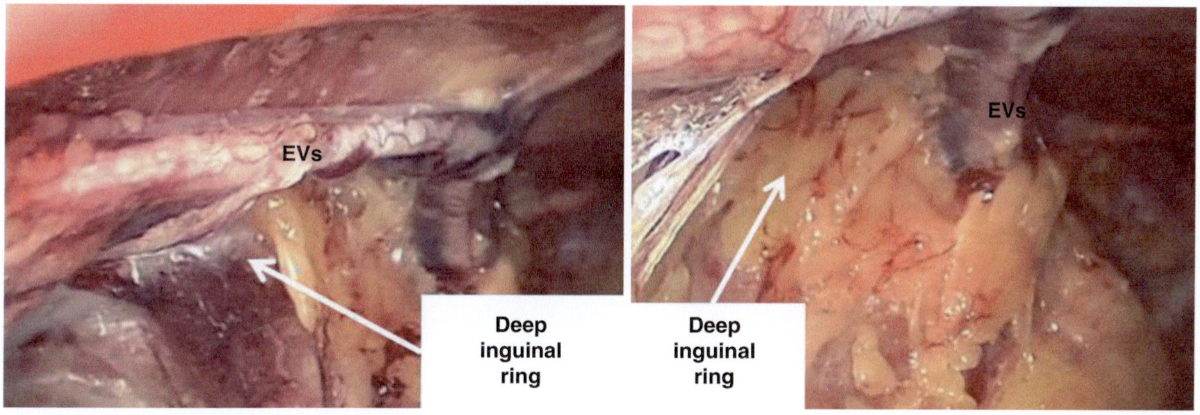

Fig. 1.6 Site of dissection in the angle between the epigastric vessels (EVs) and the peritoneal reflection at the level of the deep inguinal ring for creation of the extraperitoneal space.

During the intraperitoneal approach, the umbilical ligaments serve as major landmarks. These structures, however, are not visible during the extraperitoneal approach, with the camera placed anterior to the bladder. The pubic symphysis and the anteriorly located epigastric vessels are the main landmarks to be identified. Identification of the pubic symphysis (which can also be palpated) allows orientation during dissection of the space of Retzius. Identification of the epigastric vessels is important to avoid their injury during dissection of the lateral peritoneal reflection. The dissection should start in the angle between the epigastric vessels and the peritoneal reflection at the level of the deep inguinal ring (Fig. 1.6). The Bogros space is situated lateral and cranial to the Retzius space, corresponding to the retroinguinal preperitoneum. Anteriorly, it is limited by the deep layer of transversalis fascia enveloping the epigastric vessels. Medially, it is limited by the adherent zone of umbilico vesical fascia, transversalis fascia, and peritoneum, situated just behind the epigastrics. The lateral limits are the pelvic wall and the iliacus muscle. The psoas muscle corresponds to the inferior limit. The key point to visualize the Bogros space is the dissection of the epigastric vessels, which are superficial to the deep layer of transversalis fascia and in close relation to the peritoneum. If one penetrates the plane superficial to the deep layer of transversalis fascia, the bare epigastrics will be exposed, and the risk of bleeding increases by trauma to the small branching vessels – this is the wrong plane of dissection. By gently brushing the tissue away from the epigastric arcade, the right plane of dissection is usually easily visualized. The dissection follows a sagittal direction (the same direction as the fascia and the epigastrics) and the dissector gently separates the avascular plane that separates the peritoneum from the deep layer of transversalis fascia.[8]

1.7 Conclusions

A clear understanding of the retroperitoneal or extraperitoneal anatomy is necessary to perform most urologic operations. With laparoscopy or robot assistance, the loose areolar connective tissues covering encountered prior to reaching the peritoneum can be a source of confusion for the novice. There are specific anatomic landmarks that should be identified to facilitate a safe and expeditious procedure.

References

1. Landman J, Pattaras G. Urologic laparoscopic anatomy. In: Moore RG, Bishoff JT, Loenig S, Docimo SG, eds. *Minimally Invasive Urologic Surgery*. Oxfordshire: Taylor & Francis; 2005:11-28.
2. Chiu AW, Chen KK, Wang JH, et al. Direct needle insufflation for pneumoretroperitoneum: anatomic confirmation and clinical experience. *Urology*. 1995;46:432-437.
3. Capelouto CC, Moore RG, Silverman SG, et al. Retroperitoneoscopy: anatomical rationale for direct retroperitoneal access. *J Urol*. 1994;152:2008-2010.
4. Skandalakis PN. *Surgical Anatomy and Technique: A Pocket Manual*. 2nd ed. New York: Springer; 1995: 123-228.
5. Brams DM. Creation of working space: extraperitoneal approaches. In: Carol EH, ed. *The SAGES Manual: Fundamentals of Laparoscopy, Thoracoscopy and GI Endoscopy*. 2nd ed. New York: Springer; 2006:39-45.
6. Gill IS, Rassweiler JJ. Retroperitoneoscopic renal surgery: our approach. *Urology*. 1999;54:734-739.
7. Gill IS. Retroperitoneal laparoscopic nephrectomy. *Urol Clin North Am*. 1998;25:343-360.
8. Rosenblatt A, Bollens R, Cohen BE, eds. Extraperitoneal laparoscopic radical prostatectomy. In: *Manual of Laparoscopic Urology*. Berlin/Heidelberg: Springer, 2008: 63-89:chap 5.

Essential Instruments in Laparoscopic and Robotic Surgery

2

Ty T. Higuchi and Matthew T. Gettman

Abstract Urologic surgery has evolved to include minimally invasive and robot-assisted techniques with excellent outcomes. These techniques have been expanded to include surgery of the retroperitoneum. Currently, minimally invasive retroperitoneal surgery has been described for surgery on the adrenal, kidney, ureter, and lymph nodes. A strong working knowledge of the essential instruments in laparoscopic and robotic surgery is crucial for successful implementation and maintenance of a minimally invasive surgical practice. This chapter will review the essential equipment for laparoscopic and robot-assisted surgery with the da Vinci® Surgical System.

Keywords Access • Laparoscopic instruments • Robotic surgery • Trocar

T.T. Higuchi (✉)
Department of Urology, Mayo Clinic,
200 First St. SW, 55905 Rochester, MN, USA
e-mail: higuchi.ty@mayo.edu

Key Points

- Implementation of a minimally invasive surgery program hinges on a complete understanding of the instrumentation required for the procedures.
- There have been countless advances in laparoscopic instrumentation including the development of the da Vinci® Surgical System (Intuitive Surgical, Sunnyvale, CA) and Laparo-endoscopic single-site surgery (LESS).
- The da Vinci® Surgical System adds three-dimensional imaging and increased surgical dexterity over standard laparoscopy.
- LESS offers improved cosmetic results by using only one port and conceals the scar umbilicus, but is technically more challenging and has a larger learning curve.
- Despite the advanced instrumentation, a competent and cohesive surgical team is vital for successful outcomes.

2.1 Introduction

Since the introduction of minimally invasive surgery in the 1980s, there have been countless advances in technology to improve laparoscopic surgery. One of the major advances in minimally invasive surgery came with the development of robot-assisted surgery. Urologists have been at the forefront of robot-assisted surgery dating back to 1989, when the PROBOT was used to assist with transurethral resection of the prostate.[1,2] Further devices were designed for transrectal

J.V. Joseph and H.R.H. Patel (eds.), *Retroperitoneal Robotic and Laparoscopic Surgery*,
DOI: 10.1007/978-0-85729-485-2_2, © Springer-Verlag London Limited 2011

ultrasound-guided prostate biopsy and percutaneous nephrolithotomy.[3,4] In the early 1990s several companies began to develop "master–slave systems," where the surgeon controls the robotic instrument arms remotely from a console. The purpose of these systems was to eliminate physiologic tremor and to increase surgical dexterity and precision. Subsequent refinement in these systems led to the introduction of the da Vinci® Surgical System (Intuitive Surgical, Sunnyvale, CA). Since the first robot-assisted prostatectomy in 2000 and subsequent Federal Drug Administration approval, the da Vinci® has been used in a vast array of urologic surgeries and surgical techniques have now been described for almost every genitourinary organ.[5]

Another recent advancement in the field of minimally invasive surgery is the application of laparo-endoscopic single-site surgery (LESS) in numerous urologic procedures. In this procedure, a single multichannel port replaces the need for multiple trocars placed throughout the abdomen.[6,7] While advances in minimally invasive surgery will continue to occur at a rapid rate, a proper understanding of basic laparoscopic and robotic instrumentation is pivotal to the implementation of a successful minimally invasive program. This chapter will review the essential equipment for laparoscopic and robot-assisted surgery with the da Vinci® Surgical System.

2.2 Access

Trocar placement was originally described and designed for transperitoneal access; however, retroperitoneal and natural orifices approaches have led to the development of modified equipment and techniques to these alternative approaches. Trocars can be placed by a closed or open technique and both disposable and non-disposable equipment are available. One must weigh the cost/benefit of the reusable equipment which requires servicing versus the cost of new equipment for every procedure. Closed access is blind trocar placement and open access refers to trocar placement under direct vision. Which technique is used largely depends on the surgical approach, patients past surgical history, body habitus, and surgeon preference. Closed access is achieved by making a skin incision and bluntly dissecting down to the fascia. A Veress needle is then inserted (Fig. 2.1). The needle has a blunt tip protecting a sharp needle. Once resistance is encountered, the blunt tip retracts exposing the sharp needle which is pushed through the external oblique fascia and transversalis fascia/peritoneum. When the resistance is removed, the blunt tip is deployed to protect the intraabdominal contents.[8,9] Verification of proper placement can be performed by aspiration, hanging drop test, saline injection with aspiration, or insufflation test. The abdomen is insufflated, needle removed, and a trocar is inserted along the same track. Veress needles are also available with an audible indicator that provides a "click" when passing through the fascia, as a component of a dilating trocar system or as a component of a 2-mm trocar where a 2-mm endoscope can be inserted to confirm position.[8] Alternatively, open access is obtained as originally described by Hasson.[10,11] A skin incision is made wide enough to accommodate the trocar and the subcutaneous tissues are dissected down to the fascia. The fascia is then incised and the peritoneum is grasped and divided sharply. A finger may then be inserted to confirm positioning and the blunt tip trocar is inserted, secured to the patient and pneumoperitoneum/retroperitoneum is established.

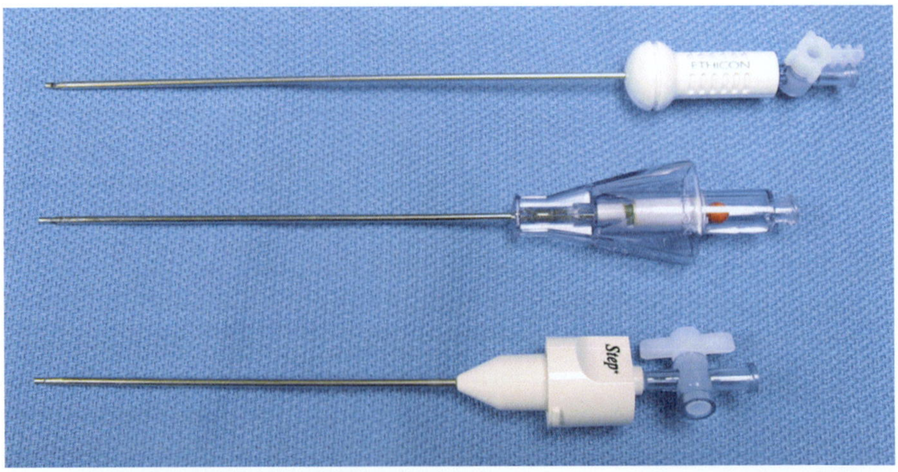

Fig. 2.1 Photograph of several Veress needles for closed laparoscopic access

Retroperitoneoscopic surgeries for renal and adrenal surgery are performed in a potential space that is created during access. Once created it has a limited working space and few anatomic landmarks.[12] The retroperitoneal space cannot be created with insufflation alone and expanding the retroperitoneum prior to insufflation using a balloon dissector was originally described by Gaur.[13] Since then several balloon dilators have been introduced to rapidly develop the retroperitoneal space (Fig. 2.2). Most of these can be easily positioned due to the rigid shaft and allow visualization of the retroperitoneum with an endoscope. The devices do not widen the original incision and most come prepackaged with a balloon trocar.[8]

Initial access is usually obtained by an open technique as described by Gill et al.[12] Briefly, the incision is made just below the tip of the 12th rib and carried down to the level of the lumbodorsal fascia. The fascia is then sharply incised and the position in the retroperitoneum is confirmed by palpating the psoas muscle posteriorly and the lower pole of the kidney superiorly. Balloon dilation can then be performed at the lower pole and mid-pole of the kidney followed by a secondary upper retroperitoneal dilation.[12] A modified blunt-tipped trocar that has a balloon at its distal end and proximal foam collar assembly, which together forms an airtight seal, can then be placed directly and insufflation started (Fig. 2.3). Additional ports can then be placed under direct vision. Alternatively, prior to placing the insufflation port, the additional ports can be placed by a bimanual technique where the nondominant hand is placed into the retroperitoneal space and the trocar is passed directly onto the surgeons hand or directed onto a retractor.[12]

2.3 Trocars

Laparoscopic trocars are composed of a hollow cannula with an obturator inserted through the cannula. The trocar is placed into the abdomen or retroperitoneum and the cannula acts as conduit to pass laparoscopic instruments or endoscopes into the operative

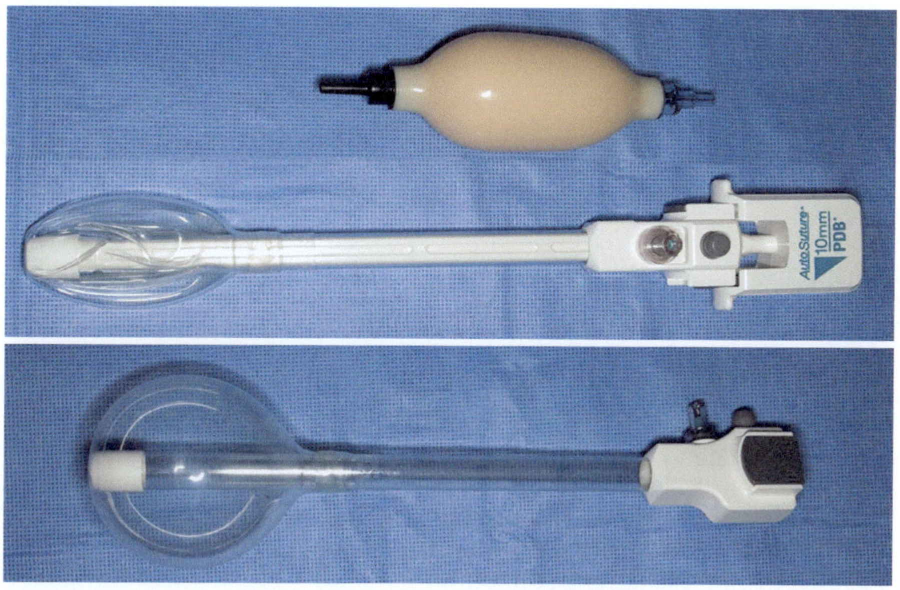

Fig. 2.2 Photograph of PDB™ (AutoSuture; Norwalk, CT) balloon dilator deflated with pump (*upper panel*) and balloon inflated with trocar removed

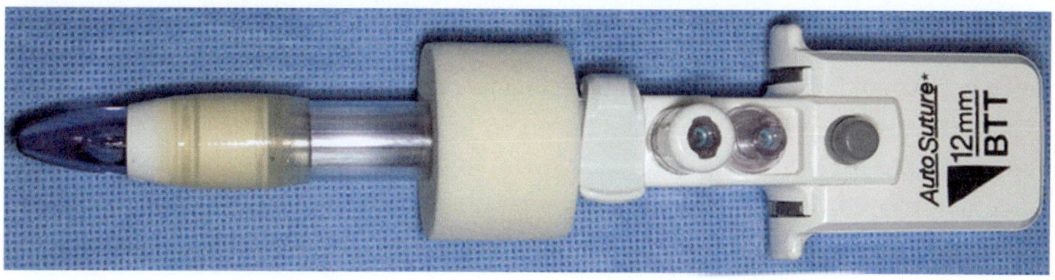

Fig. 2.3 Photograph of 12-mm blunt tipped trocar (AutoSuture; Norwalk, CT) with balloon at distal end and proximal foam collar assembly

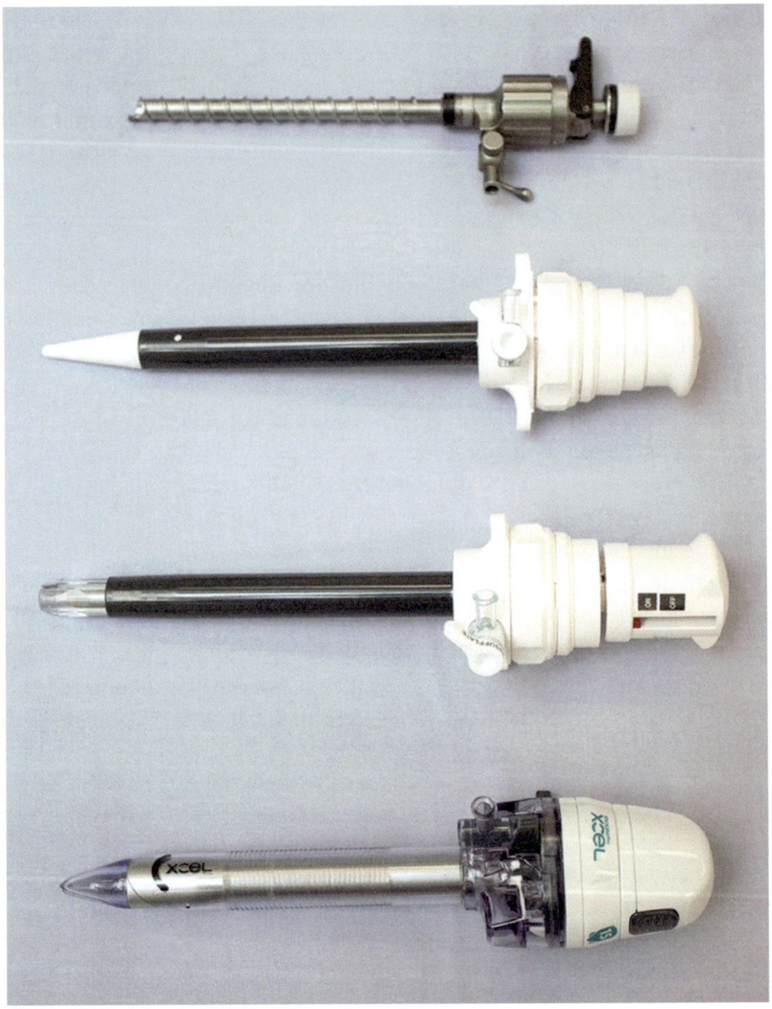

Fig. 2.4 Photograph of different trocars for laparoscopic access. From top to bottom, trocar-less rotational access cannula (TRAC), radial dilating trocar, sharp trocar with safety shield that retract when resistance is encountered at the fascia and a blunt-tipped trocar

field (Fig. 2.4). Most of them have an internal valve or seal to prevent gas leakage and loss of pneumoperitoneum/retroperitoneum with insertion or withdrawal of instruments.[8] In addition, most cannulas come with a stopcock valve that can be used for insufflation or desufflation. Trocars are available as disposable and nondisposable equipment, and come in a variety of lengths and diameters (2, 5, 8, 10, 12, and 15 mm). The obturators can be sharp or blunt (Fig. 2.4) and multiple improvements to the obturators have been implemented to try and decrease access-related complications.

A safety shield is a spring-loaded plastic shield that covers the cutting blade of the obturator until resistance is encountered. The plastic shield then retracts to expose the cutting blade to navigate through the fascia and will snap back to cover the blade once the resistance is removed. Bladeless obturators were designed to replace the sharp tip and placement is performed using a twisting motion and downward pressure to separate tissues rather than cutting through them. The VersaStep™ (Autosuture, Norwalk, CT) is a radially dilating trocar system (Fig. 2.5) that employs the use of a small expandable sleeve that is placed with a Veress needle through a small fascial incision (2–3 mm). A blunt tip obturator and trocar are then used to radially dilate the sleeve.[14,15] This system allows trocar placement through a smaller fascial incision compared to bladed trocars, allows stabilization of the abdominal wall during trocar placement, and converts the forces of entry from axial to radial.[9,14] In addition, this system allows the trocars to be easily upsized intraoperatively and obviates the need for fascial closure.[9] A trocar-less rotational access cannula (TRAC) has also been developed as a reusable threaded cannula

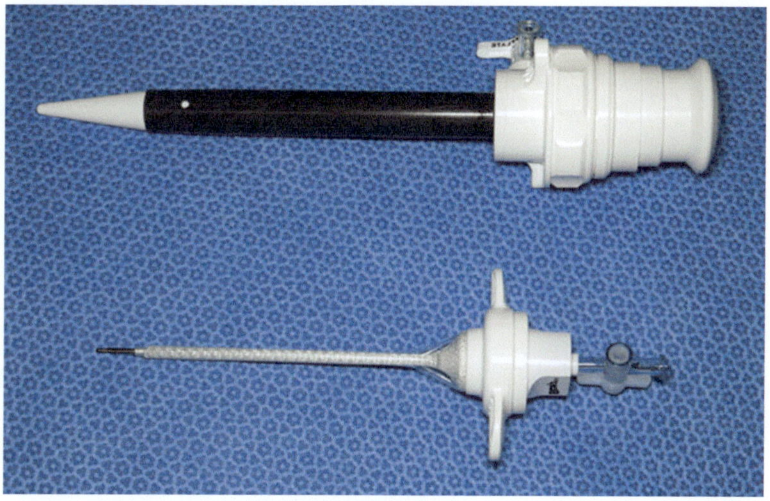

Fig. 2.5 Photograph of a VersaStep™ trocar (Autosuture, Norwalk, CT) and Step™ (Autosuture, Norwalk, CT) insufflation/access needle

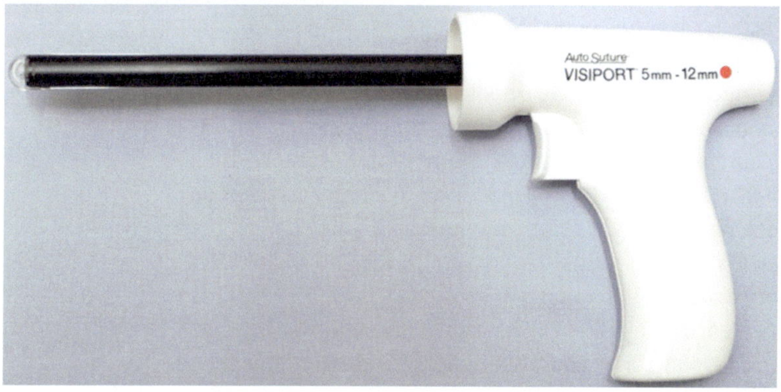

Fig. 2.6 Photograph of Visiport™ (AutoSuture; Norwalk, CT) visual trocar. The trocar is advanced under direct vision and the trigger is pulled while applying pressure to deploy a blade that cuts the tissue

that is rotated into position under laparoscopic vision (Fig. 2.4). This cannula decreases the axial forces during placement and fascial closure is often not required.[16,17]

Visual trocars (Fig. 2.6) are handled insertion devices that allow conventional trocar placement under direct laparoscopic vision.[18,19] Each device is composed of a hollow obturator with a clear dome at the distal end. A 0° laparoscope is inserted into the obturator for direct visual access. The Visiport™ (Autosuture, Norwalk, CT) has a triggered cutting mechanism at the distal end, whereas the Optiview® (Ethicon Endo-Surgical, Cincinnati, OH) has a conical tip with two cutting ridges. The visual trocars are placed after establishing pneumoperitoneum by making small skin incision and advancing the trocar through the layers of the abdominal wall under direct vision.

While there have been multiple advances in obturator and trocar design, access-related injury has been reported for all of the devices listed previously. Therefore, we typically recommend that in addition to the trocars, a laparoscope, a suction/irrigator, and a laparostomy set with vascular clamps should be readily available during access.[9]

2.4 Fascial Closure Devices

At the end of the laparoscopic procedure, the trocar sites and abdomen are inspected for any injuries and the fascial defects are repaired. It is generally recommended that fascial defects in children or >5 mm in adults be closed to prevent postoperative complications.[20] The fascia can be closed using standard open techniques, however closure of fascial defects can be difficult in obese patients. Therefore, several fascial closure devices have been developed to assist with

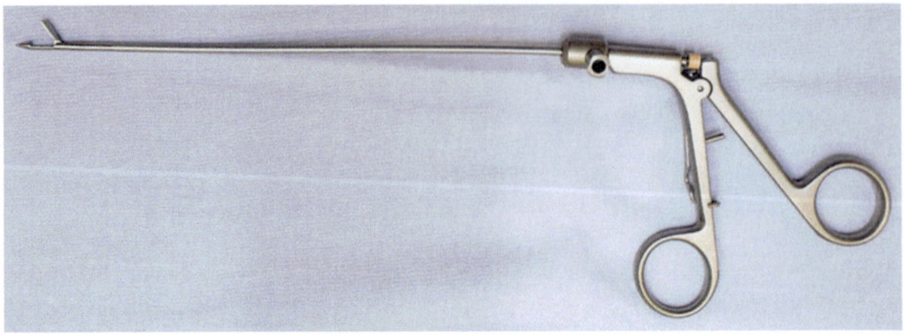

Fig. 2.7 Photograph of Berci Fascial Closure device (Karl Storz GmbH & Co. KG, Tuttlingen, Germany)

safely closing the abdomen. Most of the fascial closure devices are designed to be used with direct endoscopic vision from one of the other port sites. The Berci Fascial Closure device (Karl Storz GmbH & Co. KG, Tuttlingen, Germany) is nondisposable instrument with a sharp beak that can grasp a suture and be passed through the fascia under direct vision (Fig. 2.7). The suture is then released in the peritoneal cavity and the device is passed on the opposite side of the fascial incision and the suture is grasped and tied. The Carter-Thomason (CT) Closure System® (Inlet Medical, Inc., Eden Prairie, MN, USA) uses a similar technique but only it has a Pilot® guide that is placed into the port site. The guide has two holes located diagonally opposite to each other where the CT needle grasper is passed through one of the guides through the muscle, fascia, and peritoneum with a suture. The suture is then released and the needle is passed through the opposite guide and the suture is grasped and brought out and tied.[21] Other devices include the Endo-Judge™ (Synergistic Medical Technologies, Inc., Orlando, FL, USA) and Endo Close™ (Autosuture, Norwalk, CT) devices. All of these devices operate on the similar principle of passing a grasping needle through the fascia under direct vision of a needle and pulling a suture through the other side.

2.5 Hemostasis

Obtaining hemostasis can be one of the most challenging steps in performing laparoscopic surgery. Several open techniques – suturing, clipping, stapling – have had instruments designed to facilitate laparoscopic application of these techniques. In addition, a number of energy-based systems have been utilized to achieve hemostasis.

2.5.1 Energy Sources

Monopolar electrocautery was one of the first energy sources adapted for laparoscopy.[22] Monopolar energy uses alternating electrical current at the tip of the electrode that is passed through the body to a dispersive electrode (grounding pad). It is available on several J-hook type instruments or a variety of scissors and graspers. One disadvantage of monopolar cautery is that electrical bypass may occur at sites of low impedance or where the instrument's insulation has been damaged and cause inadvertent tissue damage. Several safety monitoring systems have been developed to actively monitor the electrode to insure there are not any breaks in the insulation.[22,23]

Bipolar cautery is similar to monopolar cautery only the current flow is between the jaws of the forceps. This potentially limits the risk of inadvertent tissue damage. Both jaws of the forceps must be in contact with the tissue for coagulation to occur. Other advanced bipolar devices – LigaSure™ (Valleylab, Boulder, CO) and PK™ technology (Gyrus Medical, Maple Grove, MN) – have the ability to coagulate larger vessels, cut following coagulation, and reduced tissue sticking. These devices are available with several different types of forceps.

The argon beam coagulator was one of the first hemostatic devices to control bleeding in renal parenchyma.[22,23] It is a monopolar electrosurgical instrument that uses high flow argon gas to deliver the energy to the tissue in a more uniform fashion. It is not used for dissection and cannot be used for controlling large vessels or significant bleeding. When using the argon beam coagulator laparoscopically, the ports must all be opened to allow sufficient gas leakage, otherwise high intraabdominal pressures may occur leading to argon gas embolism or even pneumothorax.[22,24]

The harmonic scalpel uses high frequency ultrasound between the harmonic graspers to simultaneously coagulate and cut tissue. It vibrates at a frequency >55 kHz which causes less collateral thermal damage and reduces carbonization of the tissue. However, the harmonic scalpel can only effectively coagulate vessels less than 4 mm in size.[22,24]

The use of lasers in laparoscopic urology continues to increase, but is still considered by many to be experimental. One of the advantages of lasers in partial nephrectomy is the ability to remove the tumor without hilar clamping.[25] To date the Homium:YAG (Ho:YAG),[26,27] diode,[28] potassium-titanyl-phosphate,[29] and thulium lasers[30] have been investigated for their feasibility in partial nephrectomy. Several investigators have started to use lasers in robot-assisted urologic surgery.[25,31]

2.5.2 Hemostatic Agents

There are numerous hemostatic agents available for laparoscopic surgery. Hemostatic agents act as a sealant by binding tissues together through a local polymerization reaction. The hemostatic agents can be divided into different categories based on their mechanism of action – fibrin sealants (Tisseel® (Baxter, Deerfield, IL), Vivostat® (Vivolution, Birkerod, Denmark), Costasis® (Cohesions technologies, Palo Alto, CA), Evicel® (Johnson and Johnson, New Brunswick, NJ), gelatine matrix adhesives (Floseal®, (Baxter, Deerfield, IL), hydrogel (CoSeal®, Baxter, Deerfield, IL)), methycellulose (Surgicel®; Johnson & Johnson, New Brunswick, NJ), Gelfoam® (Pfizer; New York, New York), and glutaraldehyde-based adhesive fibrin glue (BioGlue®, Cryolife; Kennesaw, GA).

2.5.3 Surgical Clips, Staplers, and Suturing

Surgical clips and staplers can be used to secure medium- to large-caliber vessels. Surgical clips are made of plastic, titanium, or steel. The clip appliers are available as automatically reloading or individually reloading devices. Endoscopic stapling devices can articulate and reticulate and stapling cartridges are available in various sizes and staple heights. Typically 2-mm stapling loads are used for vascular stapling.[8,24]

Laparoscopic suturing and knot tying in the confined space of the peritoneum or retroperitoneum is regarded by most to be the most difficult aspect of laparoscopic surgery to master.[24,32] Several refinements in needle drivers (Fig. 2.8) such as lack of finger rings, curved tips, and various jaw configurations have facilitated suturing, but the learning curve still exists. The Endostitch™ (Autosuture, Norwalk, CT) is an automated laparoscopic suture device that has two jaws and passes a needle with the suture attached to the middle of the device between the two jaws (Fig. 2.8). The suture attached to the jaw also makes intracorporeal suturing faster than conventional techniques.[24,33] Knots can be tied intracorporeal or extracorpeal. Intracorporeal knots can be performed using a variety of techniques[32] or by placing a Lapra-Ty® (Ethicon Endo-surgery, Cincinnati, OH). Extracorporeal knots are tied outside the body and a variety of knot pushers are used to push the knot down into position through the trocar or use loop ligation techniques.[32]

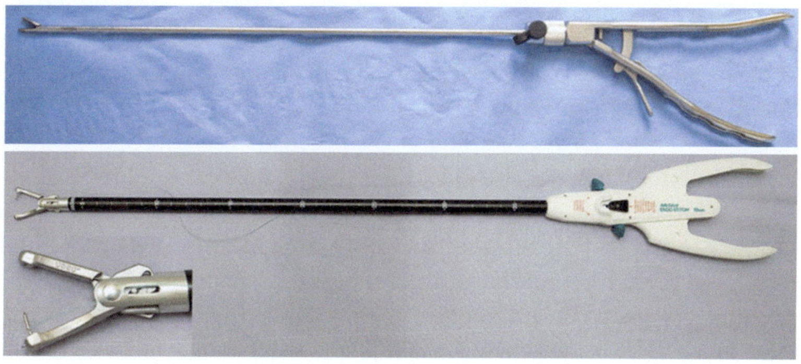

Fig. 2.8 Photograph of laparoscopic needle driver (*upper panel*) and Endo Stitch™ (AutoSuture, Norwalk, CT) (*lower panel*)

2.6 Laparoscopic Instruments

A variety of instruments are available to assist with laparoscopic surgery. Most instruments are able to be rotated 360° to adjust the tip to the proper angle. In addition, instruments are available as disposable and nondisposable products. Reusable instruments are usually modular, wherein different tips can be used with the same handle. Grasping instruments can be traumatic or atraumatic, locking or nonlocking, single or double action, and come in a variety of sizes (2–12 mm). Cutting instruments can typically be connected to monopolar electrosurgical units and are insulated down to the tips of the scissors to avoid inadvertent dispersion of electrical energy to surrounding tissues. Laparoscopic retractors may also be used to assist with retracting the bowel, liver, etc.

Several combination suction-irrigation systems are available. The irrigation system is usually connected to a pressurized solution (normal saline, antibiotic irrigation, etc.) and then the suction is connected to wall suction. The device may be used to clear the surgical field of blood, smoke, or debris or as a dissector or a retractor. To remove specimens, entrapment sacs are available and the specimen can be pulled through the laparoscopic port. If necessary, the specimen can be morcellated within an impermeable entrapment sac. However, morcellation during oncologic cases remains controversial.

2.7 Insufflation

The insufflation system (gas, pump, and tubing) is used to establish pneumoperitoneum and create the working space necessary for laparoscopic surgery. Once laparoscopic access has been established by open or closed techniques (see above and Chap. 3) the insufflation system is connected. Typically carbon dioxide (CO_2) gas is used as the insufflation gas because of its high solubility in blood.[8,34] One should be cautious when using CO_2 insufflation in patients with chronic obstructive pulmonary disease, since CO_2 may accumulate to dangerous levels. In these situations, once pneumoperitoneum is established with CO_2, helium may be used as an alternative since it is less soluble in blood.[8,35] Numerous other gases have been used for insufflation (room air, nitrous oxide, oxygen), but have been discontinued due to their risk of air embolism and combustibility. Other noble gases may be used (argon, krypton, xenon), but are typically more expensive and less absorbed in blood, increasing the risk of gas embolism.[8,24]

Insufflated CO_2 gas is 21°C and not humidified. It has been postulated that these characteristics may cause peritoneal irritation, hypothermia, and ultrastructural damage. Several accessory devices are available to heat and humidify the insufflated gas to prevent these potential side effects, but to date the benefits of heating and humidifying insufflated gas are largely unproven.[8,36] Smoke evacuators are also available as attachment filters or pumps to remove any smoke created from electrosurgical devices to keep the visual field clear.

2.8 Image System

The image system is composed of the laparoscope, camera, camera control units, light source, and monitor. Laparoscopes are available in a variety of widths (2.7–12 mm), lengths (20–45 cm), and lens angles (0–70°). The larger laparoscopes typically provide a wider field of vision with better optical resolution and a brighter image.[8] Visualization of the surgical field can be obtained by direct visualization with the naked eye or via a camera. Cameras are currently available as three-chip cameras and high definition cameras to provide superior image quality. The image obtained is filtered through the camera control units and relayed to the tele monitors. A light source is necessary to illuminate the surgical field. Image systems can be connected to digital recording devices to record the surgery or broadcast the surgery via the internet.

There are several techniques to keep the laparoscope from fogging after insertion into the surgical field. Several antifogging solutions are available. In addition, keeping the laparoscope warm with a hot water bath or scope warmer may decrease fogging. It is not unusual for the surgeon to have to remove the laparoscope several times throughout the procedure to clean or defog the laparoscope.

2.9 Instrumentation in Laparo-Endoscopic Single-Site Surgery

LESS was developed to enhance cosmetic results of laparoscopic surgery by concealing the scar within the umbilicus or minimizing it to one port incision.[6] LESS can be performed using standard laparoscopic trocars placed in close proximity or with purpose-built access devices. A variety of devices are currently available or in development. For example, a single port containing a multichannel valve with one 12 mm and two 5 mm port or three 5 mm ports and a separate stopcock valve for insufflation can be used for these procedures. In standard laparoscopic surgery, wide spacing of trocars allows proper triangulation of instruments and facilitates the dissection and intracorporeal suturing. For LESS the ports are parallel, therefore bent/flexible instruments have been designed to increase the intraabdominal/retroperitoneal working space required for intracorporeal surgery. However, several urologists have found merit in using standard laparoscopic instrumentation for LESS. LESS is technically more challenging and is associated with a steeper learning curve. To date single port laparoscopic surgery has been described for several transabdominal and retroperitoneal urologic surgeries.[7] In addition, techniques have been reported for LESS using a robotic interface.[37]

2.10 da Vinci® Surgical System

In the early 1990s several companies began to develop "master–slave systems," where the surgeon controls the robotic instrument arms remotely from a console. The purpose of these systems was to eliminate physiologic tremor and to increase surgical dexterity and precision. Subsequent refinement of these systems led to the introduction of the da Vinci® Surgical System (Intuitive Surgical, Sunnyvale, CA). To date, four different da Vinci® Surgical Systems have been released: standard, streamlined (S), S-high definition (HD), and S integrated (Si) – HD. Each system is composed of a surgeon console, a patient cart, and a vision cart.[38,39] In addition, each system requires several sterile accessories and EndoWrist® instruments. The standard system was released in 1999 and was available with one camera arm and two to three instrument arms. In 2006, the S system was introduced. This system has a similar platform to the standard system, but added a motorized patient cart, color-coded fiber-optic connections, easier instrument exchanges, quick click trocar attachments, increased range of motion and reach of instrument arms, and an interactive video touch screen display. In 2007, the S system became available with an HD camera and video system. Recently in 2009, the Si-HD system was released with an upgraded surgeon console and dual console capability. The dual console feature connects two surgeon consoles to the same patient cart. This allows two surgeons to coordinate a surgical procedure by exchanging control over the endoscope and instrument arms throughout the procedure.

2.10.1 Surgeon Console

The surgeon console (Fig. 2.9) is the driver's seat for the da Vinci® Surgical System. From here the surgeon adjusts the system using the pod controls, views a three-dimensional (3-D) image of the surgical field through the stereoviewer, and manipulates the instrument's arms using the master controllers and foot pedals.[38,39]

The surgeon is able to view a real-time magnified 3-D image of the surgical field through the stereoviewer. The 3-D image is created by capturing two independent views from two 5 mm endoscopes fitted into the stereo endoscope which are displayed into right and left optical channels in the stereoviewer.[39] For all of the da Vinci Surgical Systems®, the master controllers (Fig. 2.10) are the manual controls the surgeon uses to manipulate the robotic instrument arms and endoscope. The controllers are grasped with the index finger and thumb and movements are scaled, filtered, and relayed to the EndoWrist® (Intuitive Surgical, Sunnyvale, CA instruments). There is no measurable delay between surgeon and robotic instrument movement[38] and the system eliminates any physiologic tremor. In addition, there is a foot switch panel with five pedals – clutch, camera, focus, bipolar/auxiliary, and cautery – used in conjunction with the master controllers to drive the surgery. The different pedals allow the surgeon to move the camera, adjust the working distance of the master controllers, focus the camera, and activate bipolar or monopolar cautery.

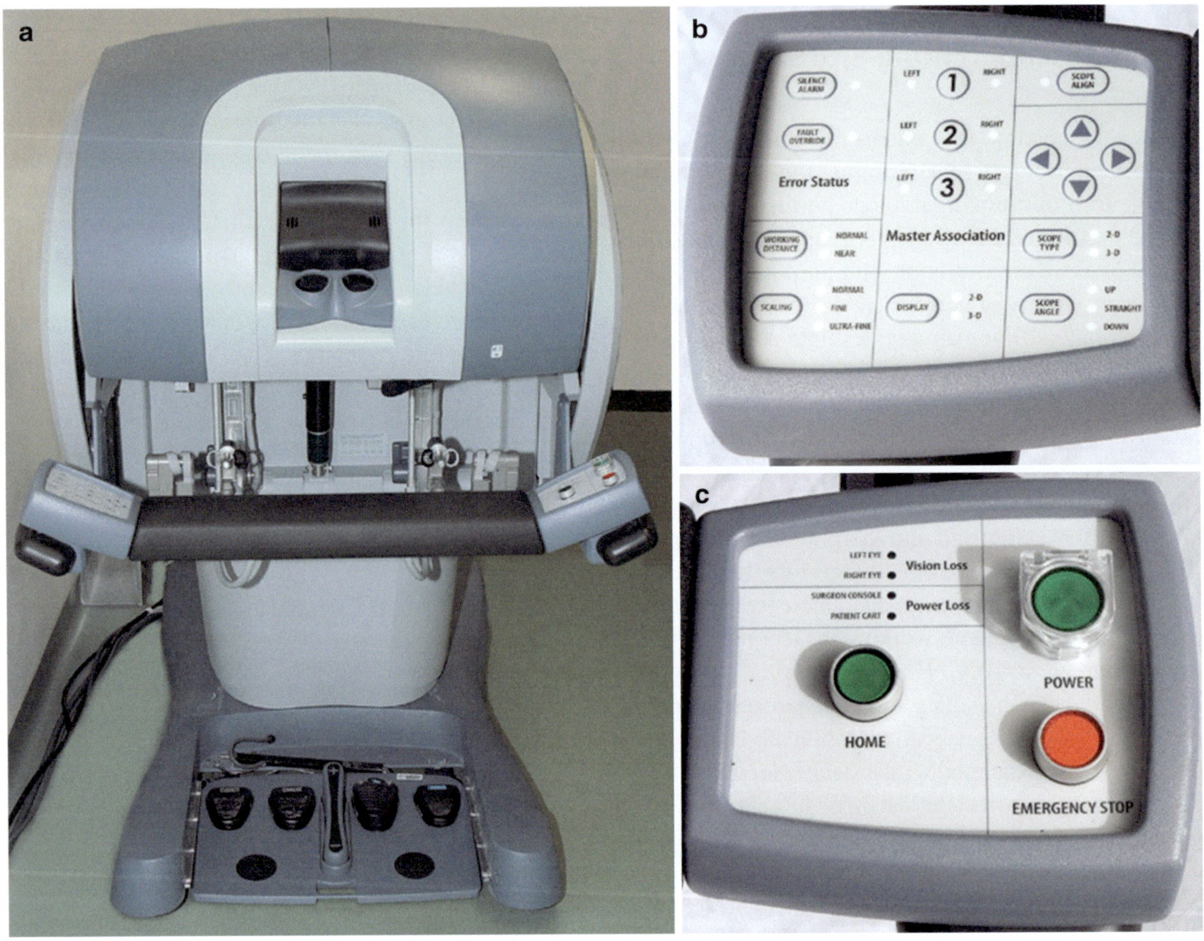

Fig. 2.9 Photograph of da Vinci® S surgeon console (**a**), left-side (**b**), and right-side (**c**) pod controls

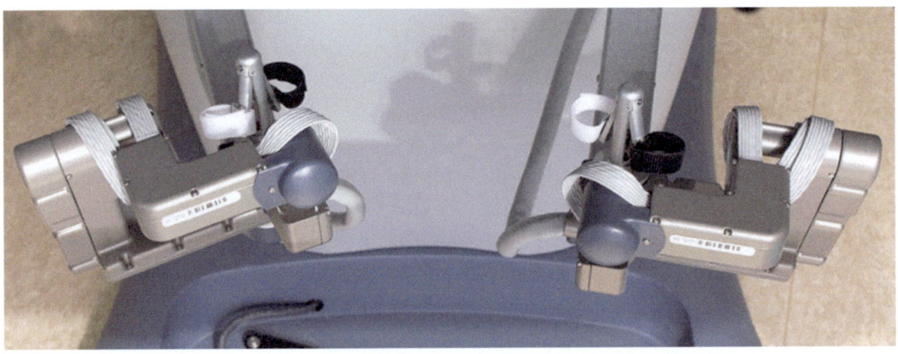

Fig. 2.10 Photograph of da Vinci® S master controllers

2.10.2 Patient Cart

The patient cart for the standard and S systems (Fig. 2.11) houses the camera and instrument arms[38,39] and is available with two or three instrument arms. Each arm has several robotic arm clutch buttons that must be depressed to move the arm, otherwise there will be resistance encountered and the arm will return to the original position. In addition, each arm also has a specific camera/instrument clutch button near the camera/instrument mounting brackets that is used to adjust the trajectory of the arm during docking and to insert or withdraw instruments.

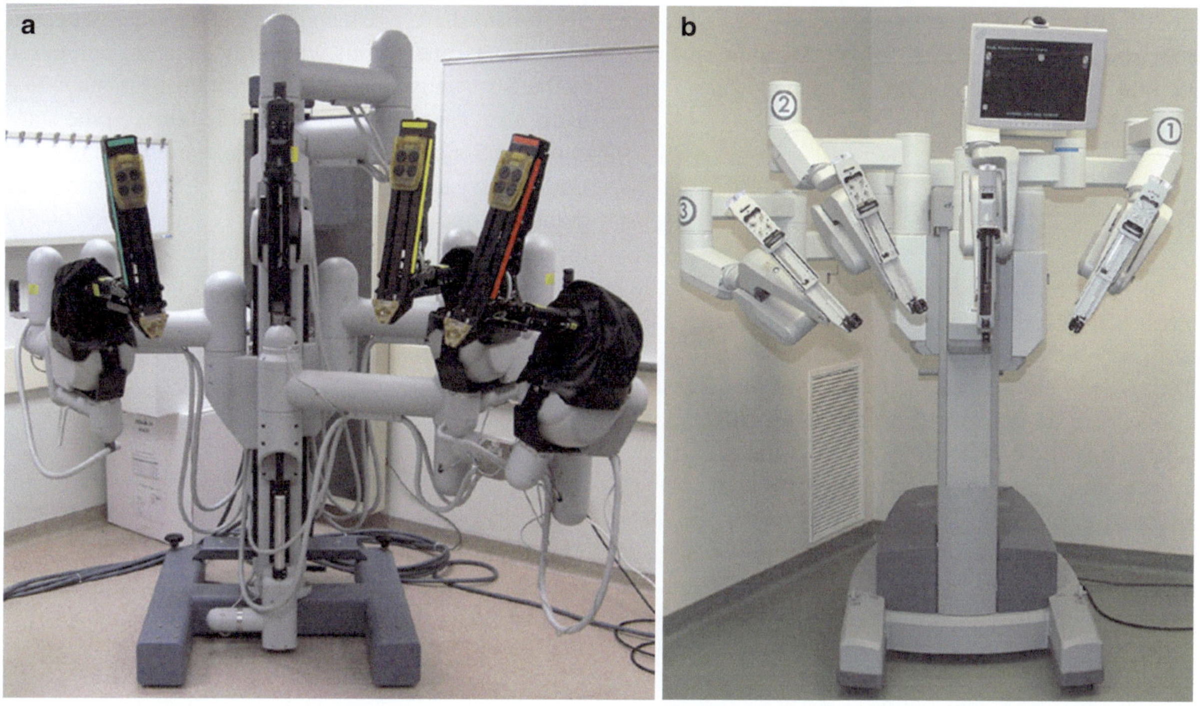

Fig. 2.11 Photograph of the da Vinci® standard patient cart with optional 3rd instrument arm (**a**) and da Vinci® S patient cart (**b**)

Each camera/instrument arm requires several sterile accessories that are placed during the draping procedure. The camera arm is compatible with most 12-mm trocars, while the instrument arms are connected to reusable 5- or 8-mm da Vinci trocars (Fig. 2.12).

2.10.3 Vision Cart

The vision cart contains the light source, video processing equipment, camera focus control, and camera storage bin.[38,39] There are also several empty storage

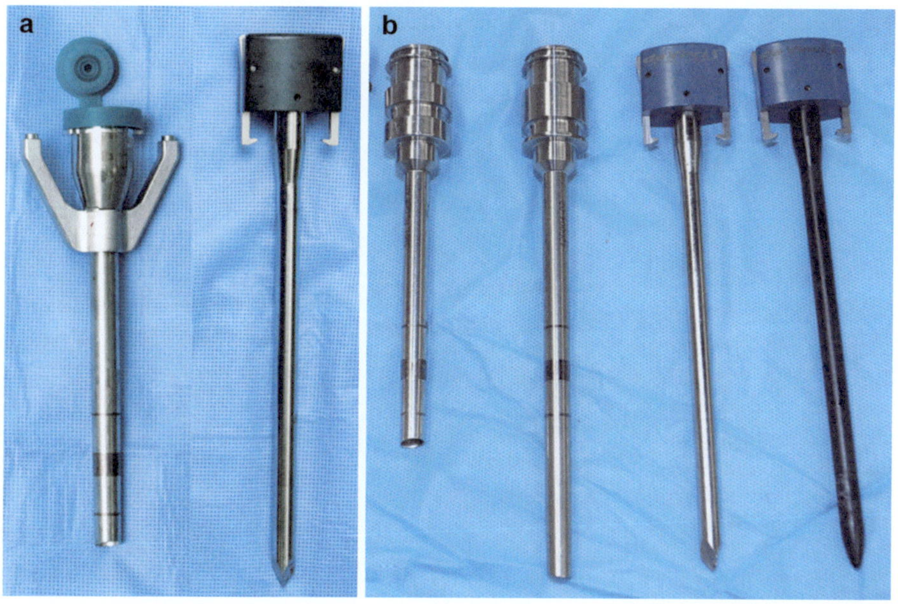

Fig. 2.12 Photograph of 8-mm trocar for the da Vinci® standard (**a**) and S systems (**b**). The trocars for the S systems also have a trocar that can be connected to the insufflator. Also shown are the sharp and blunt obturators used for trocar placement

areas that can be used for insufflators, electrosurgical units, or a DVD recording device. An additional tele monitor may be placed on the top of the tower.

2.10.4 Endowrist® Instruments

EndoWrist® (Intuitive Surgical, Sunnyvale, CA) instruments (Fig. 2.13) are connected to each instrument arm and carry out the surgeon's motions that are relayed from the master controllers. These instruments restore the degrees of freedom (DOF) lost by conventional laparoscopy by adding three DOF at the end of the instrument, giving a total of seven DOF with 180° of articulation and 540°of rotation simulating a surgeon's hand.[3] Each instrument has a fixed number of uses before being discarded.[38] EndoWrist® instruments are composed of instrument housing with release levers, instrument shaft, wrist, and tip. The da Vinci® standard instruments are 52 cm with gray housing compared to the S systems being 57 cm with blue housing. The instruments are not interchangeable between the standard and S systems. Currently, there are more than 40 EndoWrist® instruments available in 8 or 5 mm shaft diameters and several have been designed specifically for urologic surgery. The 8-mm instruments operate on an "angled joint" compared to the 5 mm on a "snake joint." The angled joint allows the tip to rotate using a shorter radius compared to the snake joint (Fig. 2.14).

2.11 Surgical Team

The surgical team is pivotal for successful implementation of a minimally invasive program. Each member must be knowledgeable in laparoscopic and robot-assisted

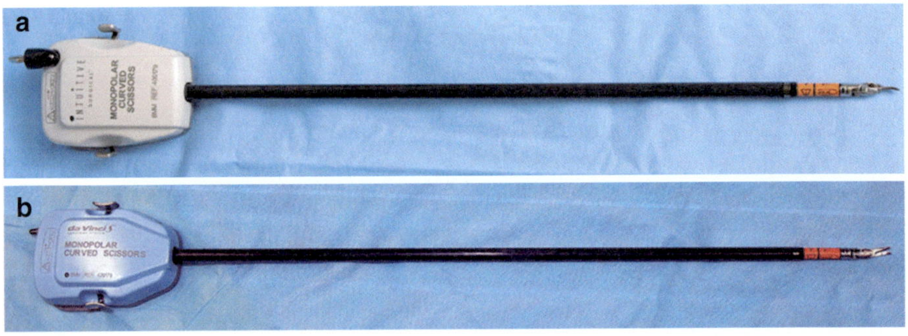

Fig. 2.13 Photograph of EndoWrist® monopolar curved scissors for the da Vinci® standard (**a**) and S (**b**) systems

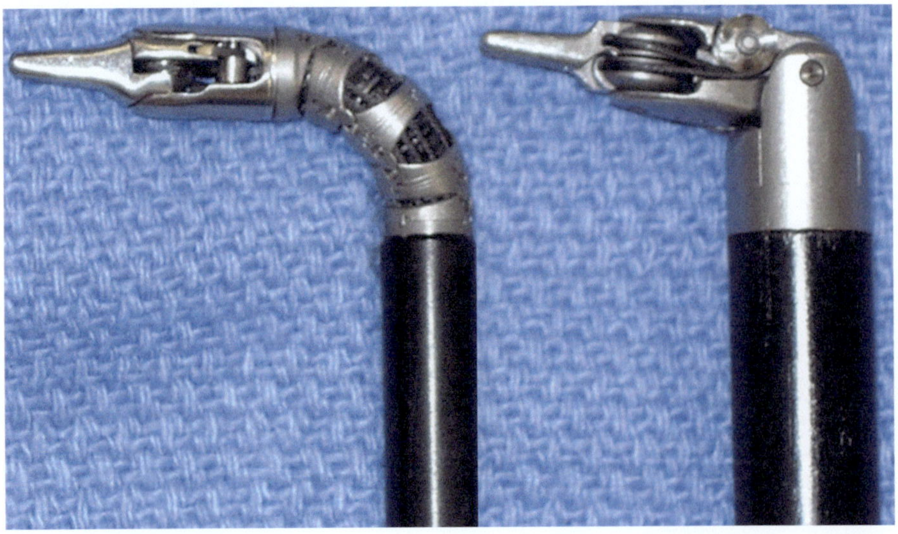

Fig. 2.14 Photograph of Endowrist® needle drivers. On the left is a 5-mm needle driver with the "snake joint" compared to the 8-mm needle driver with an "angled joint"

surgery and communication between each of these individuals is vital for successful outcomes.[40,41] For robot-assisted teams, Intuitive Surgical offers a training course for the surgical team and each member should complete the course prior to starting on the surgical team. It is also important for the surgical team to remain consistent and it is generally recommended to have a dedicated team to work through the learning curve and if possible, all robotic cases.[40]

2.12 Conclusions

Laparoscopic and robot-assisted surgeries in urologic surgery have increased significantly over the past decade. Successful implementation of a minimally invasive program hinges on a complete understanding of instrumentation required. In addition, a knowledgeable and collegial surgical team is crucial for operating room dynamics and improves patient outcomes. Minimally invasive surgery of the retroperitoneum will continue to increase with further advances in technology.

References

1. Davies BL, Hibberd RD, Coptcoat MJ, et al. A surgeon robot prostatectomy – a laboratory evaluation. *J Med Eng Technol.* 1989;13:273.
2. Davies BL, Hibberd RD, Ng WS, et al. The development of a surgeon robot for prostatectomies. *Proc Inst Mech Eng H.* 1991;205:35.
3. Dasgupta P, Rose K, Challacombe B. Equipment and technology in robotics. In: Smith JA, Tewari A, eds. *Robotics in Urologic Surgery.* Philadelphia: Saunders Elsevier; 2008:3-9.
4. Rovetta A, Sala R. Execution of robot-assisted biopsies within the clinical context. *J Image Guid Surg.* 1995;1:280.
5. Challacombe BJ, Khan MS, Murphy D, et al. The history of robotics in urology. *World J Urol.* 2006;24:120.
6. Canes D, Desai MM, Aron M, et al. Transumbilical single-port surgery: evolution and current status. *Eur Urol.* 2008;54:1020.
7. White WM, Goel RK, Kaouk JH. Single-port laparoscopic retroperitoneal surgery: initial operative experience and comparative outcomes. *Urology.* 2009;73:1279.
8. Aron M, Desai MM, Rubinstein M, Gill IS. Laparoscopic instrumentation. In: de la Rosette J, Gill I, eds. *Laparoscopic Urologic Surgery in Malignancies.* New York: Springer; 2005:271-285.
9. Gettman MT. Complications of laparoscopic access. In: Ramakumar S, Jarrett T, eds. *Complications of Urologic Laparoscopic Surgery.* New York: Informa Healthcare; 2005:13-31.
10. Hasson HM. A modified instrument and method for laparoscopy. *Am J Obstet Gynecol.* 1971;110:886.
11. Hasson HM, Rotman C, Rana N, et al. Open laparoscopy: 29-year experience. *Obstet Gynecol.* 2000;96:763.
12. Aron M, Chung B, Gill IS. Basics of retroperitoneal laparoscopy. In: Gill IS, ed. *Textbook of Laparoscopic Urology.* New York/London: Informa; 2006:119-128.
13. Gaur DD. Laparoscopic operative retroperitoneoscopy: use of a new device. *J Urol.* 1992;148:1137.
14. Schulam PG, Hedican SP, Docimo SG. Radially dilating trocar system for open laparoscopic access. *Urology.* 1999;54:727.
15. Shekarriz B, Gholami SS, Rudnick DM, et al. Radially expanding laparoscopic access for renal/adrenal surgery. *Urology.* 2001;58:683.
16. Ternamian AM. A trocarless, reusable, visual-access cannula for safer laparoscopy: an update. *J Am Assoc Gynecol Laparosc.* 1998;5:197.
17. Ternamian AM. Laparoscopy without trocars. *Surg Endosc.* 1997;11:815.
18. Marcovich R, Del Terzo MA, Wolf JS Jr. Comparison of transperitoneal laparoscopic access techniques: optiview visualizing trocar and Veress needle. *J Endourol.* 2000;14:175.
19. String A, Berber E, Foroutani A, et al. Use of the optical access trocar for safe and rapid entry in various laparoscopic procedures. *Surg Endosc.* 2001;15:570.
20. Soulie M, Seguin P, Richeux L, et al. Urological complications of laparoscopic surgery: experience with 350 procedures at a single center. *J Urol.* 2001;165:1960.
21. Shaher Z. Port closure techniques. *Surg Endosc.* 2007; 21:1264.
22. Klingler CH, Remzi M, Marberger M, et al. Haemostasis in laparoscopy. *Eur Urol.* 2006;50:948.
23. Msezane LP, Katz MH, Gofrit ON, et al. Hemostatic agents and instruments in laparoscopic renal surgery. *J Endourol.* 2008;22:403.
24. Lowry PS, Nakada SY. Laparoscopic instrumentation. In: Nakada SY, ed. *Essential Urologic Laparoscopy.* Totowa: Humana Press; 2003:9-22.
25. Lee J, Gianduzzo TR. Advances in laser technology in urology. *Urol Clin North Am.* 2009;36:189.
26. Lotan Y, Gettman MT, Lindberg G, et al. Laparoscopic partial nephrectomy using holmium laser in a porcine model. *JSLS.* 2004;8:51.
27. Lotan Y, Gettman MT, Ogan K, et al. Clinical use of the holmium: YAG laser in laparoscopic partial nephrectomy. *J Endourol.* 2002;16:289.
28. Ogan K, Jacomides L, Saboorian H, et al. Sutureless laparoscopic heminephrectomy using laser tissue soldering. *J Endourol.* 2003;17:295.
29. Moinzadeh A, Gill IS, Rubenstein M, et al. Potassium-titanyl-phosphate laser laparoscopic partial nephrectomy without hilar clamping in the survival calf model. *J Urol.* 2005;174:1110.
30. Bui MH, Breda A, Gui D, et al. Less smoke and minimal tissue carbonization using a thulium laser for laparoscopic partial nephrectomy without hilar clamping in a porcine model. *J Endourol.* 2007;21:1107.
31. Gianduzzo T, Colombo JR Jr, Haber GP, et al. Laser robotically assisted nerve-sparing radical prostatectomy: a pilot study of technical feasibility in the canine model. *BJU Int.* 2008;102:598.

32. Giorgi LJ Jr, Moran ME. Laparoscopic suturing techniques: general consideration. In: Gill IS, ed. *Textbook of Laparoscopic Urology*. New York/London: Informa Health; 2006:129-182.
33. Adams JB, Schulam PG, Moore RG, et al. New laparoscopic suturing device: initial clinical experience. *Urology*. 1995;46:242.
34. Leighton TA, Liu SY, Bongard FS. Comparative cardiopulmonary effects of carbon dioxide versus helium pneumoperitoneum. *Surgery*. 1993;113:527.
35. Ott DE. Laparoscopic hypothermia. *J Laparoendosc Surg*. 1991;1:127.
36. Margulis V, Matsumoto ED, Tunc L, et al. Effect of warmed, humidified insufflation gas and anti-inflammatory agents on cytokine response to laparoscopic nephrectomy: porcine model. *J Urol*. 2005;174:1452.
37. Haber GP, Crouzet S, Kamoi K, et al. Robotic NOTES (Natural Orifice Translumenal Endoscopic Surgery) in reconstructive urology: initial laboratory experience. *Urology*. 2008;71:996.
38. Bhandari A, Hemal A, Menon M. Instrumentation, sterilization, and preparation of robot. *Indian J Urol*. 2005;21:83.
39. Narula VK, Melvin SM. Robotic surgical systems. In: Patel VR, ed. *Robotic Urologic Surgery*. London: Springer; 2007:5-14.
40. Gettman MT, Blute ML, Peschel R, et al. Current status of robotics in urologic laparoscopy. *Eur Urol*. 2003;43:106.
41. Su LM, Smith JA Jr. Laparoscopic and robot-assisted laparoscopic radical prostatectomy and pelvic lymphadenectomy. In: Wein AJ, Kavoussi LR, Novick AC, Partin AW, Peters CA, eds. *Campbell-Walsh Urology*, vol. 3. 9th ed. Philadelphia: Saunders Elsevier; 2007:2985-3005.

3 Upper Tract Retroperitoneal Access Techniques

Ahmed E. Ghazi and Jean V. Joseph

Abstract The laparoscopic approach has been applied to a wide variety of procedures in the field of urology. Since urologists initially adopted laparoscopy from other specialties, most procedures described have been based on the traditional transperitoneal approach. Well-defined organ systems and a relative paucity of intraperitoneal fat allow the rapid identification of landmarks. Instilled gas expands the space in a predictable manner to enable optimal visualization. In contrast, it is technically difficult to develop a consistent working area in a potential retroperitoneal space occupied by areolar and fat tissues. This may explain why most initial urological laparoscopic procedures have been performed transperitoneally. Initial efforts to establish a retroperitoneal working space have been limited by inadequate distention of the retroperitoneal space, but over the last decade several techniques for retroperitoneal access have been described. We describe the increasing experience at various centers over the years, which have led to refinement of retroperitoneal laparoscopic access techniques, utilizing different access devices. Methods that take advantage of the strengths, while overcoming the perceived disadvantages of this approach have been explained.

Keywords Access • Balloon dilatation • Extraperitoneal • Laparoscopy • Retroperitoneal

Key Points

- The retroperitoneal space can be created by various techniques; balloon dilatation, blunt dissection or the use of a visual optic trocar. Each technique has its own inherent advantages and disadvantages.
- Vital points during insertion of the ports include:
  - Placing the patient in the standard flank position and flexing the operating table maximizes the limited space between the 12th rib and iliac crest, for maximal trocar spacing.
  - Placement of ports under guidance with both laparoscopic monitoring and bimanual control.
  - The initial trocar, which will hold the laparoscope, is optimally positioned anterior to the tip of the 12th rib for optimal visualization of the anterior as well as the posterior renal surface.
  - The 12 mm lower mid-axillary line surgeon port must also be located at a considerable distance (>3 cm) cephalad to the iliac bone.
  - If necessary the retroperitoneal space is further enlarged by blunt mobilization of the lateral peritoneal reflection allowing introduction of the surgeons working trocars further anterior to the axillary line.

3.1 Introduction

In 1973, Wittmoser was the first to use minimally invasive endoscopic access to the retroperitoneum. He used this technique to perform lumbar sympathectomy after

A.E. Ghazi (✉)
Department of Urology, University of Rochester Medical Center, 601 Elmwood Ave., Box 656, 14642 Rochester, NY, USA
e-mail: ahmed_ghazimd@yahoo.com, ahmed_ghazi@urmc.rochester.edu

J.V. Joseph and H.R.H. Patel (eds.), *Retroperitoneal Robotic and Laparoscopic Surgery*,
DOI: 10.1007/978-0-85729-485-2_3, © Springer-Verlag London Limited 2011

blunt dissection with a telescope and pneumatic dissection with carbon dioxide. In 1979, Wickham used a similar approach for the first retroperitoneal laparoscopic ureterolithotomy. Sommerkamp had already presented the technique of endoscopy of the retroperitoneum in 1974 as a urological variation of mediastinoscopy without using pneumoretroperitoneum to perform renal biopsies. In 1982, Bay-Nielsen and Schultz performed endoscopy of the retroperitoneum to remove upper ureteral calculi. The first attempts at retroperitoneal endoscopic nephrectomy were made by Coptcoat: Wickham and Miller, G and Weinberg and Smith in the early 1980s, and were based on the technique of percutaneous renal stone surgery.[1] However, these attempts were limited by the suboptimal pneumoretroperitoneum and inadequate working space in the retroperitoneum. The clinical breakthroughs came in 1992, when Gaur showed that distension of a balloon placed within the retroperitoneum rapidly and atraumatically displaced the adjacent fat and peritoneum, thereby creating an adequate working space for laparoscopic surgery.[2] This landmark concept has led the resurgence of interest in retroperitoneoscopy and pelvic extraperitoneoscopy.

3.2 Techniques for Retroperitoneal Access

As mentioned in the anatomy chapter, moving the patient from the supine to the lateral position leads to an enlargement of the retroperitoneal space. However, this positional enlargement is inadequate for performing retroperitoneoscopic renal manipulation and additional active enlargement of the retroperitoneum is required to create a sufficient working space. Several techniques for retroperitoneal access have been described. The most common approach is the open balloon technique, which creates an adequate working space. A variety of retroperitoneal balloons have been designed for this purpose, including the use of a laparoscopic condom and a Foley catheter.[3,4] With concerns regarding carbon dioxide gas leakage associated with access, the complications associated with balloon rupture together with the substantial costs of commercially made balloons,[5] other groups described alternative techniques for creating a sufficient working space in the retroperitoneum such as blunt finger dissection.[1,6-8] These different techniques are described in detail in this chapter.

Gill[9] described the use of the open balloon technique for creation of the retroperitoneal space. The patient is placed in the standard flank position, the kidney bridge is elevated, and the operating table is flexed to maximize the space between the lowermost rib and the iliac crest (portal for retroperitoneoscopic surgery). A horizontal 1.5- to 2-cm skin incision is created below the tip of the 12th rib, and the flank muscle fibers are bluntly separated with S-retractors. Entry is gained into the retroperitoneum by gently piercing the anterior thoracolumbar fascia with the finger tip or a hemostat. Finger dissection of the retroperitoneum is then performed in a cephalad direction, remaining immediately anterior to the psoas muscle and posterior to the Gerota's fascia/kidney to create a space for placement of the balloon dilator (Fig. 3.1). The authors published their first experience using a balloon fashioned from the two middle fingers of a sterile No. 7 surgical glove, one placed inside the other, and tied to the end of a No. 14 red rubber catheter.[10] The authors now employ a trocar-mounted balloon distension device (Origin Medsystems, Menlo Park, CA) for creating a working space in the retroperitoneum. We alternatively use the Spacemaker dissection balloon (Coviden, Autosuture, Norwalk, CT) which provides a similar dissection (Fig. 3.2). The volume of air instilled into the balloon is determined by the patient's body mass. A total of 400–600 ml is instilled in children and 800–1,000 ml in adults. Early in the

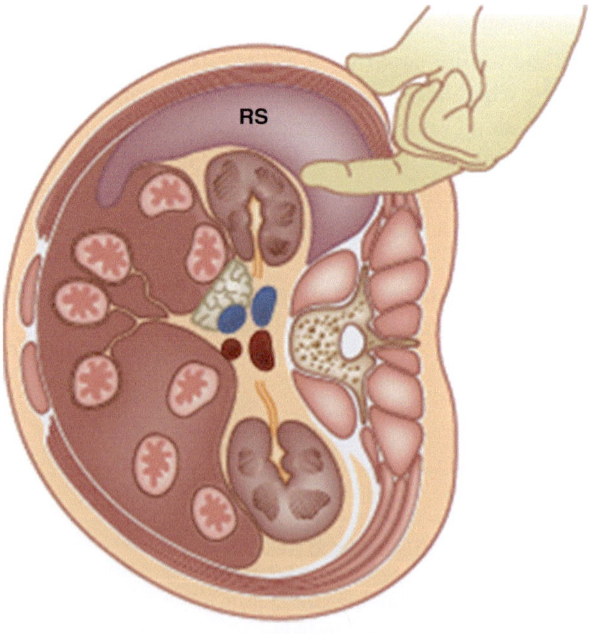

Fig. 3.1 Finger dissection of the retroperitoneum to create a space for placement of the balloon dilator. *RS*: Reroperitoneal space

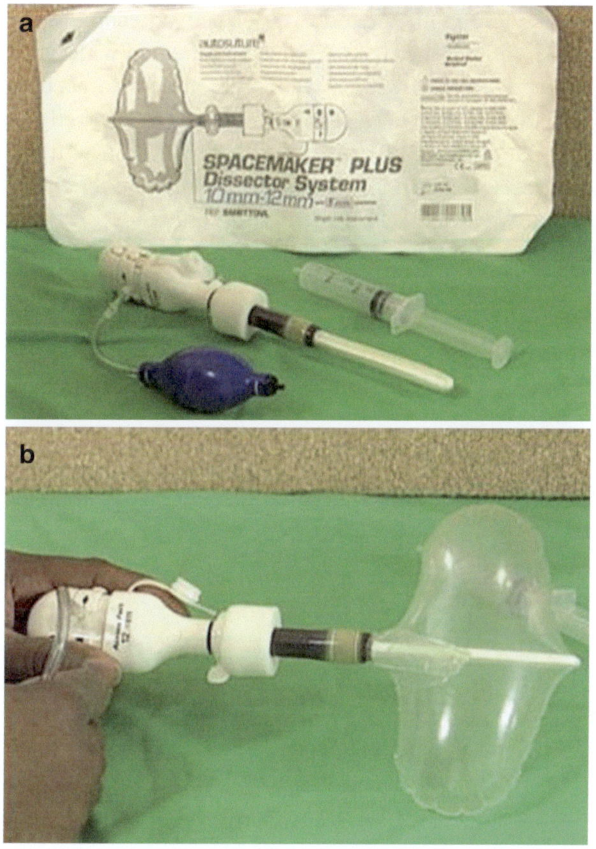

Fig. 3.2 (**a**) Spacemaker dissection balloon, (**b**) Spacemaker balloon inflated

author's experience, the balloon was placed within Gerota's fascia during all cases of retroperitoneoscopic nephrectomy in an attempt to minimize carbon dioxide leak and subcutaneous emphysema, allow safe placement of secondary ports and finally minimize peritoneal transgression. Although successful in thin patients, this maneuver was usually unsuccessful in the obese patient.[10] Based on their recent experience with retroperitoneoscopic radical surgery, intentional balloon dilation outside of Gerota's fascia was used (i.e., in the pararenal fat between the psoas muscle posteriorly and Gerota's fascia anteriorly). This effectively displaces the Gerota's fascia/kidney anteromedially (Fig. 3.3) and expedites direct access to the posterior aspect of the renal hilum and its adjacent great vessels (vena cava on the right side, aorta on the left side). Despite being obscured by fat, transmitted arterial and aortic pulsations are clearly visualized, thereby facilitating identification of the main renal artery and vein close to their origin from the aorta and vena cava, respectively. Following balloon deflation and removal, a 10-mm Blunt tip trocar (Origin Medsystems, Menlo Park, CA) is placed as the primary port. This trocar has an internal fascial retention balloon and an external adjustable foam cuff which combine to create an air-tight seal, eliminating air leakage at the primary port site. Pneumoretroperitoneum is created up to a pressure of 15 mmHg using carbon dioxide. The laparoscope is

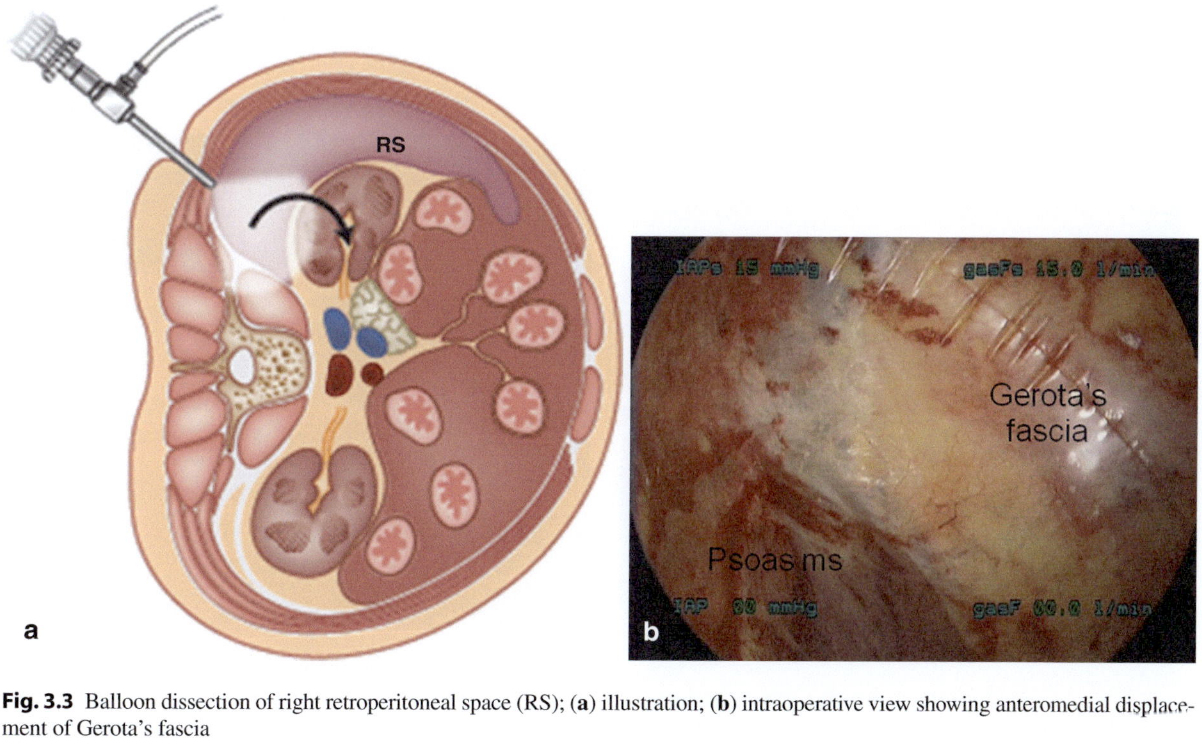

Fig. 3.3 Balloon dissection of right retroperitoneal space (RS); (**a**) illustration; (**b**) intraoperative view showing anteromedial displacement of Gerota's fascia

inserted, and the secondary ports are placed with a judicious combination of laparoscopic monitoring and bimanual control (this bimanual technique can be helpful for inserting secondary ports located in close proximity to the primary port). To insert a secondary port under bimanual control, the laparoscope and the blunt tip cannula are removed, with resultant deflation of the pneumoretroperitoneum. If necessary, the lateral peritoneal reflection is bluntly mobilized further anteromedially from the undersurface of the flank abdominal wall by the surgeon's finger inserted through the primary port incision. This maneuver enlarges the retroperitoneal space and allows greater distance between port sites. The desired secondary trocar is now inserted with bimanual guidance. The secondary trocar is inserted by the surgeon's dominant hand and guided onto the retroperitoneally positioned S retractor (Fig. 3.4).The trocar arrangement depends on the procedure to be performed.

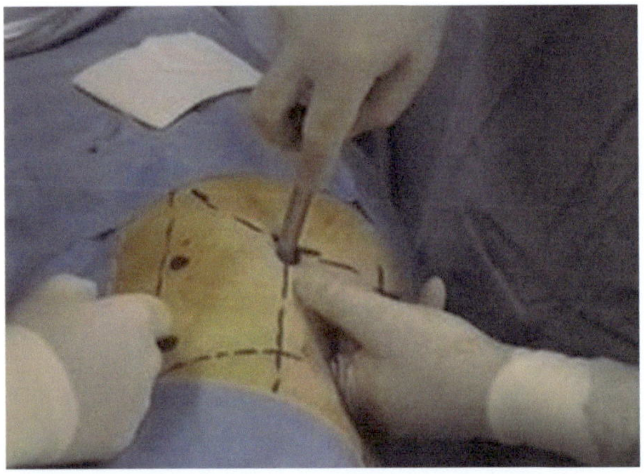

Fig. 3.4 Technique for safe introduction of secondary trocars

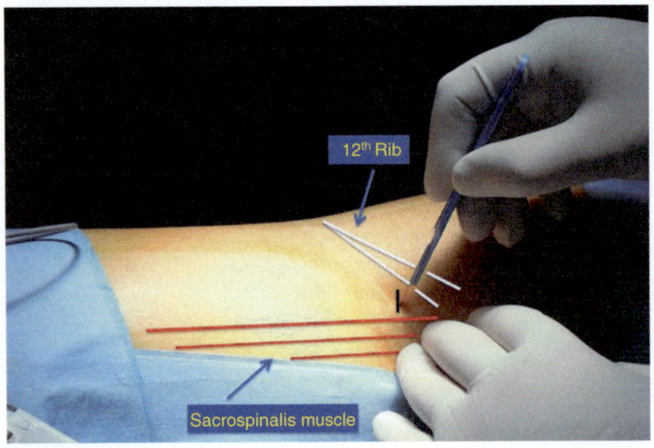

Fig. 3.5 Site of primary incision, showing surface anatomy of Sacrospinalis muscle and 12th rib

The group in Creteil[6-8] described a technique in which the retroperitoneal space was created with blunt finger dissection, which was large enough to accommodate four to five trocars according to the procedure. The patient was placed in the flank position without overextension. A 1 cm incision was made in the triangle between the 12th rib and latissimus dorsi muscle on the posterior axillary line (Fig. 3.5). A hemostat was introduced to split the muscles and the lumbodorsal fascia and create a tunnel through which an index finger could be introduced (via the incision) to push the peritoneum forward (Fig. 3.6). Two 5 mm trocars

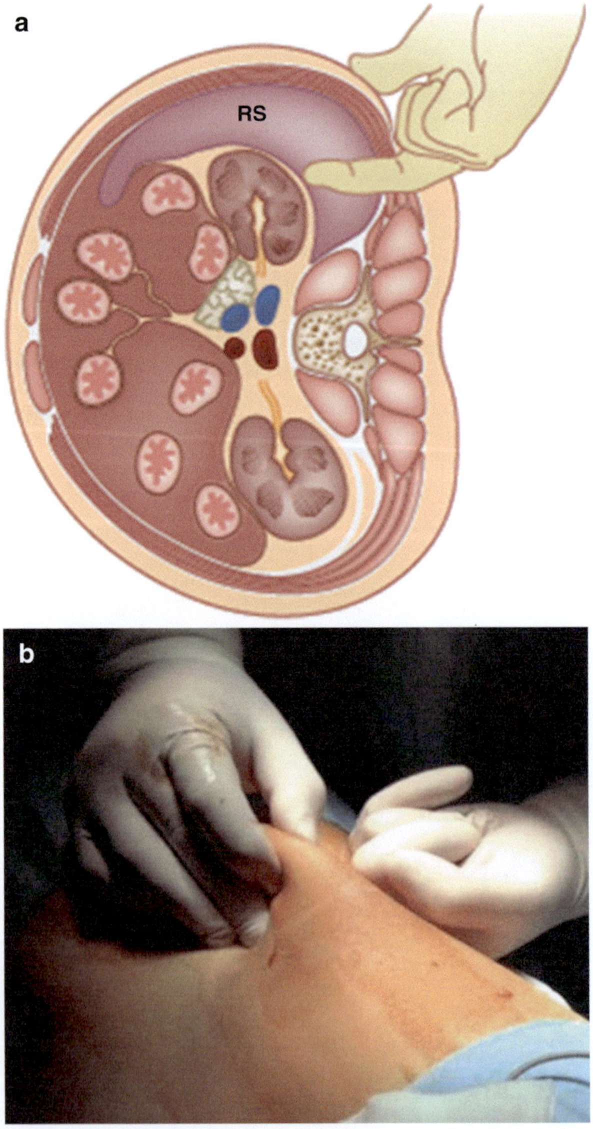

Fig. 3.6 Finger dissection of the left retroperitoneal space (RS) as an alternative to balloon dissection: (**a**) illustration of internal view and (**b**) external view

are inserted for the assistant's use on the anterior axillary line and two trocars (12 mm and 5 mm) are inserted for the surgeon's use on the posterior axillary line. A fifth trocar (10 mm) was inserted for the endoscopic lens on the midaxillary line (Fig. 3.7). Following insertion of the trocars, the working space was completed with the aid of insufflation and dissection. Gerota's fascia was then incised and the kidneys, adrenal gland with their surrounding relations were identified.

Other less than common used techniques for dissection of the retroperitoneal space include: the closed (Veress needle), direct vision, and gasless techniques. Since these are not the most commonly adopted techniques they will be briefly described. Prerequisites of the Veress needle technique include the retrograde placement of a ureteral occlusion balloon catheter and placement of the patient in the prone position on a table with fluoroscopic capability. The collecting system of the affected kidney is opacified via the catheter. A small skin incision is made at the inferior lumbar (Petit's) triangle and a Veress needle introduced perpendicularly for a distance of 3–4 cm. The needle is then advanced under fluoroscopic control until the horizontal plane of the kidney is reached. At that point the tip of the needle should reside within Gerota's fascia and just below the lower pole of the kidney. Insufflation with carbon dioxide is initiated at a pressure of 15 mmHg with a minimum flow of 2 l/min.[11] This technique is relatively blind, on the contrary to the direct vision technique in which a Visiport or Optview† trocar (Ethicon Endosurgical, Inc., Johnson-Johnson, Arlington, VA) is used to visualize the penetration of the layers at the Petit's triangle, providing a direct visual access into the retroperitoneum. Penetration of Scarpa's fascia, the flank muscles, and lumbodorsal fascia can subsequently be felt and seen in some patients.[12]

With the development of an effective, automated body-wall retractor, Etwaru et al.[13] and Hirsch et al.[14] reported a series using pre-peritoneal gasless laparoscopy. The Laprofan and Laprolift (Medsystems, Menlo Park, CA) attached to the side of the operating table is used to elevate the anterior abdominal wall, after preliminary balloon dissection of the pre-peritoneal space. An inflated Foley catheter with a stylet, placed through a separate midline incision is used to retract the peritoneum superiorly. Advantages of this technique include: eliminating the need for special trocars or endoscopic instruments, no carbon dioxide insufflation with its associated complications, and the potential for regional anesthesia. However, this technique usually results in even less exposure than low-pressure carbon dioxide insufflation. In addition, the Laprofan provides inadequate retraction in moderately obese patients. Another risk is snapping of the blades

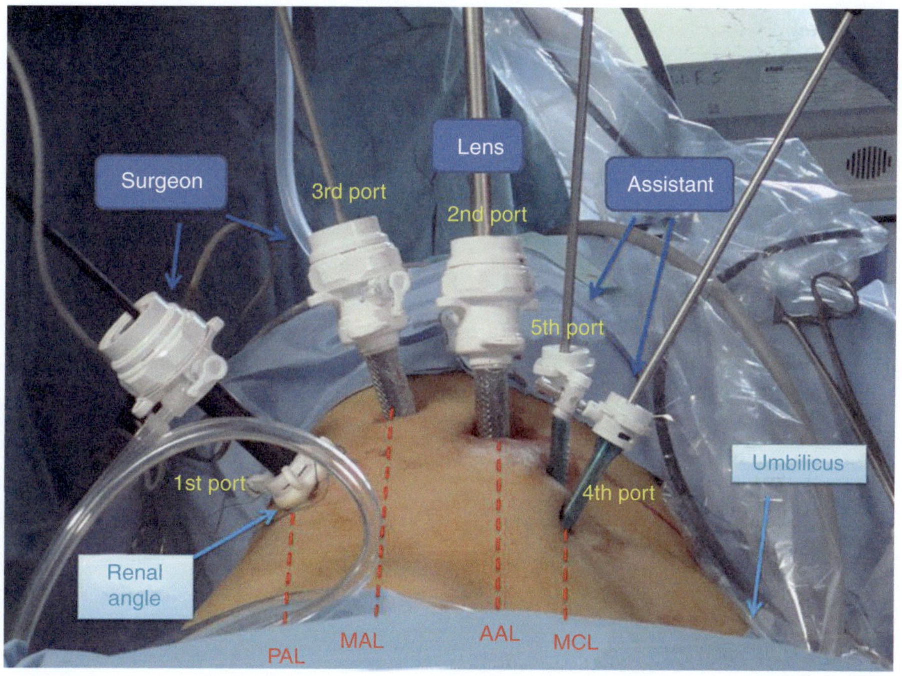

Fig. 3.7 Final five-trocar arrangement for retroperitoneal surgery. *PAL* Posterior axillary line, *MAL* Middle axillary line, *AAL* Anterior axillary line, *MCL* Middle clavicular line

of the retractor with vigorous use. Finally, a lengthy procedure increases the risk of pressure necrosis of the rectus muscle.[15]

3.3 Retroperitoneal Access in the Pediatric Population

Retroperitoneal access for renal surgery in children requires no special materials, and has been well described.[16] The patient is placed in the lateral decubitus position with flexion of the operating table sufficient to create an area as large as possible for trocar placement between the 12th rib and iliac crest. This space is particularly limited in children, rendering the working space narrower. A 1–2 cm skin incision is made at the lower border of the tip of the 12th rib (for endoscopic camera). This incision is deepened by blunt dissection using an artery forceps down to the retroperitoneal space. Gerota's fascia is opened and the perirenal fat is identified. A blunt nondisposable 5 or 10 mm trocar is introduced up in the perirenal fat, and gas insufflation initiated under laparoscopic guidance. The authors placed a purse-string suture around the skin incision to ensure an airtight seal, eliminating the need for a self-retaining disposable trocar. The suture is also attached to the trocar to prevent its exteriorization and for suspension as needed. The working space is created by gas insufflation dissection aided by a swinging movement of the laparoscope, which allowed blunt dissection of the perirenal loose tissue. The remaining operating trocars were inserted under direct vision 1 finger width from the top of the iliac crest and posteriorly in front of the lumbosacral muscle, respectively. An additional accessory trocar can be placed if needed, in front of the first trocar on top of the kidney. Insufflation pressure did not exceed 12 mmHg and in children younger than 2 years maximal pressure was 8 mmHg. Narrow retractors with long blades are used to provide deep dissection with a short incision. In addition, accurate trocar positioning was mandatory to facilitate optimal anatomical and mechanical kidney access. Patient age was not a limiting factor for this approach. In fact, young children have less fat and, thus, access is easier. The authors made all efforts to minimize the costly elements of instruments and operative time. They mainly used nondisposable instruments for retroperitoneal access and creation of the working space.

Micali described a novel closed retroperitoneal access technique in the pediatric age group.[17] The initial retroperitoneal access is obtained at the lumbar or Petit's triangle, which is formed by the intersection of the external oblique and latissimus dorsi muscles and the iliac crest. The space between the 12th rib and iliac crest was maximized by placing the patient in the standard flank position and flexing the operating table. This maneuver allowed the surgeon to identify Petit's triangle. A 12 mm incision was made within this area and a Visiport laparoscopic visual trocar was advanced directly into the retroperitoneum under direct vision. The Visiport incises each tissue layer under direct vision, allowing complete visual control to avoid blood vessels, and nerves as the retroperitoneum is entered. The penetration of Scarpa's fascia, the flank muscle, and the lumbodorsal fascia was consecutively felt and seen in some patients. The lumbodorsal fascia was visualized in all cases and it was clearly felt to give after the fascia was incised (Fig. 3.8). After the lumbodorsal fascia was transverse, the retroperitoneal space was entered and the characteristic fat was visualized. Insufflation with carbon dioxide at 15 mmHg was instituted. The laparoscope was then used to dissect bluntly the retroperitoneal space and mobilize the lateral peritoneum from the anterior abdominal wall. Care was taken when dissecting to prevent peritoneal tearing. A 5 mm trocar port was placed under direct vision in the anterior axillary line at the same level as the initial

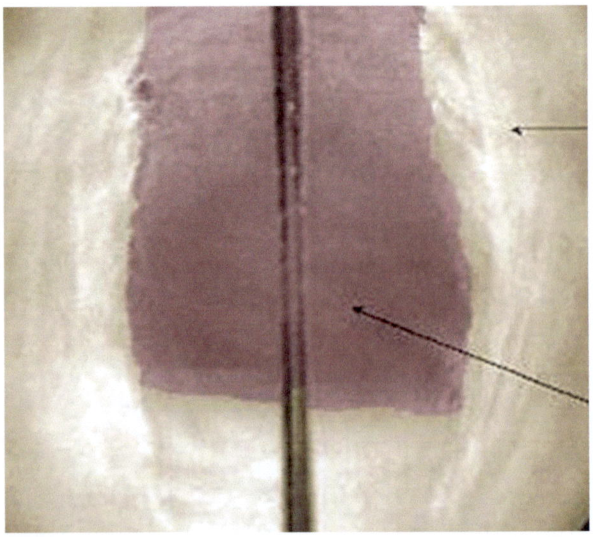

Fig. 3.8 Internal view of retroperitoneal space and lumbodorsal fascia using the Visiport device

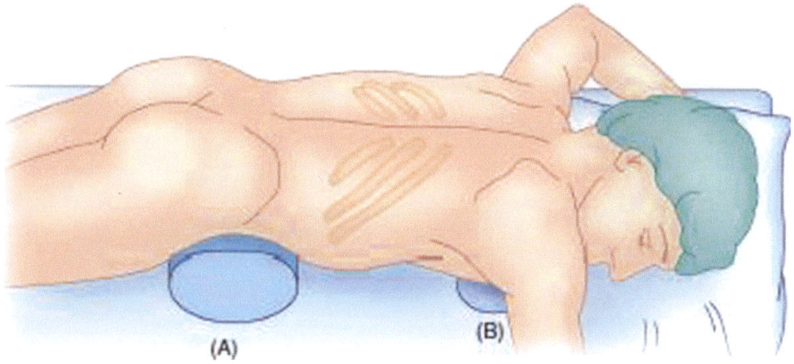

Fig. 3.9 Prone position: A-B, sites where patient is supported by sandbags; one to three sites of trocars (Reprinted from Urbanowicz et al.[18] with permission from Elsevier)

port. The autors have used this technique for procedures as renal biopsy, varicocelectomy, renal cyst ablation and pyelolithotomy, in which another 5 mm trocar was placed between the two ports. However they believe that this access technique would be effective for more complicated procedures, with the only difference being the need for a larger working space with a blunt dissection aided by a swinging movement of the laparoscope.

Urbanowicz et al.[18] described their initial experience with retroperitoneoscopic procedures in children in the prone position. The child is placed in the prone position with sandbags and protective foams used to support the shoulders, thorax and hips, allowing free excursion of the anterior abdominal wall (Fig. 3.9). Following identification of the lateral edge of the sacrospinalis muscle, tip of the 12th rib and the iliac crest, a 10 mm trocar is inserted through a 1 cm longitudinal incision in the angle of the 12th rib and the lateral edge of the sacrospinalis muscle (on the right side the incision is made 1–1.5 cm lower). This allowed a simple and comfortable entry route without risk of injuring the peritoneal reflection. A visiport (manufactured by Auto-suture) with a 0° endoscope was used to pass through the lumbodorsal fascia and the lateral aspect of the sacrospinalis muscle into the retroperitoneal space. The working space was created using carbon dioxide insufflation at a pressure of 12–15 mmHg with no use of a balloon device. At times the laparoscope can be used to push the lateral peritoneal reflection downwards below the posterior axillary line, if it was not possible to achieve this position solely by balloon insufflation. A 10 mm endoscope with a 0° lens was passed through the port and the lateral peritoneal reflection indentified. Another 5-mm port was inserted just dorsal to the peritoneal reflection halfway between the tip of the 12th rib and the iliac crest along the posterior axillary line. A third 5-mm port was inserted 1–2 cm cephalad to the iliac crest at the lateral border of the sacrospinalis muscle. The authors advocate that gravitational effect of the prone position allows the abdominal contents and peritoneum to fall ventrally. This allows for lower pressure while creating a working space, and facilitates dissection of the retroperitoneal space. In the prone position the kidney also tends to fall ventrally, exposing the renal hilum facilitating its dissection and vascular control (Fig. 3.10).

3.4 Technical Caveats

For safe and reliable retroperitoneoscopic access to the kidney and upper ureter, the surgeon must pay attention to several key technical aspects.

3.4.1 Port Positioning

The transperitoneal laparoscopic approach more closely approximates the situation encountered during open surgery. Therefore, proper placement of the port housing the laparoscope is important during retroperitoneoscopy. During port placement, every effort should be made to separate the ports as much as possible. Frustrating "clashing of swords" occurs if the trocars, and therefore the laparoscopic instruments, are located in close proximity. To overcome this, the surgeons working trocars, anterior axillary line port (surgeon working port) can be positioned further anterior to the axillary line. However, the lateral peritoneal reflection must be clearly visualized laparoscopically and avoided before this port is inserted. Furthermore, we utilize a fan retractor to bluntly peel the

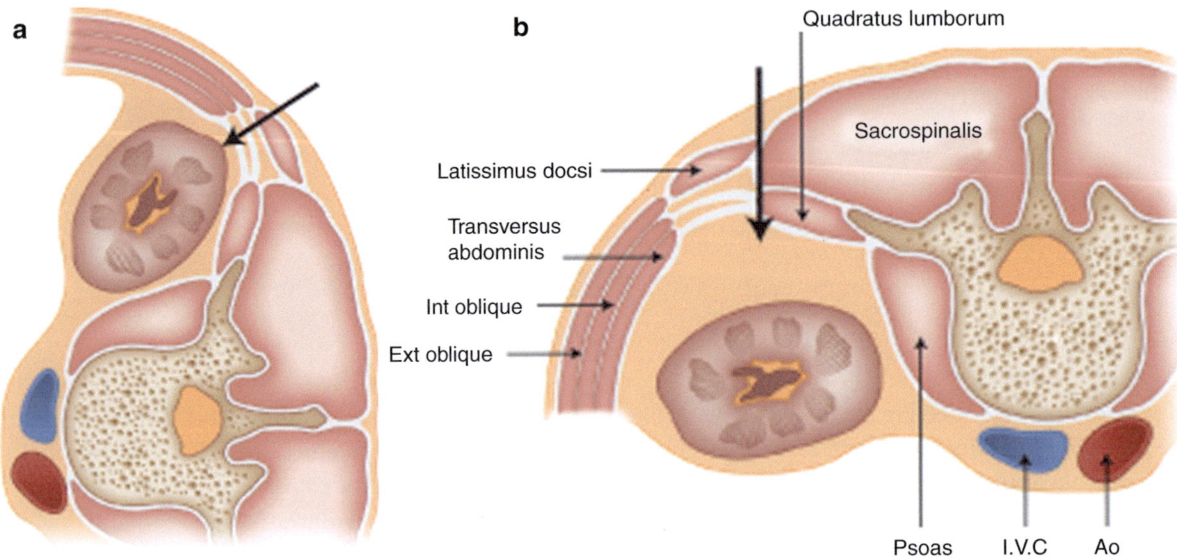

Fig. 3.10 Cross-sectional views of the kidney: arrows, trocar site no 1; (**a**) flank position, indirect access to the renal hilus; (**b**) prone position, ventral displacement of the kidney, direct view of the hilus resulting from gravitational effects (Reprinted from Urbanowicz et al.[18], with permission from Elsevier)

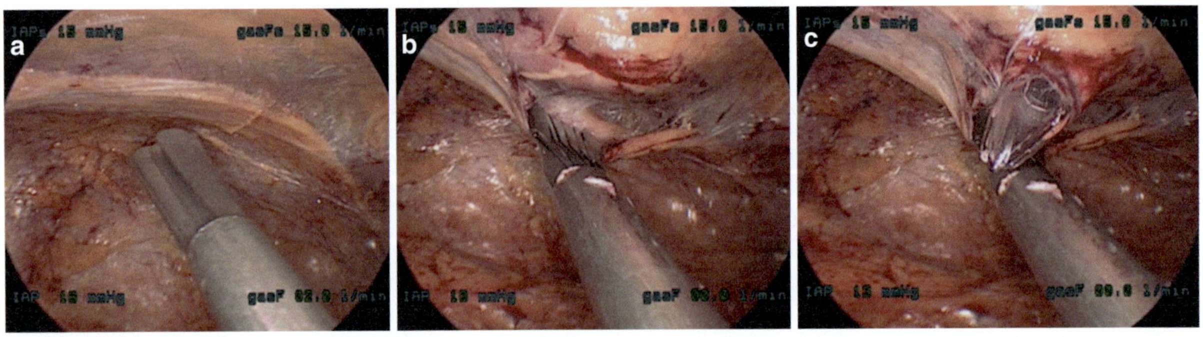

Fig. 3.11 (**a**) Fan retractor pushing peritoneum off anterior abdominal wall. (**b**, **c**) Fan retractor protecting peritoneum to avoid rent during trocar placement

peritoneal reflection anteriorly as well as protect the peritoneum during trocar insertion (Fig. 3.11). Similarly, care must be taken to avoid pleural injury during placement of the assistant port. The 12-mm lower mid-axillary line surgeon port must also be located at a considerable distance (>3 cm) cephalad to the iliac bone. The unyielding bone significantly compromises the torque capability of a trocar placed adjacent to it. The initial trocar, which will hold the laparoscope, is optimally positioned anterior to the tip of the 12th rib, which places the laparoscope in line with the lateral border of the kidney and allows good visualization of the anterior as well as the posterior renal surface.[10]

3.4.2 Orientation

It is also important to note that during retroperitoneoscopic renal procedures the kidney is approached in an end on, caudad-to-cephalad orientation where the lower renal pole is visualized first and further dissection reveals the middle and upper kidney. This event is in sharp contrast to transperitoneal laparoscopy, which is a side on approach in which the anterior surface of the kidney and the renal hilum are visualized initially. To facilitate dissection of the upper pole of the kidney, a laparoscope with a 30-degree lens is used, which provides a wider field of vision and helps to overcome some of the limitations in visualization imposed by the infracostal approach used in retroperitoneoscopy. In addition, the camera should be oriented such that the psoas muscle is always horizontal on the video monitor. The psoas muscle can be identified most easily caudal to the kidney.[10]

3.4.3 Inability to Locate the Renal Hilum

If the renal hilum cannot be located, Gerota's fascia should be incised longitudinally, along the psoas muscle. The kidney should then be retracted anterolaterally, placing the renal hilum on stretch. The laparoscope is then slowly advanced across the anterior surface of the psoas muscle from lateral to medial in a cephalad direction. With the laparoscope held steady, a search is made for pulsations along the medial border of the psoas muscle. Gentle dissection directly toward the pulsations should reveal the underlying blood vessel. Alternatively, the ureter can be followed cephalad to the renal hilum. Finally, the surface of the kidney can be identified and traced medially to its hilum.[9]

3.4.4 Peritoneal Injury

To avoid transperitoneal insertion, freeing the posterior peritoneum from the iliac fossa, is an important step in preparing the working space before inserting the accessory trocar.[10] In cases where an inadvertent peritoneotomy occurs, some advocate[9] that it does not necessarily require conversion from the retroperitoneal to a transperitoneal approach. Equilibration of pressure across the peritoneum occurs rapidly, and generally does not interfere with retroperitoneoscopic completion of the procedure. However, adequate medial retraction of the kidney by the assistant through an anteriorly placed port may be necessary to maintain operative exposure in the retroperitoneal space. In addition, thorough inspection of the intra-abdominal viscera via the laparoscope through the peritoneal rent should be carried out to assess for any injury. Care must be taken to deflate the pneumoperitoneum before terminating the procedure (a red rubber catheter introduced laparoscopically through the peritoneotomy can be helpful in this regard). Others[16] believe that when pneumoperitoneum occurs secondary to a peritoneal tear at the beginning of the procedure, the retroperitoneal working space is decreased by the effect of pneumoperitoneum. This complication can be managed by laparoscopic suturing of the tear or, if that is impossible, by insertion of a Veress needle in the peritoneal cavity to evacuate gas during the procedure. However, if the peritoneum tears after the renal vessels are ligated, or during dissection of the anterior surface of the kidney or ureter, the procedure could be completed without special management of the pneumoperitoneum.

3.4.5 Gas Leakage

A major concern of open retroperitoneal access techniques is gas leakage from the trocar access site. With this, the retroperitoneal space collapses and manipulation of instruments becomes impossible, and the likelihood of developing subcutaneous emphysema increases. This may be overcome using specially designed trocars with a fascial retention balloon and an external adjustable foam cuff (Medsystems, Menlo Park, CA). This may be preferable to the Hasson cannula, since it provides an airtight seal at the primary port site (Fig. 3.12). The fascial retention balloon is positioned within the retroperitoneal space and inflated with approximately 30 cc of air. The external foam cuff is snugly clinched down, effectively sealing the subcutaneous tissues and muscle layers around the primary port site, thus minimizing air leak. This trocar obviates the significant problem of carbon dioxide leakage and/or subcutaneous emphysema around the

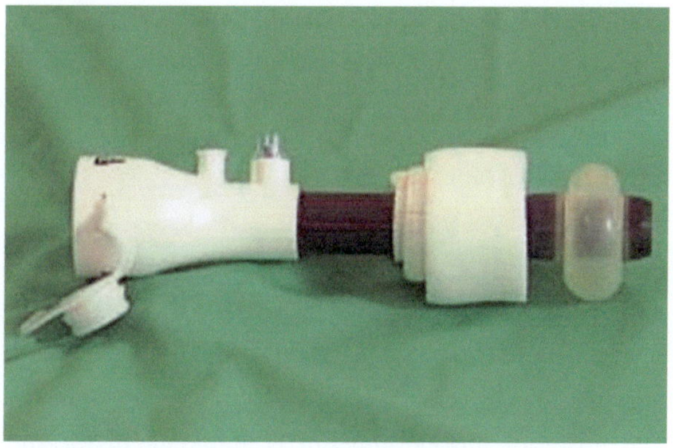

Fig. 3.12 Blunt tip trocar (Spacemaker, Autosuture) is employed to achieve an airtight seal for the primary port

Hasson cannula, which is associated with significantly greater systemic absorption of carbon dioxide.[19]

Gaur[20] described a more cost-effective technique to minimize gas leakage. A small moist gauze is tagged to a fine thread and packed around the cannula (10 mm). A 1/0 prolene purse-string suture is passed around it. The ends of the suture are passed though the plastic sheath of a disposable hypodermic needle, after cutting off its blind end. The suture is secured with a small artery forceps to make the incision air-tight.

3.4.6 Balloon Dissection

The degree of peritoneal dissection depends mostly on the distension of the balloon and to some extent on its position. If the balloon is placed toward the umbilicus, almost all the entire abdominal ureter can be clearly visualized as soon as the laparoscope is inserted. If placed toward McBurney's point, the lower part of the abdominal ureter and internal spermatic vein are easily identified. If placed toward the epigastrium it can dissect the lower pole of the kidney.[2] However, in the presence of significant adhesions, balloon dilatation may fail to mobilize the peritoneal reflection. In this situation, additional peritoneal mobilization can be achieved by gentle blunt dissection with the surgeon's finger, a swab-stick, or the laparoscope.[9]

3.4.7 Docking of the Surgical Cart

One of the crucial points of retroperitoneoscopic access is the correct placement of the surgical cart. The cart is wheeled in a 45–60° angle from the patient's head. It should be placed as closely as possible to the patient with the camera arm pointing toward the upper pole of the kidney.[21]

3.5 Devices Used for Retroperitoneal Balloon Dissection

The posterior retroperitoneum is abundant in fat and tough areolar tissue, which does not permit creation of a satisfactory pneumoretroperitoneum merely by pneumo insufflation through a needle as in the transperitoneal approach. Therefore, alternatives for creation of a retroperitoneal working space were innovated. These included, the balloon described by Gaur et al.[2]which was made at the operating table by tying a piece of surgical glove to a red rubber catheter and connected to the pneumatic pump of a standard blood pressure apparatus, with an intervening T-connector (the other end of the T-connector could be used to record pressures during balloon dissection). This was a low-pressure balloon, with the resting balloon pressure being between 10 and 40 mmHg. The balloon was placed deep to the fascia transversalis through a 2 cm incision in the lumbar region at the center of a previously marked subcostal incision after creating a space with the index finger. The dissecting balloon was inserted into this space with a pair of small retractors and a dissecting forceps. The balloon is then gradually inflated with air until a bulge appears in the abdomen. (For high-pressure balloons, normal saline and a 50 ml syringe were used for inflation to avoid any explosive balloon rupture.) It is not mandatory to record balloon pressures during inflation, but pressures in the glove below 40 mmHg indicate expansion in the right plane. The balloon was left in place for 5–7 min for hemostasis to take place and then deflated and removed. The degree of distension of the balloon depends upon the type of operative procedure to be performed.[2,22] Although the balloon creates a large retroperitoneal space and dissects the retroperitoneal organs atraumatically, there is no way of knowing that the balloon is expanding in the right plane. Gaur[3] later described a laparoscopic condom dissection as an improvement on the previously described balloon dissection technique of retroperitoneoscopy, which allowed a controlled visual dissection and creation of a space in the retroperitoneal area. The laparoscopic condom (Cook Urological, Spencer, IN) is 20 cm long and made of latex. It has a sheath of uniform diameter (0.8 cm) and a high-compliance transparent balloon (7 × 3 cm) at one end. The condom sheath is shortened to match the working length of a 10-mm laparoscopic cannula and is stretched to slide over and fit the cannula snugly (Fig. 3.13). The cannula with the condom is introduced into the retroperitoneal space by one of the two techniques; one similar to the one used for introduction of the previously mentioned balloon dissector (digital dissection). Another technique is to use an 11-mm trocar-cannula with a spring-on safety sheath introduced into the retroperitoneal space through a slightly smaller

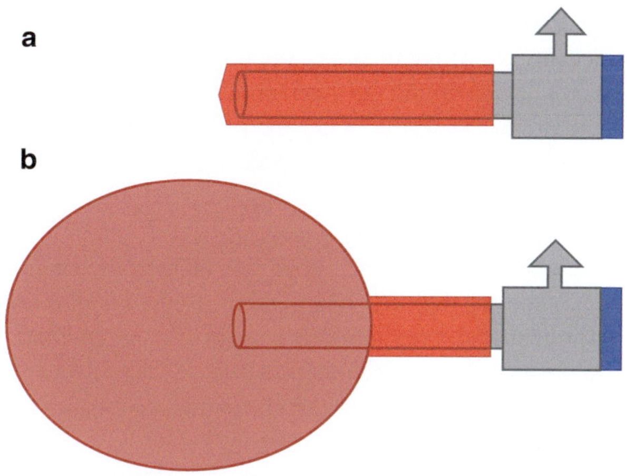

Fig. 3.13 Diagrammatic illustration of the condom cannula; (**a**) A 10 mm cannula with condom balloon. (**b**) Inflated condom balloon

incision, using a steady twisting force. Once the trocar goes through the lumbodorsal fascia (resistance disappears), the protective sheath snaps over the trocar. The tip of the cannula is removed after it is used to dissect a space in the retroperitoneum to accommodate the condom. The 10-mm cannula with the condom is then maneuvered into this space through the same track by slightly stretching the condom with a blunt dissector inserted through the cannula. The dissector is removed once the cannula is in place. A 10-mm telescope is inserted halfway into the cannula, and the condom is inflated to about 300 ml using the pneumatic pump of a standard blood pressure apparatus. The condom balloon is then connected to a pneumoinsufflator, and the balloon pressure is noted. The telescope is connected to a fiberoptic light source and is advanced further for inspection of the retroperitoneum through the transparent balloon. The pneumoinsufflator is turned on to inflate the balloon gradually to 11mmHg, and the retroperitoneal dissection by the inflating balloon is laparoscopically monitored. The condom dissection technique of retroperitoneoscopy is superior to the balloon dissection technique, as it is not a blind procedure and it allows a simultaneous laparoscopic dissection of the retroperitoneal structures. In addition, the balloon can be maneuvered with the tip of the laparoscope or the cannula. The pressure never rises above 30 mmHg, and therefore, there is less chance of balloon rupture. However, the authors concluded that the laparoscopic condom dissection was a new technique that required further evaluation.

In Gill et al.[10] preliminary experience dissecting balloon was fashioned from the two middle fingers of a sterile No. 7 surgical glove, one placed inside the other, and tied to the end of a No. 14 red rubber catheter. The catheter was introduced through 1.5–2 cm transverse skin incision made just anterior to the tip of the 12th rib, down to a 1 cm incision made in the anterior thoracolumbar fascia. Finger dissection was performed in the retroperitoneum to create a space within Gerota's fascia for placement of the balloon dilator. The index finger was introduced into the retroperitoneum in a cephalad direction to palpate the lower renal pole. Gerota's fascia is pierced with the finger and the perirenal space was entered. The catheter was inserted inside Gerota's fascia as is, or after back loading it into a 28F Amplatz dilator sheath. The balloon was gradually distended with normal saline. The balloon was kept inflated for 5 min to facilitate hemostasis. Following balloon deflation and removal, a Hasson cannula was inserted and secured with the preplaced stay sutures. To prevent loss of pneumoretroperitoneum, the conical tip of the Hasson cannula should fit snugly at the level of the anterior layer of the thoracolumbar fascia. Alternatively, a 10 mm Hasson type cannula with a fascial retention balloon and an external adjustable foam cuff can be used.

Another group[23] described a modified Metreurynter dissecting balloon (Atom Co., Ltd., Tokyo, Japan), which is used as a vaginal dilator for artificial abortion. The balloon was inserted into a space in the retroperitoneum created by blunt finger dissection toward the lower pole of the kidney and inflated with physiological saline solution using a syringe until 300 ml of inflation volume were obtained. The balloon remained inflated for 5 min, and then deflated and removed. A 10 mm trocar was inserted into the retroperitoneal space and secured with a silk stay suture to prevent carbon dioxide gas leakage, and the operating laparoscope inserted through this trocar port. Insufflation with carbon dioxide was accomplished at not more than 12 mmHg.

A Foley catheter was also described[4] to dissect the retroperitoneal space and gain access to the kidney and ureter in children. The retroperitoneum was initially accessed by blunt dissection through a 5–10 mm lumbodorsal incision, located in the angle between the lateral border of the paraspinal muscles and the 12th rib. A 16-Fr Foley catheter was introduced through the incision and the balloon was inflated with 80–100 cc of air. Inflation was maintained for 30 s; the catheter was deflated and replaced with a 5-mm port. The space created by the balloon is sufficient for placement of the initial ports for retroperitoneoscopy in children. The remaining ports were placed after creating enough working space by blunt dissection. This method can be considered both simple and effective. The firm conical tip of the Foley is useful in directing it safely into the retroperitoneum. In the event of rupture of the Foley catheter also has the added advantage of its central channel allowing the fluid to drain, preventing any compromise in vision caused by the presence of liquid in the retroperitoneal tissues.

As an alternative to the homemade balloon devices, several commercial balloon dilators have recently become available. A trocar mounted PDB balloon distension device (MedSystems, Menlo Park, CA) comprises a clear silicone balloon (capacity 1,000 ml air) mounted on a 10 mm laparoscopic trocar. The advantage of this device is that the insufflation and dissection of the retroperitoneal space can be monitored laparoscopically through the transparent balloon. The placement of the original balloon is crucial; improper placement may result in colonic injury as the peritoneal reflection is relatively fixed. The main drawback is the high additional cost and the need to insert it and the working cannula separately through the fascia defect (two-step insertion).[24] An all in one system, Spacemaker plus by AutoSuture, which includes the balloon dilator and the balloon tipped trocar has recently become available. This device eliminates the need for a two-step insertion.

3.6 Pros and Cons of Retroperitoneal Access

There are many advantages to using a retroperitoneal approach. The most obvious is the avoidance of the peritoneal cavity, minimizing the risk of postoperative ileus and other intestinal complications. The intact peritoneal barrier serves as a natural retractor, efficiently keeping the abdominal contents away from the operative field.[23]

With retroperitoneal access, the renal hilum and great vessels are easily visualized. In morbidly obese patients and in those who have undergone prior transperitoneal surgical interventions, this approach facilitates direct renal exposure.[25] The direct retroperitoneal approach may also decrease operative time particularly with upper tract surgery where there is a direct access to the vascular structures without the need for reflection of the bowel to attain access to the upper tract. Mobilization of the colon is not necessary to expose the renal hilum. In addition, the retroperitoneal approach requires fewer trocars than the transperitoneal approach, resulting in better cosmetic results. Other advantages include: a small increase in intra-abdominal pressure and minimal peritoneum stimulation, hence a weaker sympathetic response with less catecholamine release.[23] Lastly bowel herniation is also less frequent than with the transperitoneal approach.[24]

Of the main disadvantages of the retroperitoneal access compared to transperitoneal laparoscopic access is the smaller working space. However, the use of a 30-degree scope can compensate for this disadvantage. In addition, the wide longitudinal incision of the renal fascia performed at the beginning of the procedure helps to enlarge the working space.[1] Another main drawback is the close proximity of the trocar ports due to limited skin available, the retroperitoneal laparoscopic approach has essential disadvantages in that the number of usable trocars is limited, and the trocars can potentially interfere with each other. To overcome these shortcomings, mobilization of the peritoneal sac is necessary and the trocar ports should be located as far as possible from each other. Unlike the transperitoneal approach where several anatomical landmarks help the surgeon remain oriented, it can be difficult for the novice to maintain orientation in the retroperitoneum, where there are fewer visual anatomical landmarks and a significant amount of retroperitoneal fat.[23] Previous reports have also suggested that carbon dioxide absorption is higher during retroperitoneal laparoscopy than transperitoneal laparoscopy.[19] However, Ng et al.[26] demonstrated that retroperitoneoscopic renal and adrenal surgery was not associated with increased carbon dioxide absorption compared with transperitoneal laparoscopy.

3.7 Complications of Extraperitoneal Balloon Dilatation

Problems can occur with balloon misplacement in the abdominal wall musculature or fascial layers. Incorrect positioning can lead to inability to access the retroperitoneal space and make endoscopic completion of the procedure difficult. If the balloon is not completely within the retroperitoneum, the fascia and muscle can be disrupted, resulting in a hernia. Bleeding may also occur as a result of tearing of muscle fibers. Certain body habitus may put patients at risk for unsuccessful access or injury secondary to balloon misplacement. In obese patients, abundant adipose tissue (prefascial and retroperitoneal) can cause loss of anatomic landmarks and make it difficult to verify initial open placement of the balloon in the retroperitoneal space. Also, special care should be taken when performing extraperitoneal access in the pediatric and elderly population; the lax fascia in these individuals may tear if the balloon is insufflated across the fascia.

Improper placement of the balloon in the retroperitoneal space can be avoided by inspection of the potential space created before balloon dissection to help confirm correct placement. Placement of the endoscope should reveal the characteristic retroperitoneal fat. The balloon dilators equipped with a lumen to allow placement of a scope, allow the space to be developed safely under direct vision. Once secondary trocars are placed, the primary trocar site used for balloon placement should be examined to identify fascial and muscle tears.

The pressure used to fill the balloon can also cause injury. Peritoneal tears and injury to the underlying structures may occur with balloon rupture. Rupture of the balloon can be attributable to high insufflation pressures, overdistention, or a defective balloon. The balloon device should always be inspected prior to use. Balloon volumes should be monitored and inflation accomplished by filling under low pressure. If a commercially available balloon is used, volumes should not exceed the manufacturer's specifications. If resistance is encountered during filling, balloon misplacement should be suspected and filling terminated with positioning rechecked. Inflation media can affect the extent of tissue injury in the event of rupture. The use of slow inflation and a liquid medium lessens the chance of balloon failure and of problems in the event of balloon rupture. In the event of rupture, the retrieved balloon and retroperitoneum or extra-peritoneum must be carefully inspected for detached fragments. The nearby peritoneum must also be inspected for tears and if present the peritoneal cavity must also be inspected for fragments (Fig. 3.14).[5]

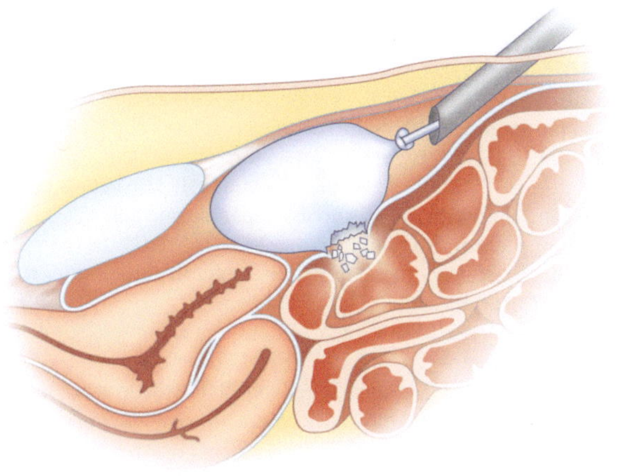

Fig. 3.14 Rupture of balloon with laceration of balloon and loss of latex fragments

3.8 Conclusions

A number of techniques have been described to allow access to the peritoneum. Virtually every open urologic procedure performed extraperitoneally can also be performed using a laparoscopic or robot-assisted technique. There are specific challenges that are unique to the extraperitoneal approach. Several recent improvements in surgical instrumentations have been helpful in overcoming these difficulties. This technique requires the surgeon to have a thorough knowledge of the retroperitoneal anatomy, to avoid disorientation, and bleeding complications, which can necessitate conversion to an open technique as reported by Gill and associates.[27] Familiarity with the access techniques is critical to the successful completion of a retroperitoneal laparoscopic or robot-assisted procedure.

References

1. Rassweiler JJ, Seemann O, Frede T, et al. Retroperitoneoscopy: experience with 200 cases. *J Urol*. 1998;160:1265.
2. Gaur DD. Laparoscopic operative retroperitonoscopy: use of a new device. *J Urol*. 1992;148:1137-1139.
3. Gaur DD, Agarwal DK, Purohit KC, Darshane AS. Laparoscopic condom dissection: new technique of retroperitoneoscopy. *J Endourol*. 1994;8:149.
4. Shah A, Chandran H. Use of Foley's catheter to gain access for retroperitoneoscopy. *ANZ J Surg*. 2004;74:1015.
5. Adams JB, Micali S, Moore RG, et al. Complications of extraperitoneal balloon dilation. *J Endourol*. 1996;10:375.

6. Gasman D, Droupy S, Koutani A, et al. Laroscopic adrenalectomy: the retroperitoneal approach. *J Urol.* 1998;159: 1816-1820.
7. Hoznek A, Salomon L, Antiphon P, Radier C, et al. Partial nephrectomy with retroperitoneal laparoscopy. *J Urol.* 1999;162:1922-1926.
8. Salomon L, Rabil R, Soulie M, Mouly P, Hoznek A, et al. Experience with retroperitoneal laparoscopic adrenalectomy for pheochromocytoma. *J Urol.* 2001;165:1871-1874.
9. Gill IS. Retroperitoneal laparoscopic nephrectomy. *Urol Clin North Am.* 1998;25:343-360.
10. Gill IS, Grune MT, Munch LC. Access technique for retroperitoneoscopy. *J Urol.* 1996;156:1120.
11. McDougall E, Clayman RV, Fadden PT. Retroperitoneoscopy: the Washington University Medical School experience. *Urology.* 1994;43:446-452.
12. Clayman RV, McDougall EM, Kerbl K, et al. Laparoscopic nephrectomy: transabdominal vs. retroperitoneal. *J Endourol.* 1993;7:S139.
13. Etwaru D, Raboy A, Ferzli G, et al. Extraperitoneal endoscopic gasless pelvic lymph node dissection. *J Laparoendosc Surg.* 1994;4:113.
14. Hirsch IH, Moreno JG, Lotfi MA, Gomella LG. Non-insufflative laparoscopic access. *J Endourol.* 1995;9:483-486.
15. Keeley FX, Tolley DA. Retroperitoneal laparoscopy. *BJU Int.* 1999;84:212-215.
16. El-ghoneimi A, Valla JS, Steyaert H, Aigrain Y. Laparoscopic renal surgery via a retroperitoneal approach in children. *J Urol.* 1998;160:1138-1141.
17. Micali S, Caione P, Virgili G, Capozza N, Scarfini M, Micali F. Retroperitoneal laparoscopic access in children using a direct vision technique. *J Urol.* 2001;165:1229-1232.
18. Urbanowicz W, Wieczorek M, Sulislawski J. Retroperitoneoscopic nephrectomy in the prone position in children (point of technique). *Eur Urol.* 2002;42:516-519.
19. Wolf JS Jr, Monk TG, McDougall EM, et al. The extraperitoneal approach and subcutaneous emphysema are associated with greater absorption of carbon dioxide during laparoscopic renal surgery. *J Urol.* 1995;154:959.
20. Gaur DD. Retroperitoneal laparoscopy: some technical modifications. *Br J Urol.* 1996;77:304-306.
21. Olsen LH, Rahwashdeh YF. Robotic pyeloplasty. In: John H, Wiklund P, eds. *Robotic Urology.* Germany: Springer; 2008:177-186.
22. Gaur DD. Retroperitoneoscopy: the balloon technique. *Ann R Coll Surg Engl.* 1994;76:259-263.
23. Takeda M, Go H, Watanabe R, Kurumada S, et al. Retroperitoneal laparoscopic adrenalectomy for functioning adrenal tumors: comparison with conventional transperitoneal laparoscopic adrenalectomy. *J Urol.* 1997; 157:19-23.
24. Moore RG, Demaree R, Sanda MG, Kavoussi LR. Retroperitoneoscopy: effects of insufflation media on surrounding tissue during balloon rupture. *J Endourol.* 1995; 9:67-71.
25. Pyo P, Chen A, Grasso M. Retroperitoneal laparoscopic partial nephrectomy: surgical experience and outcomes. *J Urol.* 2008;180:1279-1283.
26. Ng CS, Gill IS, Sung GT, et al. Retroperitoneoscopic surgery is not associated with increased carbon dioxide absorption. *J Urol.* 1999;162:1268.
27. Gill IS, Das S, Munch LC. Retroperitoneoscopy: a viable alternative (abstract). *J Endourol.* 1994;8:S91.

4 Laparoscopic and Robotic Adrenalectomy

Edmund Y. Ko, Richard T. Schlinkert,
and Mitchell R. Humphreys

Abstract Purpose: Laparoscopic adrenalectomy is a widely accepted surgical approach for treating most adrenal masses. This chapter will briefly discuss the differential diagnosis of adrenal masses, and review preoperative considerations, surgical approaches, postoperative management, and complications associated with adrenal surgery.

Method: In the era of imaging, most adrenal masses are diagnosed incidentally. A thorough endocrine evaluation is recommended for all patients with adrenal masses. A multi-specialty approach, including input from endocrinologists, anesthesiologists, and surgeons is recommended to ensure the best possible patient outcomes. Minimally invasive surgical techniques for adrenal surgery discussed include transperitoneal, robot-assisted transperitoneal, retroperitoneal, partial, needlescopic, and natural orifice approaches.

Conclusion: Laparoscopic adrenalectomy is generally considered the standard of care for treating most adrenal masses. It is safe when performed by experienced surgeons and maximizes the benefits of minimally invasive surgical approaches for patients.

Keywords Adrenalectomy • Laparoscopy • Minimally invasive surgery • Retroperitoneal laparoscopy • Robot-assisted laparoscopy

M.R. Humphreys (✉)
Department of Urology, Mayo Clinic, 5777 E. Mayo Blvd., Phoenix, AZ 85054, USA
e-mail: humphreys.mitchell@maqyo.edu

Key Points

- Laparoscopic adrenalectomy has become the standard approach to adrenal tumors at many institutions and has been demonstrated to have improved perioperative outcomes with reduced blood loss, minimal pain, improved time to recovery, and improved cosmesis when compared to the open approach.
- A multi-specialty (Anesthesia, Endocrine, Internal Medicine, Surgery/Urology, etc.) approach is paramount to minimize perioperative morbidity when approaching hormonally active adrenal tumors.
- An understanding of the retroperitoneal anatomy and desired surgical approach is crucial to performing a safe and adequate procedure and to minimize potential injury to surrounding structures.
- The two most common approaches are the transperitoneal and retroperitoneal approaches. Surgical approach is determined by surgical goals, patient medical/surgical history, and surgeon experience.
- The complication rate for laparoscopic adrenalectomy is 10.9% versus 25.2% for open adrenalectomy based on a Medline review of 98 publications. The most common laparoscopic complication is bleeding, reported at 4.7%.

J.V. Joseph and H.R.H. Patel (eds.), *Retroperitoneal Robotic and Laparoscopic Surgery*,
DOI: 10.1007/978-0-85729-485-2_4, © Springer-Verlag London Limited 2011

4.1 Introduction

Laparoscopic adrenalectomy was first described by Gagner et al. in 1992 as a viable surgical option for Cushing's syndrome and pheochromocytomas.[1] Since that time, it has evolved into a widely accepted surgical approach for adrenal lesions and has been recognized as an efficacious and well tolerated minimally invasive surgical technique.

Prior to the widespread use of imaging (ultrasonography, computed tomography, magnetic resonance imaging), most adrenal lesions were diagnosed secondary to clinical symptoms from functional hormone activity, local growth, or invasion. Most contemporary discovered adrenal lesions are diagnosed incidentally ("incidentaloma") on cross-sectional imaging. The differential diagnosis for an incidentally diagnosed adrenal mass includes benign nonfunctioning adenoma, myelolipoma, functioning cortical tumor (aldosteronoma, cortisol-producing tumor), pheochromocytoma, adrenocortical carcinoma, and adrenal metastasis.

Traditionally, open surgery has been the standard of care for the surgical management of adrenal lesions. However, minimally invasive approaches have gained rapid acceptance by patients and surgeons owing to minimal blood loss, decreased postoperative pain, shorter hospitalization, rapid recovery, improved cosmesis, and decreased overall complications.[2] Minimally invasive techniques such as the laparoscopic approach for adrenal lesions can be considered the new standard of care for the surgical treatment of adrenal pathology.

The specific steps of the laparoscopic approach to adrenal lesions will be detailed in this chapter. In addition, it will also cover important indications and contraindications for surgery, pre- and postoperative considerations, and the unique complications of laparoscopic adrenal surgery.

Table 4.1 Indications and contraindications for laparoscopic adrenalectomy[3]

Indications for laparoscopic adrenalectomy
Functioning adrenal tumor
• Aldosteronoma • Cortisol-producing adrenal tumor (Cushing's syndrome) • Pheochromocytoma • Androgen/estrogen-secreting tumor
Nonfunctioning adrenal tumor >4–5 cm
• Adenoma
Adrenocortical carcinoma
Select solitary adrenal metastasis
Contraindications to laparoscopic adrenalectomy
Absolute contraindications
• Primary adrenal carcinoma with extensive local invasion • Uncorrectable coagulopathy • Severe cardiopulmonary disease • Uncontrolled pheochromocytoma
Relative contraindications
• Tumors >10–12 cm • Pregnancy • Bowel obstruction

4.2 Indications/Contraindications

The indications for laparoscopic adrenalectomy have expanded with the refinement of surgical techniques and experience. There has been a clear shift in the treatment paradigm for adrenal tumors from open surgery to minimally invasive surgical techniques.[3] Indications for surgical extirpation include: symptomatic lesions, nonfunctioning adenomas larger than 4–5 cm, documented growth progression, suspicious adrenal cysts, hormonally active tumors, primary adrenal carcinoma, and select solitary adrenal metastasis.

There are several absolute contraindications to laparoscopic adrenalectomy. These include primary adrenal carcinoma with extensive local extension making it unresectable, uncorrectable or uncorrected coagulopathy, severe cardiopulmonary disease, and uncontrolled pheochromocytoma.[3]

Relative contraindications include tumors greater than 10–12 cm, presence of venous thrombus, bowel obstruction, massive hemoperitoneum, and pregnancy (Table 4.1). Relative contraindications have decreased over time with progressive laparoscopic experience and are generally dependent on the comfort level and skill of the surgeon.[3]

4.3 Preoperative Preparation

A thorough endocrine evaluation is warranted for all adrenal masses to determine the hormonal activity of the lesion (Table 4.2). In large retrospective studies, approximately 15% of incidentally diagnosed adrenal

Table 4.2 Initial evaluation for incidentally detected adrenal tumor

Initial evaluation
• Physical examination • Blood pressure measurement
Basic laboratory studies
• CBC • BMP • 24-h urine collection
Hyperaldosteronism (Conn's syndrome)
• Urine aldosterone level • Aldosterone:renin ratio
Cushing's syndrome
• 24-h urine cortisol
Pheochromocytoma
• 24-h urine catecholamines and metanephrines • Plasma metanephrines

masses are hormonally active.[4] Of these 15%, 9% were Cushing syndrome, 4% were pheochromocytomas, and 2% were aldosteronomas. Hormonal secretion affects surgical indications, perioperative management of electrolytes, fluid status, blood pressure, and anesthetic considerations.

Cooperation between the surgeon, anesthesiologist, and endocrinologist is paramount for accurate diagnosis and proper preoperative management in order to minimize morbidities. Patients with an aldosteronoma often are hypokalemic and require potassium repletion or initiation of a potassium sparing diuretic. Patients with Cushing syndrome require correction of their electrolyte abnormalities as well as their hyperglycemia. These patients should also receive a steroid prep preoperatively as they cannot increase cortisol levels in response to surgical stress.

Patients with pheochromocytoma can have poorly controlled hypertension, paroxysmal hypertensive episodes, tachycardia, and hypovolemia due to catecholamine release. Preoperative medical therapy is designed to blunt catecholamine response to effect blood pressure control and volume expansion.[5] Patients are treated with α(alpha)-adrenergic or calcium channel blockers preoperatively. Phenoxybenzamine, an irreversible, long-acting, nonspecific α(alpha)-adrenergic blocking agent, is our preferred drug for controlling hypertension. Doxazosin or prazosin, both α(alpha)-1-selective blockers, can also be used. Calcium channel blockers include nifedipine and verapamil. Patients are encouraged to increase their fluid and sodium intake on the second or third day of treatment to counteract the catecholamine-induced volume contraction. After adequate α(alpha)-adrenergic blockade is established, a β(beta)-blocker may be added if tachycardia is present.[3] β(beta)-blockade should never be initiated prior to α(alpha)-blockade as this may induce a paradoxical rise in blood pressure due to unopposed α(alpha)-adrenergic stimulation. Patients may be admitted 1 day prior to surgery for intravenous fluid resuscitation, if necessary.

Pre-surgical medical clearance should be obtained to evaluate the cardiopulmonary risks of the patient, and to ensure that the patient is an acceptable surgical candidate. Evaluation includes chest X-ray, electrocardiogram, and any additional diagnostic studies deemed necessary by the surgical team. Prior to surgery, all patients should receive deep vein thrombosis (DVT) and intravenous antibiotic prophylaxis.

A special consideration with minimally invasive approaches is the requirement for pneumoperitoneum. Pneumoperitoneum theoretically increases the pressure on the adrenal gland and could cause a catecholamine surge resulting in severe hypertension and tachycardia.[2] However, studies have shown these complications are no more frequent in patients undergoing laparoscopic resection than those undergoing open surgery.[6] Pneumoperitoneum can also decrease cardiac output, venous return, blood pressure, and lung capacity. It can increase carbon dioxide absorption leading to hypercapnia and acidosis. Patients with severe chronic obstructive pulmonary disease may not be able to physiologically tolerate pneumoperitoneum. Other potential complications of pneumoperitoneum include subcutaneous emphysema, venous gas embolism, pneumopericardium, pneumomediastinum, and pneumothorax.

4.4 Operative Approaches and Steps

4.4.1 Positioning and Preparation

Patients are positioned in a flank position ranging from 30° to 80° elevation from supine with all pressure points carefully padded. This may be achieved with the patient starting in the supine position with a sandbag bump placed underneath the table cushion.

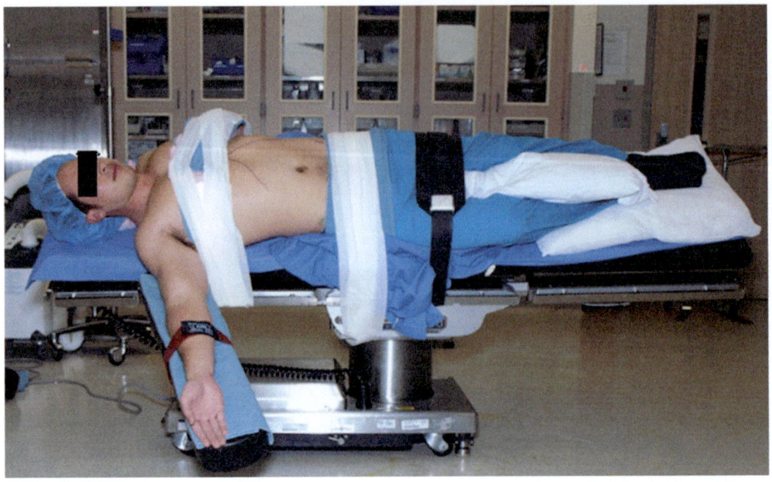

Fig. 4.1 Modified flank position for transperitoneal left laparoscopic adrenalectomy with ipsilateral arm in sling position.[7] (Photographer: D. Rose (Mayo Clinic, Phoenix, Arizona))

This effectively raises the operative flank up to 30°, known as the modified flank position (Fig. 4.1).[7] Alternatively, the patient may be placed in a lateral decubitus position and rotated slightly backward (~80°). In the modified flank position the authors place the ipsilateral arm in the "sling" position against the chest with the elbow flexed greater than 90°. The arm can also be placed on an arm board in the lateral decubitus position. In either position the contralateral arm is straight and completely extended 90° away from the body and secured to a standard arm board. An axillary roll is recommended for all patients in the lateral decubitus position. The contralateral (bottom) leg is bent and the ipsilateral (top) leg is straight ensuring that all pressure points are carefully padded and supported. Our typical method of securing the patient to the table is to use cloth tape over a towel across the chest, hips, and legs which allows for extreme table rotation while the patient is in the modified flank position. This achieves a true flank position (90°) relative to the horizontal, and permits additional mobility to increase operative exposure.

A retroperitoneal approach requires positioning the patient in the traditional 90° flank position in order to gain access to the patient's retroperitoneal space. The kidney rest is elevated and the table is flexed in order to open up the space between the ribs and the iliac crest. For a posterior retroperitoneal approach, the patient is positioned in the prone jackknife position, again utilizing appropriate padding and support.[8]

An oro- or naso-gastric tube and Foley catheter are placed to decompress the stomach and bladder prior to starting the procedure. Anesthesia may choose to place arterial and central venous lines to ensure precise blood pressure and volume monitoring during the operation. This may also be useful in perioperative monitoring and management.

4.4.2 Transperitoneal Port Placement

We employ the Veress needle technique to achieve a carbon dioxide pneumoperitoneum of 15 mmHg for the surgically naive abdomen. This is typically achieved with a small incision just lateral to the linea alba midline and cranial to the umbilicus. A 5- or 10-mm port can be placed depending on lens size. Alternatively, for patients with a history of previous abdominal surgery, the authors prefer a Hassan technique to gain access to the peritoneal cavity. The abdominal cavity is then surveyed to address any potential adhesions prior to the placement of any additional ports.

For a left-sided adrenalectomy, a 5-mm port is placed at or just medial to the mid-clavicular line (MCL), below the subcostal margin for the left-hand instruments. A 12-mm port is placed 1–1.5 (7–10 cm) hand breadths caudal to the 5-mm left-hand port along the MCL for the right-hand instruments forming a triangular port configuration (Fig. 4.2a). The 12-mm port allows the use of an endovascular stapler to secure the adrenal vasculature if necessary. A 5-mm port may be substituted if only clips are used. An additional 5-mm port may be placed in the anterior-axillary line at the

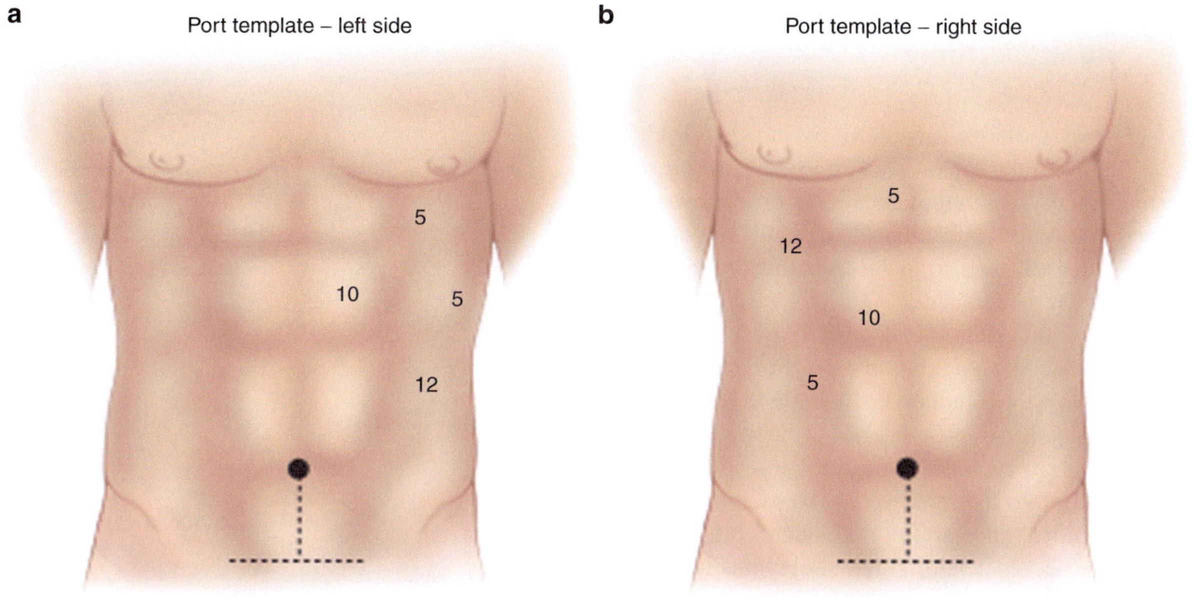

Fig. 4.2 (**a**) Left laparoscopic adrenalectomy port placement. The *dashed lines* represent possible extraction sites. The *12*, *10*, and *5* refer to the size of the trocar, in mm, used at each location. The small *5* laterally represents the site of an additional port for retraction which may not always be necessary. (**b**) Right laparoscopic adrenalectomy port placement. The *dashed lines* represent possible extraction sites. The *12*, *10*, and *5* refer to the size of the trocar, in mm, used at each location. The superior and medial *5* trocar is used for liver retraction

intersection of the right- and left-hand ports to create a diamond configuration for additional bowel retraction, if needed.

For a right-sided adrenalectomy, the port locations are a mirror image on the contralateral side (Fig. 4.2b). Differences include the placement of the 12-mm right-hand port in the subcostal position and the 5-mm left-hand port caudal to this in the MCL. Some surgeons prefer the 12-mm port in the left-hand position to achieve the angle necessary for ligation of the right main adrenal vein, which usually drains in a high posterior position on the inferior vena cava (IVC). In addition, a 5-mm sub-xiphoid port is placed for cephalad retraction of the liver, which is critical for adequate exposure of the right-sided adrenal gland. An additional port can again be placed laterally for additional bowel retraction if necessary.

The triangular positioning of the laparoscopic ports ensures that the laparoscope is kept out of line with the working instruments. It also allows the template to be easily shifted cephalad, caudal, medial, or lateral and to be rotated clockwise or counterclockwise depending on the anatomy and the size of the individual patient. Another port site configuration involves placing three to four working trocars just below the subcostal margin between the MCL and the posterior axillary line (Fig. 4.3).

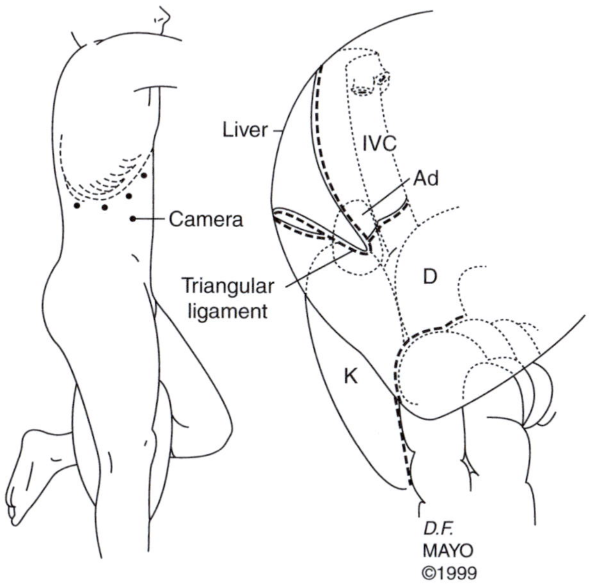

Fig. 4.3 Right subcostal port placement for laparoscopic adrenalectomy. *IVC* inferior vena cava, *Ad* adrenal gland, *D* duodenum, *K* kidney

4.4.3 Transperitoneal Left Adrenalectomy

The colon is mobilized medially by incising Toldt's white line from the splenic flexure to the pelvis using thermal energy (monopolar cautery or a harmonic scalpel) combined with blunt dissection. The spleen and the pancreas are also mobilized medially in order to expose Gerota's fascia. Gerota's fascia is then incised over the kidney and the left renal hilum is exposed. If the left renal hilum is hard to expose, one can start below the hilum by first identifying the ureter and gonadal vein complex anterior to the psoas muscle and following it cephalad toward the insertion of the gonadal vein into the renal vein. The main left renal vein is identified and carefully skeletonized to expose the main left adrenal vein. This vessel typically drains from the inferomedial border of the left adrenal gland into the superior aspect of the left main renal vein. Once the main adrenal vein is identified, it can be secured and divided with clips or an endovascular stapler. Conventional wisdom dictates that the venous drainage be controlled prior to excessive adrenal gland manipulation to prevent catecholamine release during the surgical treatment of pheochromocytoma, although this has been recently called into question.[9]

Gerota's fascia is then incised over the upper pole of the kidney, if not already done, and the adrenal gland, encased in periadrenal fat, is exposed. The adrenal gland is then retracted anterolaterally and the posterior attachments along with the vessels are individually ligated and transected with clips, harmonic scalpel, and/or an endovascular stapler. The variable arterial supply to the adrenal gland includes branches from the inferior phrenic artery, aorta, and the renal artery. The dissection is completed by separating the adrenal gland from the upper pole of the left kidney and surrounding tissues (Fig. 4.4).

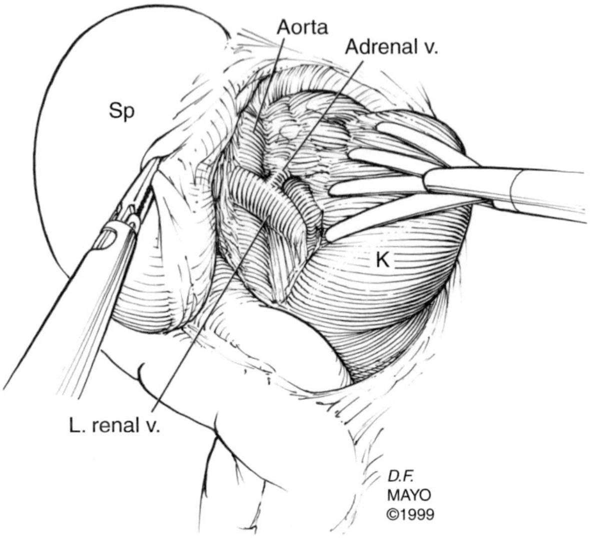

Fig. 4.4 Left laparoscopic adrenalectomy anatomic associations. *Sp* spleen, *K* kidney, *L. renal v.* left renal vein, *Adrenal v.* adrenal vein

4.4.4 Transperitoneal Right Adrenalectomy

The right adrenal gland is usually located more medial to the upper pole of the kidney compared to the left adrenal gland. The upper pole of the kidney and liver may interfere with adrenal exposure because of this. We use a locking grasper through the 5 mm subxiphoid laparoscopic port to retract the liver cephalad. The peritoneum is incised using a combination of thermal energy and blunt dissection starting caudal to the undersurface of the liver and extending down the posterior peritoneum to expose the lateral aspect of the IVC. The triangular ligament can be ligated to gain additional liver retraction and provide exposure for high-riding or very large adrenal tumors (Fig. 4.3). Unlike the left side, the ascending colon and the hepatic flexure do not have to be routinely mobilized.[2] For large adrenal masses or those that involve the kidney, the standard exposure for a right-sided laparoscopic nephrectomy is achieved by mobilizing the ascending colon along with the hepatic flexure and then reflecting the duodenum medially by incising Toldt's white line and employing the Kocher maneuver respectively.[10]

A plane is then developed between the medial border of the adrenal gland and the IVC using careful traction and countertraction to expose the adrenal vein (Fig. 4.5). Care is taken to minimize aggressive lateral retraction of the adrenal gland to prevent inadvertent avulsion of the main adrenal vein or veins. The right adrenal vein is typically short and empties directly into the posterolateral aspect of the IVC and can be difficult to control if injured during the dissection. Identification of the right adrenal vein can be especially challenging with large tumors, and profuse, life-threatening bleeding can occur

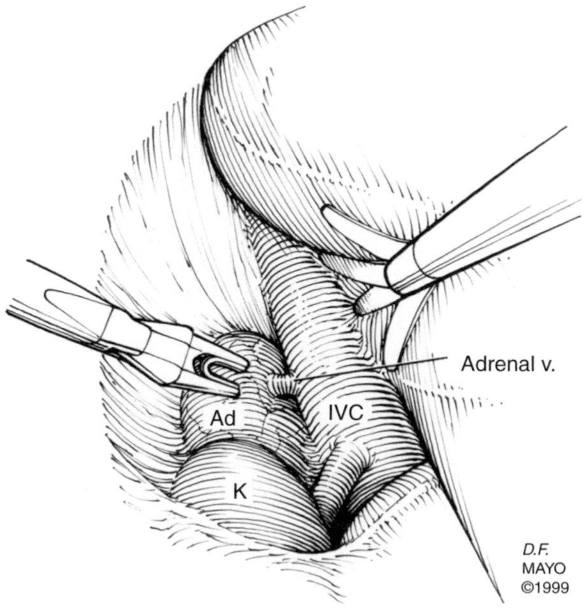

Fig. 4.5 Right laparoscopic adrenalectomy anatomic associations. *IVC* inferior vena cava, *Ad* adrenal gland, *K* kidney

if it is not identified and controlled early during the dissection.[3] Once the vein is identified and skeletonized, it is secured and transected with clips and scissors or an endovascular stapler. The remaining attachments to the adrenal gland are then dissected free using care to control the blood supply of the adrenal gland.

4.4.5 Retroperitoneal Approach

A retroperitoneal adrenalectomy can be performed with the lateral or posterior approach. The lateral approach is more commonly utilized although the posterior approach has been championed by some due to its direct approach to the adrenal glands.[8,11]

4.4.6 Lateral Retroperitoneal Approach

The patient is positioned in the 90° full flank position as previously described. A small 1.5 cm incision is made 1–2 cm below the tip of the 12th rib in the midaxillary line and is used to access the retroperitoneal space. Blunt finger dissection is useful to create the working space anterior to the psoas muscle. Caution is recommended to avoid inadvertent entry into the peritoneal cavity. The operative space in the retroperitoneum is then developed with a balloon dilator. By generating this space, critical intraperitoneal structures such as the liver, spleen, and colon are deflected medially.[12] A 30° 10-mm laparoscope is then placed to inspect the retroperitoneal space. Two secondary working 5-mm ports are then placed under direct vision, one in the anterior axillary line and the other posteriorly just under the 12th rib at the junction of the erector spinae muscle. The right hand port can be upsized to 12-mm if an endovascular stapler is to be used for vascular control.

4.4.7 Lateral Retroperitoneal Left Adrenalectomy

Dissection differences between a left versus right laparoscopic retroperitoneal adrenalectomy stems from the anatomical differences in venous anatomy. Because the longer, inferiorly located left main adrenal vein usually drains directly into the left renal vein, the dissection on this side begins by incising Gerota's fascia posteriorly at the upper pole of the kidney. The avascular plane between the inferolateral adrenal edge and the upper pole of the kidney is developed to mobilize the adrenal gland. The dissection is then carried caudally along the medial edge of the kidney until the renal hilum along with the main left adrenal vein is identified and can be secured with an endovascular stapler or clips. The border between the medial aspect of the adrenal gland and the aorta is then carefully developed in order to carefully secure and ligate the adrenal arteries. The superior edge of the adrenal gland is then developed from the diaphragm with care not to avulse any vasculature from the inferior phrenic vessels. At this point, the adrenal gland is completely mobilized and is placed into a laparoscopic bag.

4.4.8 Lateral Retroperitoneal Right Adrenalectomy

The right laparoscopic retroperitoneal adrenalectomy dissection is dictated by the short and superolateral location of the right adrenal vein draining directly into the IVC. The dissection begins first by identifying the right renal artery. By freeing up the cephalad edge of the renal artery, the edge of the IVC can be identified. Dissection is then carried cephalad along the edge of the IVC until the main adrenal vein is identified draining into the posterolateral edge of the IVC where it can be secured with clips or an endovascular stapler. Because of the short nature of the vein, care must be taken to not retract the gland aggressively during the dissection. The superior edge of the adrenal is then dissected off of the diaphragm ligating all vessels carefully. The gland is then carefully separated from the upper pole of the right kidney.

4.4.9 Posterior Retroperitoneal Approach

The posterior retroperitoneal laparoscopic approach is less popular than the transperitoneal approach. However, it has its distinct advantages including a direct approach to the adrenal gland. This tactic has been demonstrated to be safe and associated with short operative times and quick patient recovery.[8,11]

General endotracheal anesthesia is achieved in the supine position, and then the patient is re-positioned in the prone jackknife position. This requires the knees and hips to be positioned at 90° angles in relation to the spine and femur, on a rectangular support table or a Cloward table saddle (Cloward Surgical Saddle, surgical Equipment International, Honolulu, HI). This allows the ventral abdominal wall to hang dependently without restriction or compression on the great vessels.

A 1.5-cm transverse incision is made just off of the tip of the 12th rib and the retroperitoneal space is entered with blunt and sharp dissection. The space deep to the ribs and diaphragm is bluntly developed in the retroperitoneum with the index finger. Generally digital direction is used within the space in order for two additional ports to be placed. A medial 10-mm port is placed along the paraspinal musculature approximately 3 cm below the 12th rib with a cephalad angle at 45° pointing toward the adrenal gland. A lateral 5-mm port is placed in a similar fashion approximately 5 cm from the initial incision below the 11th rib. A blunt trocar with an inflatable balloon and adjustable sleeve is placed into the initial incision and pneumoperitoneum is maintained at a pressure of 20–28 mmHg.[11] A higher pressure is required to develop the retroperitoneal space, maintain an adequate pneumoperitoneum, and keep a bloodless field. It is well tolerated and noted to have minimal adverse cardiovascular effects.[8] A fourth port can be placed caudal to the first line of ports for retraction.

The adrenal gland is exposed below the diaphragm after mobilizing the kidney. Gerota's fascia is entered and the upper pole of the kidney is identified. Landmarks include the upper pole of the kidney, the paraspinous muscles medially, and the posterior surface of the spleen or liver through the peritoneum. Mobilization of the adrenal gland starts caudally and medially using blunt and thermal dissection. The caudal aspect of the adrenal gland is separated off the upper pole of the kidney. Medial mobilization involves identifying the adrenal vein and ligating it. Adrenal arteries are then identified and ligated. The posterior approach to the IVC facilitates identification of the right renal vein which is located posterolaterally. After the vessels have been ligated, the adrenal gland is then separated from the remaining retroperitoneal attachments.

4.4.10 Robot-Assisted Laparoscopic Adrenalectomy

Da Vinci (Intuitive Surgical, Mountain View, CA) robot-assisted laparoscopic adrenalectomy in a human subject was first described in 2001.[13] Safety and feasibility for this robot-assisted laparoscopic adjunct has been demonstrated in multiple small studies.[14,15] There have been no documented advantages for this approach compared to other minimally invasive techniques.

Theoretical advantages of robot-assisted surgery compared to traditional laparoscopic techniques include three-dimensional vision, improved magnification, tremor minimization, instrument articulation, greater range of motion, and improved ergonomics. Disadvantages include the lack of tactile feedback, absence of the surgeon at the operative field, and the added cost of utilizing the robot.[14]

The patient is placed in a lateral decubitus position as previously described. Port placement is dictated by the ability to bring the robot in from behind the patient and docking it as close to the bed as possible in order to capitalize on the full range of motion of the robotic arms. Insufflation is achieved through a 12-mm incision at the midpoint between the xiphoid and the umbilicus at or just lateral to the linea alba. The 8-mm robotic arm ports (the newer 5-mm ports may also be used depending on the model of the Da Vinci used) are placed 1–1.5 hand breaths away with the left arm placed just below the subcostal margin cephalad to the camera, and the right arm placed in the anterior axillary line to complete a triangular template. Two assistant ports (5 and 12-mm) are also placed under direct vision in the mid to lower abdomen to allow suctioning, retraction, or the passage of suture or an endovascular stapler. The procedure is performed in the same fashion as previously described for the transperitoneal approach.

4.4.11 Needlescopic Adrenalectomy

The needlescopic adrenalectomy approach uses instrumentation measuring ≤3 mm. Although scarring is kept to a minimum due to the use of puncture sites rather than formal incisions for port placement, the procedure can be complicated by diminished visualization through the 2-mm needlescope, decreased tensile strength of thinner instrumentation, and limited instrument availability and variety.[16] However, improved visualization can be achieved by hiding a 5- or 10-mm camera port in the umbilicus. The needlescopic procedure is again accomplished in the same manner as the transperitoneal approach.

4.4.12 NOTES/LESS Adrenalectomy

Natural orifice transluminal surgery (NOTES™) is the latest frontier in minimally invasive surgery. By utilizing natural orifices (mouth, rectum, vagina, urethra) for port placement and extraction the morbidity, pain, and scarring of skin incisions are theoretically eliminated. Although there have been no published human subject studies at this time, it has been demonstrated to be feasible in both porcine and human cadaver studies.[17] Laparoendoscopic single-site surgery (LESS) is a hybrid technique in which articulated instruments are employed to overcome the lack of external triangulation so that the procedure can be accomplished through one small incision.[18] The outcomes and clinical benefits to patients have yet to be fully elucidated for these procedures and are still considered experimental at this time.

4.4.13 Laparoscopic Partial Adrenalectomy

Laparoscopic partial adrenalectomy can be considered for patients with solitary glands or bilateral benign adrenal tumors. Patients at risk for developing multiple adrenal tumors, such as those with multiple endocrine neoplasia (MEN 2A and 2B) and von Hippel-Landau (VHL) disease, are also candidates. Preserving at least one-third of the adrenal gland spares the patient from requiring chronic steroid replacement.[19] Despite the potential benefits, there are currently no guidelines regarding the applications of laparoscopic partial adrenalectomy.[20]

4.4.14 Extraction and Closure

Once the adrenal gland has been completely freed, it can be placed into a retrieval bag and extracted through the 12-mm port site. If it is a large mass (>4–5 cm) the 12-mm port site can be enlarged, or an infraumbilical abdominal extraction site can be created via a midline or pfannenstiel incision using a muscle sparing technique to extract the specimen.

The surgical bed should always be examined under low pneumoperitoneum to ensure that complete hemostasis has been achieved. If there is any oozing from the surgical bed, topical hemostasic agents can be utilized.

The fascia of the extraction site and port sites greater than 5 mm should be closed. At our institution, we do not routinely close the 5-mm port sites as few cases of 5-mm port site hernias have been reported. Skin incisions are reapproximated with 4-0 absorbable suture in a running subcuticular fashion. We routinely use local anesthetic, such as 0.25% bipuvicaine, at the surgical sites.

4.5 Postoperative Management

The oro- or naso-gastric tube is removed by anesthesia at the end of the procedure. The foley catheter is kept until the patient is ambulatory. Most foley catheters are removed on or before postoperative day 1.

Postoperative pain can be treated with IV and oral narcotics and analgesics as needed. A clear liquid diet is started immediately in the postoperative period and advanced to a regular diet as tolerated. Once the patient is tolerating adequate oral intake, they are quickly transitioned exclusively to oral narcotics for pain control.

Early ambulation (postoperative day 0) and aggressive incentive spirometry use is encouraged by the surgeon and nursing staff to prevent pulmonary and thromboembolic (DVT) complications.

A complete blood count (CBC) and basic metabolic panel (BMP) is obtained on the morning after surgery to identify any residual electrolyte abnormalities.

Most patients are discharged home 1 day after surgery. Patients with underlying medical comorbidities or volume or pressure concerns due to the treatment of select lesions may be kept an extra day.

Patients lacking adrenal glands will require corticosteroid and mineralocorticoid replacement therapy. Pre- and postoperative consultation with an endocrinologist should be considered for lifelong medical management of these patients.

4.6 Complications

The overall complication rate for laparoscopic adrenalectomy is 10.9% versus 25.2% for the open approach ($p \leq 0.0001$) as reported by Brunt in a Medline meta-analysis comparing 50 laparoscopic studies (1,633 adrenalectomies in 1,522 patients) with 48 open surgical studies (2,747 adrenalectomies in 2,273 patients).[21] Bleeding is the most common overall complication encountered in laparoscopic adrenalectomy, and was found in 4.7% of patients with 1.8% requiring transfusion. Bleeding resulting in open conversion occurred in 1.6% of patients, which accounted for 30% of all conversions identified in this Medline review. Wound complications occurred in 1.4% of patients. Pulmonary (0.9%), gastrointestinal (0.7%), surrounding organ injury (0.7%), urinary (0.5%), thromboembolic (0.5%), endocrine (0.5%), neurologic (0.3%), and cardiac (0.3%) complications all occurred in less than 1% of the reported laparoscopic populations. Infectious complications, including wound (0.6%), urinary tract (0.5%), and pulmonary (0.2%) infections occurred in <1% of patients. Overall mortality rate for laparoscopic versus open adrenalectomy was 0.3% and 0.9% respectively, which was not statistically significant.

In a recent publication by Tessier et al., previously unreported high-grade complications of adrenalectomy were reviewed and discussed.[22] Complications include: transection of the porta hepatis during right laparoscopic adrenalectomy leading to liver failure requiring emergent transplantation; hepatic artery ligation during right open adrenalectomy leading to recurrent cholangitis and bile duct sclerosis ultimately requiring liver transplantation; left ureter ligation during laparoscopic adrenalectomy resulting in eventual loss of renal function; renal artery ligation during open adrenalectomy resulting in eventual renal unit loss requiring laparoscopic nephrectomy; and laparoscopic adrenalectomy for a 6-cm hypervascular mass in the left retroperitoneum with postoperative imaging demonstrating persistence of the mass in the left upper pole of the kidney, necessitating a left hand-assisted laparoscopic nephrectomy.

Laparoscopic adrenalectomy is one of the least commonly performed of all laparoscopic operations due to the low prevalence of disease. The morbidity of adrenalectomy is low in high-volume tertiary centers, however serious and life-threatening complications can occur at least in part due to less experienced surgeons treating an uncommon adrenal disease.[21,22]

4.7 Advantages and Pitfalls of the Technique

Laparoscopic adrenalectomy has been demonstrated to provide superior results for patients.[23] Laparoscopic adrenalectomy has become the procedure of choice due to minimal blood loss, decreased analgesic requirement, improved return of bowel function and advancement to regular diet, shorter hospitalization, rapid recovery, improved cosmesis, and decreased overall complications when compared to the traditional open approach.

Initial operative times may be longer early in the laparoscopic adrenalectomy learning curve, although they do decrease markedly with increasing repetition and surgeon experience.[24] Open adrenalectomy is still an excellent choice for larger or invasive tumors and, like the laparoscopic approach, requires a thorough knowledge of the anatomy and surgical technique.

4.8 Summary

Laparoscopic adrenalectomy has become the standard approach for the resection of most adrenal tumors. There are many different minimally invasive approaches for adrenalectomy and each has its own unique advantages. In the hands of experienced surgeons, the indications for laparoscopic adrenalectomy have increased to include most pathology. It is imperative that the surgeon understand the anatomical associations in the retroperitoneum and be prepared for any untoward events to minimize potential complications.

References

1. Gagner M, Lacroix A, Bolte E. Laparoscopic adrenalectomy in Cushing's syndrome and pheochromocytoma. *N Engl J Med*. 1992;327(14):1033.
2. Sung GT, Gill IS. Laparoscopic adrenalectomy. *Semin Laparosc Surg*. 2000;7(3):211-222.
3. Wang SD, Terashi T. Laparoscopic adrenalectomy. *Urol Clin North Am*. 2008;35(3):351-363.
4. Mantero F, Terzolo M, Arnaldi G, et al. A survey on adrenal incidentaloma in Italy. Study Group on Adrenal Tumors of the Italian Society of Endocrinology. *J Clin Endocrinol Metab*. 2000;85(2):637-644.
5. Pacak K, Linehan WM, Eisenhofer G, et al. Recent advances in genetics, diagnosis, localization, and treatment of pheochromocytoma. *Ann Intern Med*. 2001;134:315-329.
6. Gill IS. The case for laparoscopic adrenalectomy. *J Urol*. 2001;166(2):429-436.
7. Martin GL, Nunez RN, Martin AD, et al. A novel and ergonomic patient position for laparoscopic kidney surgery. *Can J Urol*. 2009;16(2):4580-4583.
8. Perrier ND, Kennamer DL, Bao R, et al. Posterior retroperitoneoscopic adrenalectomy: preferred technique for removal of benign tumors and isolated metastases. *Ann Surg*. 2008;248(4):666-674.
9. Vassiliou MC, Laycock WS. Laparoscopic adrenalectomy for pheochromocytoma: take the vein last? *Surg Endosc*. 2009;23(5):965-968.
10. Rosoff JS, Raman JD, Del Pizzo JJ. Laparoscopic adrenalectomy for large adrenal masses. *Curr Urol Rep*. 2008;9(1): 73-79.
11. Walz MK, Alesina PF, Wenger FA, et al. Posterior retroperitoneoscopic adrenalectomy-results of 560 procedures in 520 patients. *Surgery*. 2006;140:943-950.
12. Munver R, Ilbeigi P. Retroperitoneal laparoscopic adrenalectomy. *Curr Urol Rep*. 2005;6(1):72-77.
13. Horgan S, Vanuno D. Robotics in laparoscopic surgery. *J Laparoendosc Adv Surg Tech A*. 2001;11:415-419.
14. Hyams ES, Stifelman MD. The role of robotics for adrenal pathology. *Curr Opin Urol*. 2009;19(1):89-96.
15. Wu JC, Wu HS, Lin MS, et al. Comparison of robot-assisted laparoscopic adrenalectomy with traditional laparoscopic adrenalectomy – 1 year follow-up. *Surg Endosc*. 2008;22(2): 463-466.
16. Gill IS. Needlescopic urology: current status. *Urol Clin North Am*. 2001;28(1):71-83.
17. Allemann P, Perreta S, Marescaux J. Surgical access to the adrenal gland: the quest for a "no visible scar" approach. *Surg Oncol*. 2009;18(2):131-137.
18. Tracy CR, Raman JD, Cadeddu JA, et al. Laparoendoscopic single-site surgery in urology: where have we been and where are we heading? *Nat Clin Pract Urol*. 2008;5(10): 561-568.
19. Walz MK, Peitgen K, Diesing D, et al. Partial versus total adrenalectomy by the posterior retroperitoneoscopic approach: early and long-term results of 325 consecutive procedures in primary adrenal neoplasias. *World J Surg*. 2004;28(12):1323-1329.
20. Disick GI, Munver R. Adrenal-preserving minimally invasive surgery: update on the current status of laparoscopic partial adrenalectomy. *Curr Urol Rep*. 2008;9(1):67-72.
21. Brunt LM. The positive impact of laparoscopic adrenalectomy on complications of adrenal surgery. *Surg Endosc*. 2002;16:252-257.
22. Tessier DJ, Iglesias R, Chapman WC, et al. Previously unreported high-grade complications of adrenalectomy. *Surg Endosc*. 2009;23:97-102.
23. Haveran LA, Novitsky YW, Czerniach DR, et al. Benefits of laparoscopic adrenalectomy: a 10-year single institution experience. *Surg Laparosc Endosc Percutan Tech*. 2006;16:217-221.
24. Barreco M, Presenti L, Renzi C, et al. Expectations and outcomes when moving from open to laparoscopic adrenalectomy: multivariate analysis. *World J Surg*. 2003;27:223-228.

5 Retroperitoneoscopic Simple and Radical Nephrectomy

Guillaume Ploussard, Andras Hoznek, Laurent Salomon, Claude C. Abbou, and Alexandre de la Taille

Abstract The first retroperitoneoscopy was performed by Gaur who had constructed a simple device consisting of a No. 7 surgical glove mounted on a red-rubber catheter and created the workspace of the retroperitoneal laparoscopy by inflating the glove. Since this first report, retroperitoneoscopic nephrectomy has become a safe and efficient procedure. Retroperitoneoscopy can be the technique of choice for accessing and carrying out surgery of the upper urinary tract. Surgeons who want to perform laparoscopic nephrectomy should know how to do both approaches (retroperitoneal and transperitoneal) because some patients will require retroperitoneal approach. This approach is preferable in patients with a history of abdominal surgery because it eliminates risky and tiresome lysis of the adhesions. Retroperitoneoscopy respects the principles of oncological surgery and most complications are minor and easily managed.

Keywords Kidney cancer • Laparoscopy • Nephrectomy • Retroperitoneoscopy • Surgical technique

Key Points

- The indications for retroperitoneoscopic nephrectomy are the same as those for laparoscopic transperitoneal nephrectomy.
- Working space: finger dissection and creation of the working space is done in the posterior pararenal space, identification of the psoas muscle
- Anatomic landmarks:
  - Left: Internal spermatic vein, ureter
  - Right: Inferior vena cava
- Advantages of retroperitoneoscopy:
  - Direct approach to the retroperitoneum
  - Reduced risk of visceral and vascular injury
  - Limited postoperative adhesions, ileus and peritonitis
  - Elective approach in patients with a history of multiple abdominal surgical procedures or peritonitis
  - Easy quick access
  - Direct approach to the renal hilum (early control)
- Most complications are minor and easily managed.

5.1 Introduction

The introduction of laparoscopy in urology has been slow due to technical limitations. This approach was adopted from gynecologists and general surgeons who generally use a transabdominal or a transperitoneal approach. The clinical step forward was a transperitoneal

A. de la Taille (✉)
Department of Urology, CHU Mondor, 51 avenue du Maréchal de Lattre de Tassigny, Créteil 94000, France
e-mail: adelataille@hotmail.com

J.V. Joseph and H.R.H. Patel (eds.), *Retroperitoneal Robotic and Laparoscopic Surgery*,
DOI: 10.1007/978-0-85729-485-2_5, © Springer-Verlag London Limited 2011

laparoscopic nephrectomy performed by Clayman et al. in 1991.[1] Although retroperitoneoscopic surgery was described in 1973 by Wittmoser, who performed a lumbar sympathectomy, and in 1979 by Wickham who performed a retroperitoneoscopic ureterolithotomy, the full scope of retroperitoneoscopy was realized only after 1990 when Gaur constructed a simple device consisting of a No. 7 surgical glove mounted on a red-rubber catheter and created the workspace of the retroperitoneal laparoscopy. He inflated the glove to 110 mmHg using a pneumatic pump and manometer.[2-4] He successfully used this approach for multiple retroperitoneal procedures including simple nephrectomy, renal biopsy, ureterolithotomy, and pyelolithotomy.[5]

To date, retroperitoneal laparoscopy, also known as retroperitoneoscopy or lumboscopy, has been described by numerous centers for a variety of procedures, including pelvic lymph node dissection, ureterolithotomy, partial nephrectomy, adrenal surgery and a variety of renal procedures.[6-11]

Many centers around the world have reported their experience with endoscopic radical nephrectomy and consistently this has been shown to be better than the open surgical approach in terms of perioperative morbidity, convalescence, and cosmesis.[12] The long-term follow-up after laparoscopic radical nephrectomy (LRN) has also been reported and is considered to confer the same oncologic effectiveness as open radical nephrectomy.[13]

Initial reports described as disadvantages of the retroperitoneal laparoscopic approach the increased operative duration, poor visualization secondary to inadequate insufflation of the retroperitoneum, and considerable experience and training needed.[14]

Subsequent comparative studies have demonstrated equivalence between laparoscopic transperitoneal approach and retroperitoneoscopy.[15,16] Many surgical teams have reported considerable experience using this technique.[17] For simple and radical nephrectomy, laparoscopic approaches using transperitoneal, transperitoneal hand assisted, retroperitoneal and retroperitoneal hand assisted methods are mainly applied. We prefer to keep the term LRN for the transperitoneal approach and to use retroperitoneoscopic radical nephrectomy (RPRN) for the retroperitoneal approach, because "laparoscopy" by definition is the inspection of the peritoneal cavity. The choice of the approach depends on the individual surgeon's preference, training and comfort level with the approach.

5.2 Indications and Contraindications

The indications for retroperitoneoscopic nephrectomy are the same as those for laparoscopic transperitoneal nephrectomy.

LRN has now become an established surgical procedure with lower morbidity when compared to open surgery. The laparoscopic approach (transperitoneal or retroperitoneal) duplicates established open surgical oncologic principles, that is, with early control of the renal vessels before tumor manipulation, wide specimen mobilization external to Gerota's fascia, avoidance of specimen trauma or rupture and intact specimen extraction. The laparoscopy (by transperitoneal or retroperitoneal approach) has become the reference procedure and the standard of care for radical nephrectomy for stage T1-T2 tumors.[18]

Laparoscopy is feasible for treatment of T3-T4 cancers and remains an option for these locally advanced cancers.

Laparoscopic simple nephrectomy is indicated in the treatment of most benign renal diseases which cause renal dysfunction and/or repeated pyelonephritis.

5.3 Preoperative Management

Informed consent should be obtained with a discussion of possible complications. The patient has to be informed that conversion to open surgery might be necessary to safely complete the planned procedure. Laboratory studies and electrocardiogram depend on the medical history of the patient.

A computed tomography (CT) scan of the abdomen and pelvis, without and with injection of contrast medium, is necessary for diagnosis, assessing the tumor size and location, local and regional extension, possible thrombi, the condition of the contralateral kidney and the possible presence of hepatic or lymph node metastases (clinical staging of the tumor). A chest X-ray is usually performed. A magnetic resonance imaging (MRI) study may be indicated when there is doubt concerning the presence of an angiomyolipoma, or to evaluate the extension of a caval thrombus more precisely. If the patient presents with other symptoms in case of kidney cancer, a brain scan, bone scan or chest scan can be included in the workup.

The patient must fast, starting from the previous night of the surgery. Determination of blood type and a cross match are carried out. No bowel preparation is needed.

When inducing the general anesthesia, prophylactic antibiotic therapy with a second generation cephalosporin is administered. Prophylactic treatment with low molecular weight heparin is begun on the day of surgery.

5.4 Operative Steps

We present a standardized procedure which has been used in our department since 2001. Globally, the retroperitoneal approach mimics open surgery and avoids the entry into the peritoneal cavity.

5.4.1 Patient Positioning and Setting

In the beginning the patient is positioned decubitus and general anesthesia is induced followed by placement of a nasogastric or orogastric tube and a Foley urinary catheter.

Then the patient is placed in standard full flank lateral decubitus (lumbotomy) position. The anatomic access site for retroperitoneoscopy is the space between the lowermost (12th) rib superiorly, the iliac crest inferiorly, the lateral border of the paraspinal muscles posterolaterally and the lateral peritoneal reflection anteromedially. The tumor side is hyperextended to make a space between the costal margin and the iliac crest. The dimensions of this access field are maximized by elevating the kidney rest and flexing the operating table with the lumbar support raised to its maximum height; the calves and the thighs (always with compression stockings/tights) are bent 20°, flexed slightly forward and placed on the anterior leg rest. All pressure points, including head and neck, hips, knees, and ankles, are protected with silicone pillows and padded. The axilla is supported with an axillary roll. The posterior leg rest is removed to leave room for the assistant who holds the laparoscope.

The patient is secured and scrubbed from above the costal margin to below the iliac crest.

The operating surgeon and the first assistant (camera operator) are positioned facing the back of the patient, the second assistant is positioned facing the patient's abdomen, opposite the operating surgeon and the scrub nurse next to the first assistant (or on the other side of the surgeon).

There are preferably two laparoscopic towers with the monitors, facing the surgeons from both sides of the patient's head.

5.4.2 Instrument Set Up

The following is a list of the instruments used:

- 1 Cold light cable
- 1 laparoscope optics 0° of 10 mm
- Trocars (5): 1 of 5–12 mm, 2 of 12 mm with the Step 14G needle, 2 of 5 mm
- An irrigation–aspiration device nozzle 5 mm
- 2 Needle-holders
- 1 pair of laparoscopic scissors 5 mm with monopolar cautery
- 1 Monopolar cable
- 1 Bipolar grasping forceps
- 1 Bipolar cable
- 1 toothed (crocodile) grasper
- 1 atraumatic fenestrated grasper double
- 1 atraumatic fenestrated grasper double curved
- 2 atraumatic fenestrated simple graspers
- 1 laparoscopic dissector
- 1 lapsack 15 mm
- Hem-o-lock clip applicator 10 mm with clips
- Ligaclip ERCA (medium-large) with 5 mm titanium clips
- A refillable automatic cutting stapler – Linear stapler
- Liga-sure V 5 mm
- 1 set for extracorporeal suturing
- Instrumentation necessary for the realization of a Pfannenstiel incision or the lumbotomy and its closing
- 1 drain Redon

5.4.3 Trocar Placement and Creation of the Retroperitoneal Space

First trocar: A minimal (1 cm) lumbotomy cutaneous incision is performed 1 cm subcostally and in parallel with the 12th rib, on the lateral border of the paraspinal

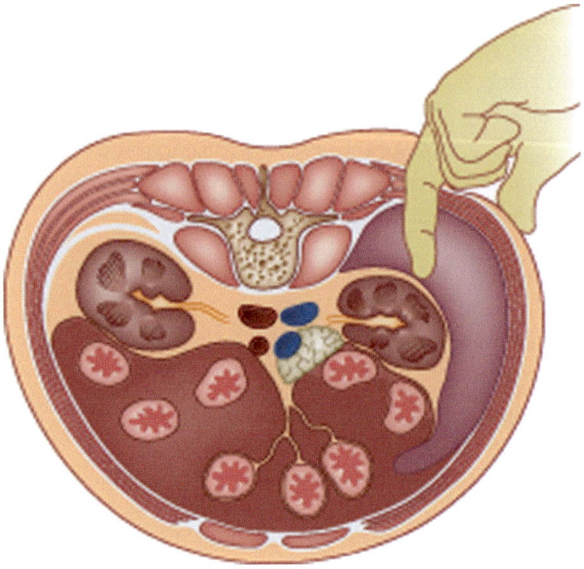

Fig. 5.1 Finger dissection and creation of the working space

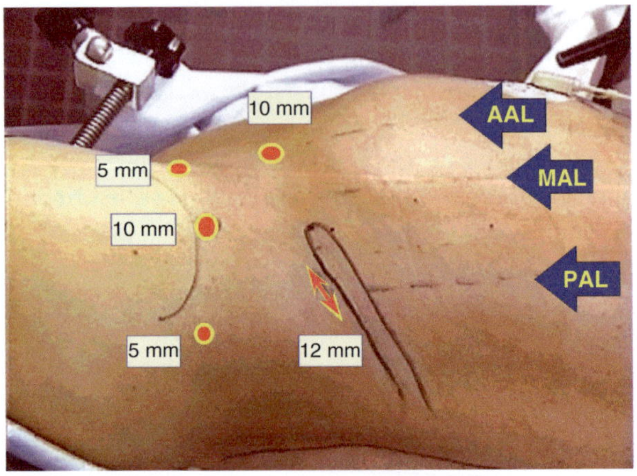

Fig. 5.2 Trocar placement

muscles that projects roughly onto the posterior axillary line (Fig. 5.1).

The surgeon pierces the muscles and fascias with a Kelly clamp or using a hemostat all the way to the retroperitoneal posterior pararenal space with impunity. Then he creates an orifice by opening the clamp. At this point, there is not any significant vessel involving risk of vascular wound. To our knowledge, no vascular wound was described during the creation of the retroperitoneal workspace. Care should be taken that this fascial opening is snug around the index finger and no larger, so that intraoperative air leak is minimized. Index finger palpation of the belly of the psoas muscle posteriorly and the Gerota's fascia-covered inferior pole of the kidney anteriorly confirms proper entry into the retroperitoneal space (Fig. 5.2). Then finger dissection and creation of the working space is done in the posterior pararenal space. This space is located between the fascia transversalis and the fascia of Gerota. The peritoneum is mobilized from the abdominal wall anteriorly toward midline allowing the insertion of the trocars under digital control. Care must be taken to digitally dissect in an anterior plane and in a 180° angle so as not to traumatize the paraspinal muscles.

This particular incision is closed later (after placing the second and third trocars) by fixing a 5–12 mm trocar with sealing ring and the skin and subcutaneous tissue closed tightly with two no. 2 absorbable sutures. Through this trocar the surgeon interchangeably uses the monopolar scissors, bipolar grasping forceps, suction device, needle holder and various large-caliber instruments, including a 12-mm EndoGIA stapler, a 10-mm right-angle dissector, clip appliers and specimen retrieval bag.

Second trocar: A 12 mm trocar with the Step 14G needle is placed (under digital control), 2 cm above the iliac crest and 2 cm anterior to level of the first trocar in order to allow good mobility of the trocar and instruments. Through this trocar the surgeon can use the same instruments as through the first one.

Third trocar: A 12 mm trocar with the Step 14G needle is placed (under digital control), at the same level as the second trocar but 4 cm anteriorly (roughly at the medial axillary line). This port is reserved for the 0° optics handled by the first assistant.

Then the trocar with the foam grip is introduced through the initial lumbotomy incision. Insufflation is begun with the maximum CO_2 pressure set at 12 mmHg and the optics is introduced through the second port. Under vision the pneumo-dissection proceeds. The first reference mark is the psoas muscle, easily identifiable in the lower part of the workspace. The pneumo-dissection pushes back the peritoneum attachment and its contents forward, allows a progressive separation of perirenal fat, through which we can identify the renal capsule. Using the fenestrated grasper, +/– bipolar the surgeon frees the anterior abdominal wall from the peritoneum or fatty tissue in order to introduce the next two secondary ports.

Fourth trocar: A 5 mm trocar is placed (under laparoscopic control) at the anterior axillary line across the first port. This trocar will be used by the second assistant for aspiration and various graspers during the operation.

Fifth trocar: A 5 mm trocar is placed (under laparoscopic control) at the anterior axillary line across the second port, 2–3 fingerbreadths above and medial to the antero-superior iliac spine. This trocar is used by the assistants for aspiration and various graspers during the operation and for placement of a drain at the end of the procedure.

Hereafter the laparoscope is introduced through the third trocar.

We do not use balloon distension to create the workspace. Since we standardized our technique, the single digital dissection proved to be sufficient for adequate exposure of the retroperitoneal space. Thus, we could reduce our operating time by 5–15 min, which was usually required for balloon dissection. Additionally, severe adhesions, such as those after previous renal surgeries, can be lysed sufficiently by endoscopic incision. The peritoneum is separated from the abdominal wall by the index finger of the surgeon introduced through the subcostal incision. The first two trocars are placed under digital control. The wide longitudinal incision of the renal fascia performed at the beginning of the procedure helps to enlarge the working space. An important factor is optimal exposure of the entire surgical field before starting dissection at the renal hilum.

5.4.4 Orientation and Landmarks

The trocars being set up, the optics is placed into the third trocar. The anatomical reference marks are always the same ones: The first anatomical landmark is the psoas major muscle. To find it, the third assistant (standing opposite the surgeon) pulls the paranephric fat and the peritoneum toward himself/herself with two atraumatic forceps and the fatty tissue overlying that structure is gently swept away.

The best orientation is to have the psoas muscle along and parallel to the base of the television monitor so, for the left kidney, the cephalad direction is to the right side of the screen and the caudal to the left. When the operation is for the right kidney, the cephalad direction is to the left side of the monitor and the caudal to the right.

The lateral surface of the muscle is freed cephalad and caudally, to create a sufficient working space. Using this reference mark, the fascia of Gerota can be easily highlighted.

On the left side, the dissection is pursued cephalad with the scissors and the suction through the first and second trocars. Very often, the ureter and the genital vein, which run parallel to the psoas major muscle, are exposed at this point (Fig. 5.3). By following them cephalad, the renal pedicle can be identified by the deep pulsations of its artery under the lower renal pole.

On the right side, the psoas major muscle is followed medially. Sometimes the dissection is facilitated with graspers through the anterior trocars. The inferior vena cava is recognized running parallel with psoas. The dissection that is pursued along the inferior vena cava cephalad (to the left of the screen) sometimes exposes the ureter or the genital vein medially to vena cava and finally leads to the right renal pedicle. The fragile genital vein is divided between two clips near the vena cava to avoid tearing during maneuvers, which could result in bleeding that is hard to control.

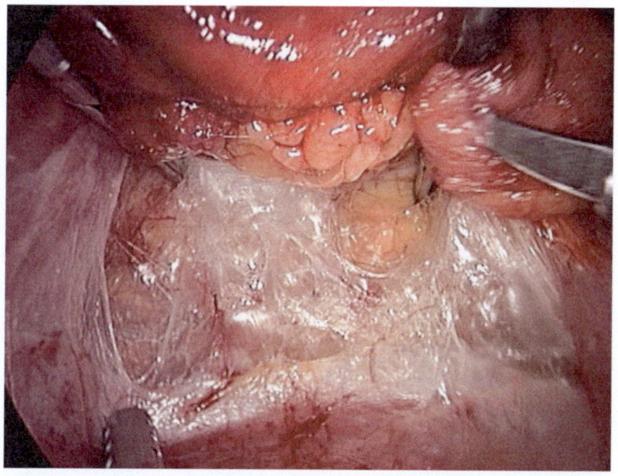

Fig. 5.3 The first anatomical landmark is the psoas major muscle: the best orientation is to have the psoas muscle along and parallel to the base of the television monitor. The lateral surface of the muscle is freed cephalad and caudally, to create a sufficient working space. Using this reference mark, the fascia of Gerota can be easily highlighted

5.4.5 Renal Hilum Dissection and Pedicle Ligation

For the left kidney, when the fatty tissue is freed from the lower pole and the assistant is pushing the kidney toward the peritoneum, the branches of the renal vein are exposed. The genital (internal spermatic) vein drains into the proximal portion of the renal vein and its direction is toward the left side of the screen when the psoas muscle is at the base of the screen. Posteriorly, the second azygo-lumbar vein forms a bridge above the aorta and courses toward the psoas major muscle. On the superior border of the renal vein, the renal artery appears (right side of the screen).

The renal pedicle being discovered, a 2 cm portion of the renal artery is freed completely with the suction in the left hand and the scissors or the dissector in the right hand (Fig. 5.4). The renal artery is ligated with three or five 9 mm hem-o-clips and divided, leaving two clips on the remaining stump. (The hem-o-lock is inserted through the first trocar.) The left adrenal vein, now exposed, is heading cephalad under the renal artery to the right of the screen.

The lumbar vein is ligated with metal clips or hem-o-clips if necessary and divided.

Under the divided azygos vein the proximal portion of the renal vein must then be completely dissected to make it easily twist and not to have any tissue within contact for a free zone at least 1–2 cm all around the vein in order to set up easily the Endo GIA® (Fig. 5.5).

The draining to-the-renal-vein vessels (genital +/– adrenal veins) are ligated with metal clips and divided.

A linear stapler is positioned through the first trocar. Its tip must go beyond the renal vein, without catching the deep tissue layers in its jaws. The benchmarks of Endo GIA® are well checked and the linear stapler is then closed and activated to staple and divide the renal vein.

For the right kidney, following vena cava cephalad the surgeon finds the gonadal vein, the renal vein and artery and the adrenal vein. The renal vein is dissected free and the renal artery on the superior border of the renal vein (on the left side of the screen) is exposed as it crosses the inferior vena cava posteriorly, and is entirely freed as well. The renal artery first and vein second are clipped and divided following the same principles as those described for the left kidney. The vena cava may be seen collapsed because of the pneumo-retro-peritoneum but it is better to push downward with the suction (left hand) during the stapling of the right renal vein to avoid trauma to the vena cava.

If an adrenalectomy is combined with the radical nephrectomy, the freeing of the vena cava is pursued cephalad until the adrenal vein is found near the junction of the renal vein and the vena cava. The adrenal vein is then clipped and divided with hem-o-clips.

Regional lymph node dissection is carried out if indicated. It is carried out by removing the lymphatic tissue of the renal pedicle. If one wishes to carry out a more extensive dissection, it will have to be done at the

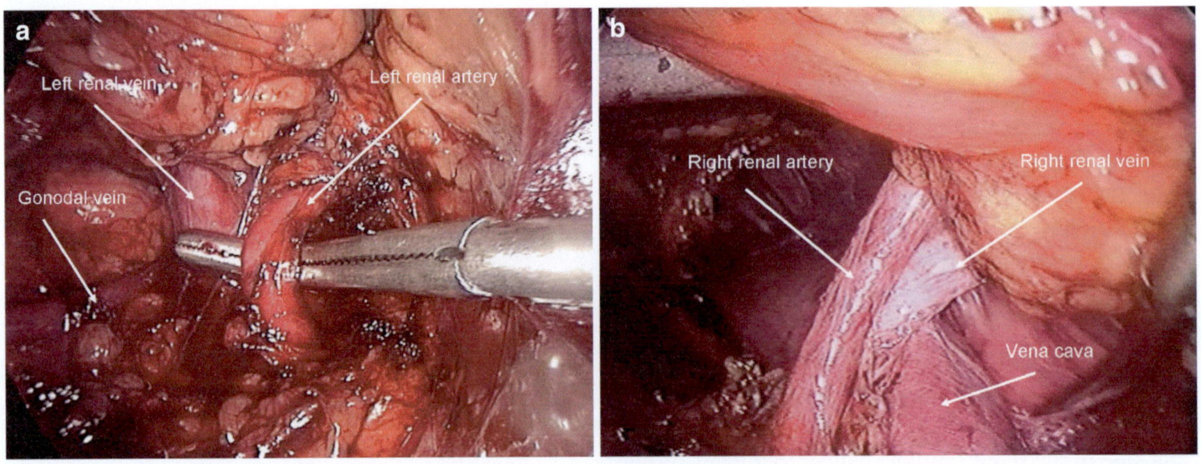

Fig. 5.4 (**a**) Left and (**b**) right renal pedicles

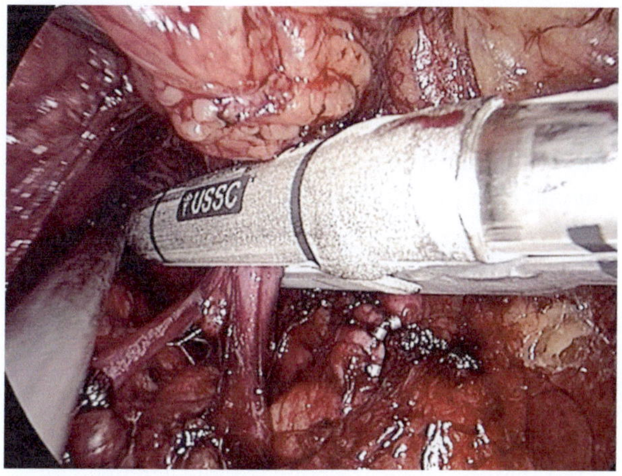

Fig. 5.5 Section of the renal vein

time of the access of the renal pedicle in the beginning of the intervention. Indeed, with the kidney fully mobilized, it may be more difficult to perform the lymph node dissection.

5.4.6 Kidney Mobilization

After the renal pedicle is controlled and the hilar area is dissected, complete mobilization of the kidney is performed. It is necessary to dissect the kidney by separating the fascia of Gerota from the peritoneum and the abdominal wall. Most of the dissection is performed bluntly.

The use of the liga-sure is indicated when there is considerable bleeding during the dissection, or when there is remarkable neo-vascularization due to tumor. In this setting it is advisable to raise the gas pressure as well.

The mobilization of the kidney surrounded by perirenal fat and Gerota's fascia begins at its posterior surface and begins from the renal hilum and is extended cephalad, while the assistant pulls the kidney to the abdominal wall. The adrenal artery is identified, ligated and divided if necessary.

At this point, the anterior attachments are left intact. They keep the kidney suspended and, along with the "retraction" effect of the pneumo-retro-peritoneum, facilitate the posterior cleavage. The surgeon then reaches the diaphragm and can free the superior pole entirely. In order to perform this the surgeon uses the instruments (scissors, bipolar, liga-sure, suction or atraumatic forceps) through opposed trocars (the second and fifth or the first and fourth) so as to have a better working axis.

The adrenalectomy can be considered at the same time according to the indications. In the event of an obligatory adrenalectomy, it is necessary to be performed en-block with the kidney specimen during the separation of the upper pole of the kidney. When associated on the right side, after having controlled the renal pedicle and dissecting along the vena cava, we recognize the adrenal vein which is clipped and divided. On the left side, the adrenal vein drains at the beginning of the renal vein as already mentioned.

Then the anterior leaflet of Gerota's fascia is separated from the peritoneum cephalad to caudal including the renal hilum. The kidney and peritoneum are tensioned by the second assistant who pushes the peritoneum medially to the abdominal wall. During this procedure, a peritoneal tear can sometimes occur. It is of no consequence if the peritoneum tears and sometimes, it will facilitate cleavage because it will be better visible. However, the surgeon must avoid using intensive cauterization with the monopolar scissors because of the close proximity of the digestive tract and the tail of the pancreas on the left side.

The inferior pole of the kidney is then freed.

The ureter can be divided at the end of intervention at the time of the access of the lower pole. It is freed up to the iliac crest and divided between two clips.

The specimen is reflected caudally so as the last attachments are divided.

5.4.7 Specimen Extraction

The kidney is reflected cephalad to the diaphragm and toward the abdominal wall with the assistant's grasping forceps. The pressure of the retroperitoneum is decreased to 5 mmHg to check for possible bleeding.

The first trocar is removed. A purse string suture is placed around the edges of the minimal lumbotomy.

The retrieval bag is placed in the retroperitoneal space. The suture is tightened, enabling a reestablishment of the pneumo-retro-peritoneum.

The bag is deployed under laparoscopic control. The kidney is released by the assistant, and the whole operative specimen, including the fatty covering, lymph tissue, adrenal gland and the ureter, is pushed into the bag.

The bag is then extracted through the wall, after enlarging the initial lumbotomy incision so that it should measure between 4 and 6 cm. If the specimen is too big there is always the option to extract it through a flank incision of 5–6 cm beginning at the level of the fifth trocar. This presupposes the pass of the lapsac string through the fifth trocar before the final incision (by putting a grasper through the fifth trocar to the lumbotomy to snatch the string).

5.4.8 *Wound Closure*

The trocars are removed. A drain (Redon) is inserted through the second trocar in the mid axillary line. The muscular and fascial planes of the lumbotomy incision and/or the flank incision are closed. The other trocar wounds do not require fascial closure. The skin is sutured using an intradermic running suture with rapidly absorbable 4.0 polyglycolic suture.

5.4.9 *Summary of Surgical Steps*

1. Working space: posterior pararenal space, identification of the psoas muscle
2. Incision of Gerota's fascia
3. Anatomic landmarks:
   (a) Left: Internal spermatic vein ureter
   (b) Right: Inferior vena cava
4. Renal pedicle:
   (a) Section of the artery (clips)
   (b) Section of the vein (Endo-GIA)
5. Adrenalectomy (if necessary)
6. Radical nephrectomy
7. Section of the ureter
8. Specimen extraction

5.5 Postoperative Management

The orogastric tube is removed at the end of the surgical procedure. Liquid intake is allowed on the operative day. The drain is removed the day after the surgery. Serum creatinine is measured postoperatively and intravenous line is removed. Intravenous analgesia is relayed by oral analgesia. At 1 day after nephrectomy, patient is allowed to stand and encouraged to walk. Urine is collected through the Foley catheter during the first 24 h. Mean duration of hospital stay (including the day before the surgery and the day of the nephrectomy) is 5 days. Postoperative visit is planned at 1 month after the surgery.

5.6 Complications

It has been demonstrated in worldwide series that all the surgery of the upper urinary tract can be carried out by retroperitoneal laparoscopy: simple nephrectomies, radical nephrectomies, partial nephrectomies, adrenalectomies, lymphadenectomies, renal cyst ablation, diverticulectomies, pyelolithotomy, ureterolysis, ureterolithotomy, and retrocaval ureters.[8,9,19,20]

The main causes of conversion from the lumboscopy to open surgery are complex anatomical situations or gross obesity which does not allow proper dissection, or patients presenting with perinephric adhesions, due to infectious side effects, or previous surgery in the area. Indeed, these fibrous adhesions obstruct the creation of the workspace and complicate this approach. The retroperitoneal laparoscopy makes it technically possible to extract bulky masses.

The conversions undertaken as an emergency are usually secondary to a major complication such as bleeding. With experience, the vascular traumas which occur at the time of the dissection of the renal pedicle can be managed by endoscopy. The urgent conversion rate in our experience is less than 1%[17]; it is related primarily with the radical nephrectomies and often results from difficulties of dissection related to the presence of loco-regional adenopathies. To avoid these complications, it is imperative that there is minimal handling or probing of the region of the renal hilum. Rassweiller et al. reported a total conversion rate of 7.5% including 3% for peri-operative hemorrhages.[10] Desai et al. reported an experience of 404 retroperitoneoscopies and a conversion rate due to hemorrhage of 1.7%.[15] In a series of 274 urologic operations of the upper urinary tract, Thiel et al. reported a hemorrhagic accident rate of 1.7% mentioning that only 0.3% has been converted.[21]

Life-threatening vascular injuries can occur during the dissection of the renal hilum. The vascular injuries are generally venous because of their brittleness. They relate to the renal vein, the vena cava and, sometimes, the avulsion of the genital vein. Most cases can be treated endoscopically by clamping and suturing of the bleeding area.[17] Bleeding from gonadal vessels and their retro-peritoneal branch vessels can occur toward the end of the procedure, during blunt dissection of the kidney and ureter.

In retroperitoneoscopy, it is rare to traumatize a vessel at the time of the insertion of the trocars. Indeed, there are no important vessels along the posterior abdominal wall. The digitally guided insertion protects the large abdominal vessels.[22] Complete transection of the vena cava, however, has been reported.[23]

Careful inspection of the retroperitoneum must be systematical to minimize postoperative bleeding.

The digestive tract injuries during retroperitoneal surgery seem to be attributed to the use of monopolar coagulation and the diffusion of heat energy at the time of the dissection of the kidney and the peritoneum near the intestine and the pancreas. Theoretically, the rate of injuries of intraperitoneal organs by laparoscopic transperitoneal approach is higher. Of 20 digestive injuries, Fahlenkamp et al. indexed 15 during the transperitoneal approach.[24] It generally results from the handling of the digestive tract and lysis of adhesions in the event of postsurgical fibrosis. By the transperitoneal approach, Parsons et al. mentioned a rate of 2.13% and Vallancien et al. reported a rate of 1.2% for 206 operations of the upper urinary tract.[25,26] In his series comparing 50 nephrectomies for cancer carried out by transperitoneal laparoscopy with 52 nephrectomies for cancer carried out by retroperitoneal laparoscopy, Desai et al. counted four injuries transperitoneally against none retroperitoneally.[15] Bishoff et al., in a series of 915 laparoscopies, however, found only 0.2% of digestive tract perforations; half of them resulted from electrocoagulation.[27] He insists on the difficulty of such a diagnosis in the postoperative period; the digestive wound presents with diarrhea, ileus, leucopenia and especially with persistent pain on the site of trocar nearest to the wound.

A tear at the peritoneum is considered as a minor complication and if it does occur, the problem can be managed using a variety of techniques. An intravenous cannula can be inserted into the peritoneum to vent the CO_2. This helps to increase the retroperitoneal space by reducing the intraperitoneal pressure. Another option is to widen the tear intentionally to equalize the pressure on the two sides. These techniques are usually sufficient to overcome the problem.

Other surgical complications are very rare. A hernia from 12 mm trocar opening is rarely noted. Indeed, the retroperitoneal laparoscopy decreases morbidity related to the large incisions of lumbotomy (often by extracting the specimen through a small incision in the iliac fossa). Elashry et al. reported incisional hernia in five of 29 patients (17%) after transperitoneal laparoscopic nephrectomy.[28] In our experience, all specimens were removed intact, either by enlarging the primary port site or by a small 5 cm iliac incision. Retroperitoneal access provides protection against hernia formation and intact specimen retrieval is safe with this approach, especially when the wound is closed in layers.

The retroperitoneal laparoscopic approach technically makes it possible to remove large masses even if the workspace is limited. Nevertheless, in the event of bulky tumors and/or of lymphadenopathies solidifying the pedicle, the interest of another way initially can be discussed. Higher dimensions would increase the risk of capsular invasion and loco-regional relapses. Nevertheless, the laparoscopic results are comparable with those of the conventional surgery.[29]

In theory, retroperitoneal laparoscopy, while remaining apart from the peritoneum, allows a faster approach to the retroperitoneal organs and prevents completely the risk of fibrous adhesion formation intraperitoneally and thus of later occlusions. In addition, the scapular pain of the pneumoperitoneum is less frequent with retroperitoneoscopy, which may be associated with less postoperative pain.[30] Nevertheless, in his comparative series, Desai et al. did not find significant differences in terms of hospital stay and consumption of analgesics between the two approaches.[15]

Insufflation-related complications are subcutaneous emphysema and gas embolism. Diaphragm injury is rare but has to be treated to prevent major pneumothorax. The thoracic complications, such as pulmonary infections, are generally infrequent.

Globally, the retroperitoneal approach offers similar results compared with transperitoneal laparoscopic nephrectomy in terms of complications and postoperative parameters.[15,16,30]

5.7 Advantages and Pitfalls

The retroperitoneal laparoscopy (or retroperitoneoscopy or lumboscopy) is a relatively recent way of approaching the retroperitoneum. Today this technique is well standardized and reported in almost all the relevant articles for retroperitoneal space.

The advantages of retroperitoneoscopy are the direct approach to the retroperitoneum despite the difficulties associated with the smaller operating chamber. By avoiding the peritoneal cavity the risk of visceral and vascular injury may be reduced. Retroperitoneal organs and certain landmarks can be visualized directly. Intestinal retraction is made easier as the peritoneal envelope surrounds the intestines and individual bowel loops need not be retracted. Postoperative adhesions and peritonitis if there is spillage of infected renal contents are minimized. Moreover, lumboscopy meets all the criteria of open renal surgery, given all urologic interventions are performed via the retroperitoneal route without transgressing the abdominal cavity. Thus, patients with a history of multiple abdominal surgical procedures or peritonitis may benefit from retroperitoneoscopy.

In addition, the retroperitoneal approach provides easy quick access and direct approach to the renal hilum (early control) and a lower incidence of intra-abdominal organ injuries, ileus, etc., and these could balance the relatively limited working space.

A liquid collection in the retroperitoneum is spontaneously controlled by the limited workspace and natural tamponade thus caused. This is a potential advantage of the retroperitoneal approach.

As McDougall and Clayman indicated, our experience with retroperitoneal laparoscopic nephrectomy resulted in a greater decrease in operative time compared to transperitoneal laparoscopic nephrectomy and open surgery.[30] In the randomized trial of Desai et al., the retroperitoneal approach had a shorter operative time compared with the operative time in transperitoneal surgery (150 vs. 207 min, $p<0.001$).[15] In a second randomized series (retro- vs. transperitoneal nephrectomy), Nambirajan found no difference in terms of operative and postoperative parameters.[16]

Limitations of the retroperitoneal approach include the possible obliteration of this potential space by previous surgical procedures or inflammatory processes. A more common problem is that excessive fat may obscure the retroperitoneal anatomy. Obesity is not a contraindication to retroperitoneoscopy but fatty tissue can make identification of the anatomy challenging. Obesity is also a risk factor for postoperative complications in both open and laparoscopic surgery. Landmarks in the retroperitoneum are relatively few compared with the peritoneal cavity. In addition, the limited skin area available may make port placement more difficult. Improper placement may result in colonic injury, as the peritoneal reflection is relatively fixed.

Even if the working space in RPRN is limited it is very rare to have difficulties to deploy and use the endobag for specimen entrapment. We believe that the size of the tumor is not a contraindication for RPRN. However, adequate laparoscopic experience is necessary when performing RPRN for larger tumors. Furthermore, in RPRN, the intercostal flank incision is avoided and the specimen is removed via a small incision, sparing the cutaneous and muscle nerves. Since tumor size is no longer a limiting factor to perform laparoscopic surgery, for many surgeons the most important factor is to make this technique simpler. The technique has to be standardized through detailed simple steps trying to overcome the difficulty in orientation.

5.8 Summary

To conclude, numerous studies have confirmed that RPRN is a safe and efficient procedure. At the beginning of the third millennium, it is possible to state that retroperitoneoscopy can be the technique of choice for accessing and carrying out all the surgery of the upper urinary tract. Surgeons who want to perform renal laparoscopic surgery should know how to do both approaches (retroperitoneal and transperitoneal) because some patients will require retroperitoneal approach, for instance if they had previous major intraperitoneal surgeries or if it is a urinary upper tract tumors. Retroperitoneoscopy respects the principles of oncological surgery. This approach is interesting in the event of previous history of abdominal surgery because it makes it possible to avoid risky and tiresome lysis of the adhesions. Most complications are minor and easily managed.

References

1. Clayman RV, Kavoussi LR, Soper NJ, et al. Laparoscopic nephrectomy: initial case report. *J Urol*. 1991;146:278-282.
2. Wittmoser R. Die Retroperitoneoskopie als neue Methode der lumbalen Sympathikotomie. *Fortschr Endoskopie*. 1973;4:219.
3. Wickham JEA. The surgical treatment of renal lithiasis. In: Wickham JEA, ed. *Urinary Calculus Disease*. New York: Churchill Livingstone; 1979:145-198.

4. Gaur D. Laparoscopic operative retroperitoneoscopy: use of a new device. *J Urol*. 1992;148:1137-1138.
5. Gaur DD, Agarwal DK, Purohit KC. Retroperitoneal laparoscopic nephrectomy: initial case report. *J Urol*. 1993; 149:103-105.
6. Kavoussi LR, Sosa E, Chandhoke P, et al. Complications of laparoscopic pelvic lymph node dissection. *J Urol*. 1993;149:322-325.
7. Munch LC, Delworth MG, Gill IS. Retroperitoneal laparoscopic ureterolithotomy. *J Endourol*. 1993;7:137-138.
8. Cicco A, Salomon L, Hoznek A, et al. Results of retroperitoneal laparoscopic radical nephrectomy. *J Endourol*. 2001;154:355-359.
9. Salomon L, Soulie M, Mouly P, et al. Experience with retroperitoneal laparoscopic adrenalectomy in 115 procedures. *J Urol*. 2001;1661:38-41.
10. Rassweiler JJ, Seemann O, Frede T, Henkel TO, Alken P. Retroperitoneoscopy: experience with 200 cases. *J Urol*. 1998;160:1265-1268.
11. McDougall EM, Dayman RV, Fadden PT. Retroperitoneoscopy: the Washington University Medical School experience. *Urology*. 1994;43:446-450.
12. Rassweiler J, Frede T, Henkel TO, Stock C, Alken P. Nephrectomy: a comparative study between the transperitoneal and retroperitoneal laparoscopic versus the open approach. *Eur Urol*. 1998;33:489-496.
13. Portis AJ, Yan Y, Landman J, et al. Long-term followup after laparoscopic radical nephrectomy. *J Urol*. 2002;167(3): 1257-1262.
14. Gill IS, Dayman RV, Albala DM, Aso Y, et al. Retroperitoneal and pelvic extraperitoneal laparoscopy: an international perspective. *Urology*. 1998;52:566-571.
15. Desai MM, Strzempkowski B, Matin SF, et al. Prospective randomized comparison of transperitoneal versus retroperitoneal laparoscopic radical nephrectomy. *J Urol*. 2005; 173:38-41.
16. Nambirajan T, Jeschke S, Al-Zahrani H, Vrabec G, Leeb K, Janetschek G. Prospective, randomized controlled study: transperitoneal laparoscopic versus retroperitoneoscopic radical nephrectomy. *Urology*. 2004;64:919-924.
17. Liapis D, de la Taille A, Ploussard G, et al. Analysis of complications from 600 retroperitoneoscopic procedures of the upper urinary tract during the last 10 years. *World J Urol*. 2008;26(6):523-530.
18. Ljungberg B, Hanbury DC, Kuczyk MA, et al. European Association of Urology Guideline Group for renal cell carcinoma renal cell carcinoma guideline. *Eur Urol*. 2007;51:1502-10.
19. Gill IS, Schweizer D, Hobart MG, Sung GT, Klein EA, Novick AC. Retroperitoneal laparoscopic radical nephrectomy: the Cleveland clinic experience. *J Urol*. 2000; 163:1665-1670.
20. Hoznek A, Salomon L, Antiphon P, et al. Partial nephrectomy with retroperitoneal laparoscopy. *J Urol*. 1999;1626:1922-1926.
21. Thiel R, Adams JB, Schulam PG, Moore RG, Kavoussi LR. Venous dissection injuries during laparoscopic urological surgery. *J Urol*. 1996;155:1874-1876.
22. Yiou R, Delmas V, Chopin D, Abbou CC. Anatomical basis of lumboscopy. *Surg Radiol Anat*. 2001;233:179-184.
23. McAllister M, Bhayani SB, Ong A, et al. Vena caval transection during retroperitoneoscopic nephrectomy: report of the complication and review of the literature. *J Urol*. 2004;172:183-185.
24. Fahlenkamp D, Rassweiler J, Fornara P, Frede T, Loening SA. Complications of laparoscopic procedures in urology. Experience with 2407 procedures at 4 German centers. *J Urol*. 1999;162:765-768.
25. Parsons JK, Varkarakis I, Rha KH, Jarrett TW, Pinto PA, Kavoussi LR. Complications of abdominal urologic laparoscopy: longitudinal five-years analysis. *Urology*. 2004;63:27-32.
26. Vallancien G, Cathelineau X, Baumert H, Doublet JD, Guillonneau B. Complications of transperitoneal laparoscopic surgery in urology: review of 1, 311 procedures at a single center. *J Urol*. 2002;168:23-26.
27. Bishoff JT, Allaf ME, Kirkels W, Moore RG, Kavoussi LR, Schroder F. Laparoscopic bowel injury: incidence and clinical presentation. *J Urol*. 1999;161:887-890.
28. Elashry OM, Giusti G, Nadler RB, McDoughall EM, Dayman RV. Incisional hernia after laparoscopic nephrectomy with intact specimen removal: caveat emptor. *J Urol*. 1997;158:363-369.
29. Permpongkosol S, Chan DY, Link RE, et al. Long-term survival analysis after laparoscopic radical nephrectomy. *J Urol*. 2005;174:1222-1225.
30. McDougall EM, Clayman RV. Laparoscopic nephrectomy for benign disease: comparison of the transperitoneal and retroperitoneal approach. *J Endourol*. 1996;10:45-47.

6 Laparoscopic and Robotic Partial Nephrectomy

Lori M. Dulabon and Michael D. Stifelman

Abstract Over the past decade, there has been a change in the management of newly diagnosed renal cortical tumors, shifting away from radical nephrectomy (RN) toward the application of partial nephrectomy (PN). Minimally invasive surgical approaches have been increasingly used in patients with small renal masses over the last several years with equivalent oncologic outcomes.[1] Minimally invasive extirpative surgical approaches used to treat small renal masses include: laparoscopic partial nephrectomy (LPN) (both transperitoneal and retroperitoneal approaches) and robot-assisted laparoscopic partial nephrectomy (RLPN). The focus of this chapter will be on transperitoneal and retroperitoneal approaches to LPN and robotic PN.

Keywords Kidney cancer • Laparoscopic • Nephron-sparing • Partial nephrectomy • Renal tumor • Robot-assisted

Key Points

- Study preoperative imaging thoroughly. Understand renal vascular anatomy (number and locations of veins, arteries).
- Use endoscopic ultrasound to mark out tumor borders intraoperatively.
- Utilize laparoscopic Doppler probe to confirm ischemia prior to tumor excision.
- Perform venous clamping (in addition to arterial clamping) to prevent back-bleeding during difficult/complex tumor resections (endophytic, hilar tumors, etc.).
- Bed-side assistant surgeon is essential to optimize successful outcomes during robot-assisted PN.

6.1 Introduction

With nearly 60,000 new cases diagnosed annually, kidney cancer ranks among the top three most common genitourinary malignancies in the USA.[2] Surgical extirpation, mainly by radical nephrectomy (RN), has been the standard of care for localized renal tumors for nearly 50 years. Since Clayman et al. described the first laparoscopic RN in 1991, the application of laparoscopy and minimally invasive surgery has revolutionized field of urologic oncology.[3] Recently, data has emerged which has challenged the notion of RN as the standard of care for the treatment of localized renal masses. Due to a multitude of factors, including the downward stage migration of kidney cancer and a better appreciation of the negative impact of radical surgery on kidney function and other co-morbid conditions,

M.D. Stifelman (✉)
Department of Urology, NYU Langone Medical Center, New York University School of Medicine, 150 E. 32nd Street, 2nd Floor, New York 10016, NY, USA
e-mail: michael.stifelman@nyumc.org

J.V. Joseph and H.R.H. Patel (eds.), *Retroperitoneal Robotic and Laparoscopic Surgery*,
DOI: 10.1007/978-0-85729-485-2_6,

there has been a recent trend toward the application of nephron-sparing surgery (NSS), mainly through the use of partial nephrectomy (PN).[1,4-6] Numerous reviews of PN have proven its previously equivocal oncologic outcomes while preserving maximal renal function.[7,8] Additionally, PN is no longer reserved for patients with essential indications (solitary kidney, bilateral renal tumors, etc.) but is now applied to patients with elective indications as well. PN may now be regarded as the standard of care for patients with localized renal masses up to 7 cm in size in order to preserve optimal renal function.[8,9] Despite this, analysis of the Surveillance, Epidemiology and End Results (SEER) cancer registry up to 2001 demonstrated that only 20% of renal tumors ranging from 2 to 4 cm in size were treated with PN.[10]

The first laparoscopic partial nephrectomy (LPN) was described by Winfield in 1993, in an attempt to reduce the morbidity associated with open PN.[11] Data suggests that application of LPN permits patients to recover from surgery faster with less pain and blood loss.[12] However, LPN remains an advanced surgical procedure that requires a great deal of technical skill to perform, often keeping LPN in the hands of only the most experienced surgeons.[13] The difficulty associated with LPN has prevented the widespread adoption of this procedure within the urologic community.

Recently, robotic-assistance has been embraced by the urologic community to perform radical prostatectomy. Reported advantages of robotic assistance over open surgery and pure laparoscopic prostatectomy include: decreased positive margin rate, decrease morbidity, and less blood loss.[14] It has been suggested that these same advantages may be realized when employing robotics to PN. Robot-assisted laparoscopic partial nephrectomy (RLPN) has been demonstrated to be a safe and feasible option for NSS.[15] Most recent studies have comparable or improved results to the traditional laparoscopic approach.[16,17] Robotic-assistance may allow for more precise, accurate, and efficient tumor resection and renal reconstruction while reducing some of the technical surgical challenges often encountered in traditional laparoscopy. Technical advantages of robotics include: high definition 10x magnified stereoscopic image, increased surgeon control with four-arm approach, and computer-assisted dampening of tremor. Furthermore, a recent multi-institutional retrospective study suggested that robotic assistance may facilitate the extirpation of complex renal tumors, reducing warm-ischemia times and blood loss when compared to laparoscopy.[16]

There has been much debate regarding the merits of a retroperitoneal versus transperitoneal approach to laparoscopic renal surgery. A prospective, randomized comparison of transperitoneal laparoscopic radical nephrectomy (LRN) and retroperitoneal LRN by Desai et al. showed an advantage of the retroperitoneal approach regarding decreased time to renal hilar control and overall operative time. In this particular study, there was no significant difference in blood loss, hospital length of stay, complications, or analgesic requirements.[18] There has been additional data documenting the benefit of the retroperitoneal approach in obese ($BMI \geq 30$ kg/m^2) and extremely obese patients ($BMI \geq 40$ kg/m^2) with a trend for less estimated blood loss (EBL) and open conversion rates, and shorter operative times and length of hospital stay.[19]

After the first transperitoneal LPN described by Winfield et al. in 1993 and the first published report of retroperitoneal LPN described by Gill et al. in 1994, albeit both for benign disease, the same benefits of retroperitoneal LRN were found to hold true for retroperitoneal LPN.[11,20] A retrospective comparison of transperitoneal and retroperitoneal LPN by Wright and Porter found that mean operative times and estimated blood loss were significantly less ($p < 0.001$) for the retroperitoneal approach.[21] Additionally, the patients who underwent the retroperitoneal approach were able to tolerate a regular diet significantly sooner and were discharged home sooner than their transperitoneal LPN counterparts. Warm-ischemia times were not significantly different between the two groups. Advocates of the retroperitoneal laparoscopic approach for renal tumors also argue that there is improved access for posteriorly located tumors. In this chapter we will review the technique of transperitoneal and retroperitoneal LPN.

In terms of robotic PN, though there is evidence that this technique may have certain significant advantages over LPN including facilitating the removal of complex renal tumors and further reduction in warm-ischemia times and blood loss,[16] there is no published literature on a retroperitoneal approach. At our own institution, in the last 100 consecutive robot-assisted PNs, we performed only two via the retroperitoneal approach secondary to surgeon preference. Therefore, we will focus mainly on the technique, advantages, complications and postoperative care associated with transperitoneal robot-assisted laparoscopic PN (RALPN), but the retroperitoneal approach will also be discussed.

6.2 Indications/Contraindications

The indications for PN have been expanded beyond the absolute, essential indications (solitary kidney, bilateral tumors, chronic renal insufficiency, etc.) and now include the elective use of PN for patients with otherwise normal contralateral kidneys. In the early published literature, large tumor size was a relative contraindication to PN. However, more recent studies have shown equivalent oncologic outcomes of PN when compared to traditional RN in tumors ≤4 cm as well as select tumors up to 7 cm.[8,9]

The application of laparoscopic and robot-assisted PN is now routinely used in patients with localized renal masses. Initially, only employed to small, exophytic tumors, LPN and RLPN are now utilized for patients with increasingly complex renal tumor location (i.e., tumors abutting the renal sinus, multiple tumors within the same renal unit, and renal hilar lesions). Successful outcomes of LPN and RLPN for complex renal masses have been well documented in the literature.[22-24] At our institution, we do not use LPN or RLPN for patients with significant renal insufficiency or solitary kidneys in which the lesion is complex, as clamp-time may reach >30 min. In these selected patients, we prefer to perform open PN with cold ischemia. However, a comparative analysis by Gill et al. evaluated patients with solitary kidneys who underwent LPN versus open PN. The mean change in serum creatinine in the group who underwent LPN was found to only be 0.07 mg/dL at 30 days post-op, despite significantly longer warm-ischemia times in the laparoscopic group compared to the open group, at 27.8 min versus 17.5 min respectively.[12]

Other relative contraindications to laparoscopic or robotic PN include: renal vein thrombus, >2 renal tumors on affected side (again, due to prolonged warm-ischemia time), and those patients with a history of prior ipsilateral renal surgery (especially previous ablative procedures) secondary to significant potential for dense adhesions.

In terms of the retroperitoneal approach to PN, we would reserve this for patients with an extensive history of prior intra-abdominal surgeries/adhesions or those on peritoneal dialysis in order to avoid adhesions and potential bowel injury. However, there are surgeons who routinely utilize the retroperitoneal approach for any lateral to posteriorly located tumors, and may be particularly useful when applied to morbidly obese patients. Again, there is no current literature on retroperitoneal robotic PN.

6.3 Preoperative Preparation

All patients considered for PN are evaluated preoperatively with a metastatic work-up including abdominal magnetic resonance imaging (MRI) with and without intravenous contrast or computerized tomography (CT) with and without intravenous contrast (Figs. 6.1 and 6.2). This also serves to fully elucidate renal anatomy (location of tumor and number and location of renal arteries/veins). All patients also have a chest X-ray performed and full laboratory assessment of liver function, renal function with basic metabolic panel, preoperative hematocrit with complete blood count, and coagulation panel. Further studies including head CT, chest CT, and bone scan are ordered on an individual basis depending on clinical symptoms.

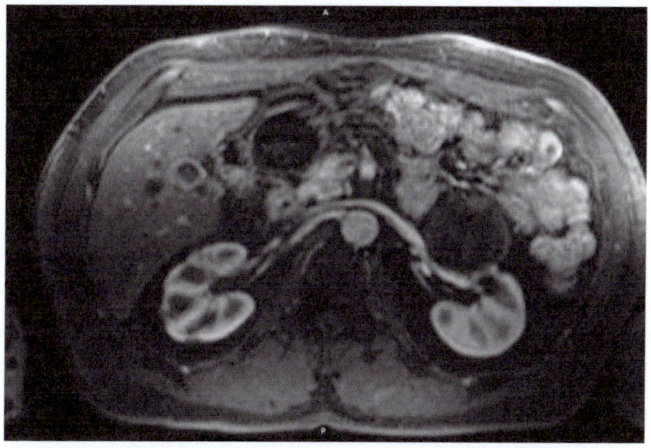

Fig. 6.1 MRI of left renal hilar renal lesion that was successfully removed by robot-assisted PN

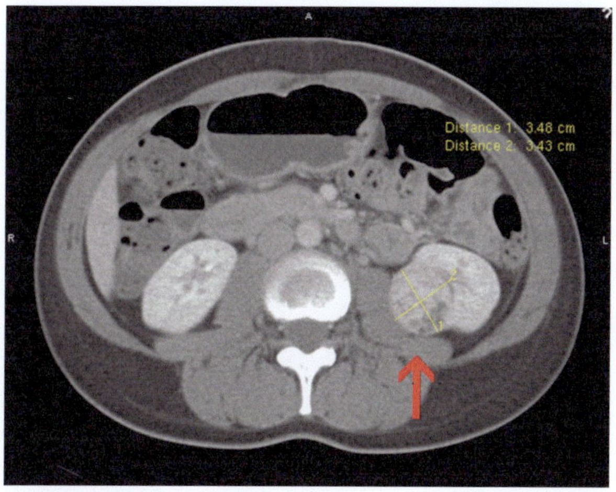

Fig. 6.2 CT scan of left endophytic, complex renal tumor (*arrow*) that was successfully removed via RPLN

All patients receive a modified mechanical bowel prep and consume only clear liquids the day before surgery. All patients provide informed consent for possible conversion to open surgery and possible RN.

6.4 Operative Steps

6.4.1 Robot-assisted Transperitoneal Partial Nephrectomy: Patient Positioning

After preoperative prophylactic intravenous antibiotic (usually a first generation cephalosporin) is administered, pneumatic compression devices are applied to the patient's lower extremities, and general anesthesia is induced. Complete paralysis is essential to obtaining an effective pneumoperitoneum. The patient is then shaved/prepped in the standard fashion and the bladder is drained with a Foley catheter. The patient is then repositioned in the modified semi-lateral decubitus position with gel-roll lumbar and sufficient axillary support. The table is then gently flexed. All bony prominences and pressure points are carefully padded (Fig. 6.3).

6.4.2 Robot-assisted Transperitoneal Partial Nephrectomy: Port Placement

We prefer to obtain transperitoneal access via a Hasson-technique. The initial 12-mm Hasson trocar is placed in the midline, superior to the umbilicus under direct vision. This is also the port we use to retrieve the specimen. The abdomen is insufflated with CO_2 until 15 mmHg of pneumoperitoneum is achieved. We then proceed to place the remainder of the trocars. For transperitoneal RLPN, there are two main port placement strategies: medial and lateral. We prefer to use the medial approach, as it more closely resembles our previous traditional laparoscopic experience and allow a more global view of the operating field. With the medial approach, we place two–three 8 mm robotic working ports under direct vision. An additional 12-mm assistant port is placed inferior to the umbilicus (Fig. 6.4). The Hasson port is used to introduce the robotic camera with a 30° "down" lens. Three additional, 10-mm robotic working ports are placed under direct vision and an additional 8-mm assistant port is placed inferior to the umbilicus. The robot is then docked posterior to the patient.

6.4.3 Patient Positioning and Port Placement Retroperitoneal LPN

For patients undergoing a retroperitoneal LPN, a standard modified flank position with pathologic side up is used (Fig. 6.5). Full flexion and a slight anterior rotation of the operative table optimize the retroperitoneal working space. Access to the retroperitoneum is obtained using an open technique. A 1.2-cm skin incision is made just below the tip of the 12th rib. The flank muscle fibers are bluntly split, and the thoracolumbar fascia is then exposed and bluntly entered

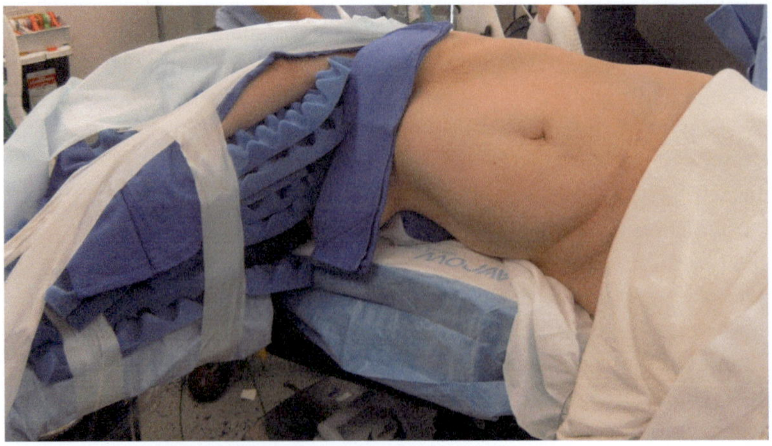

Fig. 6.3 Example of modified semi-lateral decubitus position for left-sided renal tumor

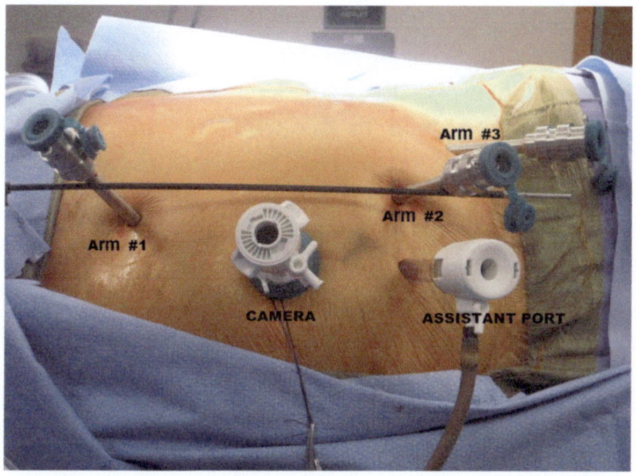

Fig. 6.4 Transperitoneal robotic port placement for left RLPN. Patient is in 45° modified flank position

with a fingertip. The surgeon's finger is then used to bluntly develop the potential space anterior to the psoas muscle and posterior to Gerota's fascia. A balloon dilator is utilized to create a retroperitoneal working-space as previously described by Gill et al.[25] The balloon dilator is used to inflate the retroperitoneal space with approximately 800 mL of air to displace the kidney anteromedially, provide adequate working space, and to expose the psoas muscle. This maneuver also provides direct access to the renal hilum.

The primary camera port is then placed at the site of the balloon dilator, just below the tip of the 12th rib. Two robotic trocars are utilized and placed 4 cm lateral and medial to the balloon trocar and one assistant post is placed in the lower quadrant. Typically only two additional working ports are required which are placed in such a way that the angle between them and camera port is obtuse, thus preventing clashing of instruments. Proposed port placement for laparoscopic retroperitoneal access is demonstrated in Fig. 6.6.

6.4.4 Robot-assisted Transperitoneal Partial Nephrectomy: Initial Dissection

The peritoneum is inspected for any significant adhesions. If required, they are taken down using the 30° up lens ensuring against injury to the bowel. We then switch to a 30° down approach.

With PK bipolar forceps in the left hand and hot scissors in the right hand (Table 6.1), the dissection begins by incising the peritoneum sharply along the Line of Toldt and the bowel is mobilized medially, thus developing the plane between Gerota's fascia and the posterior mesocolon. Please note, for right-sided

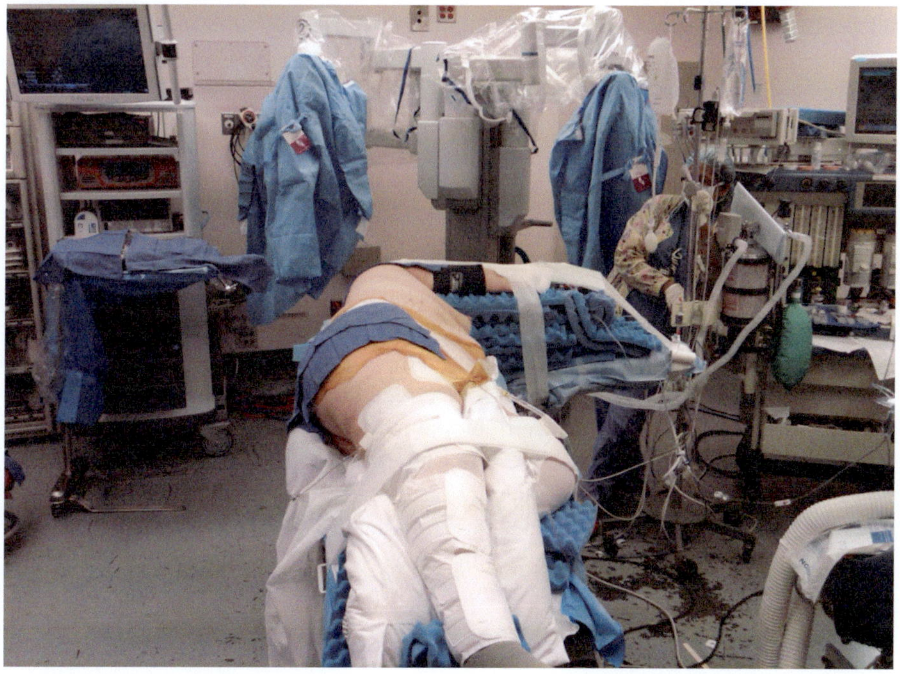

Fig. 6.5 Example of patient positioning for right retroperitoneal LPN. Of note, the camera port is typically placed below the tip of the 12th rib

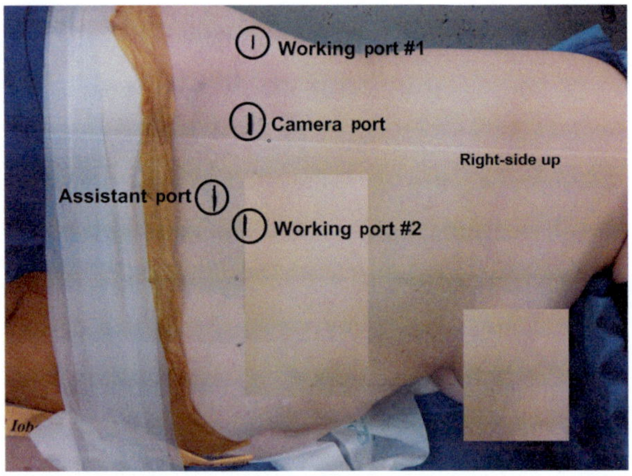

Fig. 6.6 Example of right retroperitoneal robotic PN port placement

Table 6.1 Key instruments used in robotic partial nephrectomy

Instrument	Use
PK Maryland forceps	Left hand
Monopolar "Hot" cautery scissors	Right hand
Prograsp forceps	Left hand (3rd arm)
2, large needle drivers	Renorrhaphy/suturing
Tissuelink®	Renorrhaphy/coagulation (assistant)
Laparoscopic ultrasound	Tumor identification
Laparoscopic Doppler probe	Confirm ischemia after renal artery clamping (assistant)

tumors, gentle mobilization of the duodenum may be required. Attachments between the upper pole of the kidney and the liver/spleen are taken down with cautery. The liver is then retracted superiorly using a self-retaining triangular retractor placed percutaneously.

We continue medial reflection of the colon inferiorly to the bifurcation of the iliac vessels and cephalad to the liver/spleen. The goal is to expose the vena cava on the right and medialize intra-abdominal organs to the aorta. Following this, the gonadal vessel is identified and traced back to the vena cava on the right and the renal vein on the left. An incision is made just lateral to the gonadal vein. The gonadal vein is then retracted medially to allow exposure and access to the ureter. The ureter is identified and retracted with the lower-pole attachments anteriorly off the psoas muscle. The posterior attachments of the kidney are dissected off the psoas muscle, while the gonadal vein is retracted medially and ureter and lower-pole attachments are gently retracted anteriorly. The gonadal vein can be used as a "highway" to the hilum, especially on the left.

Attention is paid to dissecting out all posterior attachment of the kidney from the lower to upper pole. Whenever possible, we utilize the fourth arm to retract the kidney anteriorly by placing it in the space between the psoas and posterior aspect of the kidney. With the hilum on stretch, we utilize the laparoscopic Doppler probe to identify the renal artery and any accessory branches. The renal arteries are dissected free enough to allow placement of a bulldog clamp on each vessel individually. We do not use a Satinsky clamp for fear of inadvertent collisions inside and outside the body. Attention is then turned toward identifying the tumor seen on preoperative imaging. Intraoperative, real-time laparoscopic ultrasound is used to facilitate identification of tumor borders/depth in order to ensure negative margins. When possible, we like to leave the fat overlying the tumor, and clear off the normal renal capsule of fat circumferentially around the tumor. It is crucial to ensure normal capsule is exposed around the tumor for at least 2–3 cm from the tumor edge as this facilitates reconstruction later. The ultrasound is brought back into the patient and the lateral margins of the tumor are scored with the electrocautery device on the capsule. (Note, if fat overlying the tumor is removed, it is sent separately for pathologic analysis to evaluate for potential pT3a disease). Twenty minutes prior to clamping, we administer 12.5 g of Mannitol intravenously and the entire surgical team confirms that hemostatic agents are available, reviews the back table, ensures all equipment/sutures are available for renorrhaphy, and makes certain the CO_2 tank does not need to be changed prior to the tumor resection. For exophytic renal lesions, we place a bulldog clamp only on the renal artery; however, for largely endophytic tumors and hilar lesions, we will often also clamp the renal vein separately to prevent excessive back bleeding. Notably, we utilize a laparoscopic Doppler probe on the kidney prior to and after clamping to confirm adequate ischemia.

6.4.5 Tumor Excision

Sharp tumor excision then begins under warm ischemia. Keys to success include: incising the capsule widely prior to excision, utilizing the fourth arm to elevate the tumor, and utilizing the bed-side surgeon to assist with suction and to place countertraction on the renal bed to keep the field clear. If bleeding obscures vision, choices include: re-clamping, increasing pneumoperitoneum, or performing pin-point suturing to control bleeding. Excision should never be performed in a field obscured by blood. The tumor resection plane is constantly inspected and adjusted to ensure negative surgical margins. The bed-side surgeon is especially important during this part of the operation, to provide optimal exposure, visualization, suction and retraction for the console surgeon during tumor resection and renal parenchymal reconstruction. We do not routinely send frozen sections; however, if violation is of concern, deep margins from the tumor base are sent for pathologic analysis to ensure negative deep tumor margins. Once the tumor is free, it is placed in an endoscopic specimen retrieval bag.

6.4.6 Renorrhaphy Technique

The robotic instruments are exchanged for robotic needle drivers, and the defect of the resection bed is inspected carefully and repaired. If entry is made in the collecting system, we will close this with a 3–0 Vicryl suture on an RB1 needle. This is followed by 1–3 running sutures in the base, depending upon the size and depth of the defect. We use 2–0 Vicryl suture on an SH needle for the deep renal reconstruction. The renal cortex is then cauterized with the TissueLink® device being careful to avoid the deep sutures. Interrupted bolster sutures with Hem-o-Lock® clips (Teleflex, Research Triangle Park, NC) are placed along the capsular defect in a running fashion 1 cm apart. FloSeal™ and a Surgicel® bolster are placed under these sutures. The sutures are then individually tightened using a "sliding-clip" renorrhaphy technique described by Benway et al.[26] Of note, all sutures are pre-prepared on the back tables. First, a knot is tied at the end of a 15 cm 2–0 Vicryl at one end on the suture. Above the knot, a LapraTy® (Ethicon, Cincinnati, OH, USA) clip is placed, and then a 10-mm Hem-o-Lock® clip is placed. The suture is then placed through the renal capsule, over the bolster, and through the other side of the renal defect. The suture is then cinched-down until slight dimpling is noted within the renal capsule. The contralateral side of the suture is then secured with another Hem-o-Lok® clip and LapraTy®. Once adequate compression is visualized, the venous clamp is removed. Another 12.5 g of intravenous Mannitol is administered and the arterial bulldog clamps are removed. Close inspection of the tumor base is done for bleeding. If necessary, the Hem-o-Lok® clip sutures are tightened and/or additional parenchymal compression sutures are placed. Further hemostatic agents, such as FloSeal™ may also be applied to the defect. As the surgical site is inspected again for hemostasis, the pneumoperitoneum is reduced and the mean-arterial pressure increased to at least 90 mmHg.

Following this, the renal hilum is also inspected for hemostasis. A Jackson-Pratt® (JP) drain is then placed posterior to the kidney, and the kidney is re-attached to the lateral abdominal wall using a running 2–0 Vicryl suture or Hem-o-Lok® clips on Gerota's fascia. The robot is then un-docked and all ports are removed under direct vision. The specimen is removed through the camera port. All significant fascial openings are closed with interrupted 0 Vicryl and the skin is approximately with 4–0 Monocryl and steri-strips.

6.4.7 Retroperitoneal LPN: Initial Dissection

The only difference between the retroperitoneal and transperitoneal technique is initial access and dissection. Access is as described above. Once all ports are placed, the psoas muscle is identified and an incision is created 2 cm anterior to the psoas muscle in Gerota's fascia. This incision is carried along the length of the kidney. The latter is placed on stretch, and using either visual cues or the Doppler probe, the renal artery is identified. At this point the same hilar dissection techniques, tumor preparation, tumor excision, and reconstructive techniques are utilized as described above. We utilize this technique very selectively because of the limited working space and fewer anatomic landmarks this approach affords. We find this approach most appropriate for posterior/medial tumors. We have not experienced any difficulty using the transperitoneal approach for all other tumor excisions, even in the setting of previous abdominal surgery. In contrast to the transperitoneal approach, the retroperitoneal approach allows rapid access to the renal hilum.

6.5 Postoperative Management

Mean hospital length of stay after RLPN is 2 days at our institution. Patients are given a PCA pump for analgesia immediately postoperatively, but this is converted to oral narcotic pills the morning of postoperative day (POD) one with advancement of diet to full clear liquids. Serial hematocrits are drawn every 4 h after surgery × 3 to assess for postoperative bleeding. The patient also remains on bed-rest for the first 12 h post-op. Intravenous prophylactic antibiotics are administered for 24 h only.

The patient continues on clear liquids until flatus is passed. If the patient has not passed flatus by POD two a Dulcolax® suppository is administered. The patient is also encouraged to ambulate as much as possible 12 h after surgery. The patient's Foley catheter is removed on POD two. After the patient voids, the JP fluid is sent for creatinine level. If equal to serum, the JP drain is removed prior to discharge home.

6.6 Complications/Pitfalls

Numerous studies have presented the complications LPN and RLPN. Urine leak/fistula is the most frequent complication suffered by PN. This is more common in patients undergoing resection of large, endophytic tumors which are abutting the collecting system. We do not preoperatively place an open-ended 5-French ipsilateral ureteral catheter for methylene blue injection nor do we inject intravenous indigo carmine intraoperatively to evaluate the integrity of the collecting system. Although these may be useful tools, we do not routinely employ them at our institution as entry into the collecting system is usually readily apparent on gross inspection. Any obvious entry sites are then closed with 3–0 vicryl suture. In order to maximize healing of any collecting system entry, the Foley catheter remains in place for 48 h postoperatively. Additionally, the JP drain fluid is analyzed for creatinine level after the Foley catheter is removed. If there is evidence of urine leak on POD two (i.e., elevated drain outputs, JP creatinine higher than serum) the drain is not removed and the treatment algorithm for urine leak is initiated. Usually, a urine leak self-resolves within 1 week of prolonged JP drainage. If persistent drainage continues, a CT urogram may be obtained to assess for proper drain position, possible urinoma collection, or any evidence of distal obstruction. It can then be evaluated if the patient requires additional percutaneous drainage of a urinoma collection, if the JP drain is not positioned properly. If the leak persists beyond 1 week, the drain is usually placed on gravity drainage (versus self-suction) and withdrawn in small increments on a bi-weekly basis to ensure the fistulous tract collapses slowly upon itself. Prior to complete drain removal, the fluid is sent for culture and the patient is placed on culture-specific antibiotics. We find that all prolonged urine leaks resolved without the placement of a ureteral stent. If stenting is required; however, a Foley catheter should also be placed in the bladder to prevent retrograde reflux.

Postoperative hemorrhage or delayed bleeding secondary to pseudoaneurysm formation are known complications of LPN and RLPN. In a recent review of 259 consecutive patients who underwent LPN, six (2.3%) patients were found to develop an intrarenal artery pseudoaneurysm. Patients in this cohort presented at a mean of 12.6 days post-op (range 5–23 days) and all were successfully managed with selective angioembolization.[27] Immediate postoperative bleeding is usually secondary to inadequate closure of the renal defect or unrecognized vessel injury. Diminishing the pneumoperitoneum and increasing the mean-arterial pressure to 90 mmHg prior to undocking the robot is a good way to reveal subtle, yet potentially clinically significant bleeding. This may then be managed with intra-corporal sutures or application of commercial hemostatic agent, like Floseal®. Immediately post-op the patient's hematocrit is obtained and compared to the pre-op value. We keep our patients on strict bed-rest for the first 12 h post-op, closely monitor their hemodynamics, and obtain serial hematocrits every 4 h × 3 to further assess for post-op hemorrhage. Hematuria is the most common presentation of delayed hemorrhage due to pseudoaneurysm/arterio-venous malformation. Postoperative bleeding may require supportive therapies, such as blood transfusion, or may require more invasive means like arterial embolization for resolution. Potential injury to surrounding structures is avoided by constant recognition of surgical landmarks and meticulous dissection techniques. However, specific vascular complications associated with dissection of the renal hilum have been known to occur, requiring conversion to open. In one large multi-institutional series of 771 LPNs is performed, 16 (2.1%) patients underwent open conversion mostly due to bleeding and an additional seven (0.9%) underwent RN due to positive margin, vascular or bowel injury, or tumor fracture.[13]

Acute renal failure, urinary tract infection, ileus, and deep venous thrombosis/pulmonary embolism are also known to potentially occur after PN. In attempts to prevent these complications, we administer periclamping Mannitol, keep our warm-ischemia times <20 min whenever possible, administer peri-operative antibiotics for 24 h, encourage early ambulation, and preoperatively place pneumatic compression stockings. Additionally, bowel injury is a potential complication of LPN/RLPN, especially in patients with significant intra-abdominal adhesions. A high index of suspicion is needed for intra-operative recognition of bowel injury in order to prevent future morbidity. In fact, one large series reported that 69% of bowel injuries incurred during laparoscopic urologic procedures went unrecognized at the time of initial surgery.[28]

Due to its technical complexity, mechanical failures of the da Vinci® robotic-system or instruments may be encountered. Although the reported rate is low (2.6%), it is imperative that surgeons fully counsel their patients regarding the possibility of robotic mechanic failures and potential conversion to a pure laparoscopic or open procedure.[29] In a series of nearly 100 consecutive RLPN at our institution, we experienced only one unrecoverable fault requiring us to undock the robot and complete the operation using a traditional laparoscopic approach (unpublished data).

6.7 Summary

Laparoscopic and robot-assisted PN has been demonstrated to be a safe and feasible option for nephron-sparing renal surgery. Studies have reported comparable oncologic results to the traditional open approach, with less blood loss, pain, and decreased hospital stays. Advocates of the robotic approach to PN may argue that its use further facilitates the extirpation of complex renal tumors.

References

1. Lane BR, Gill IS. 5-Year outcomes of laparoscopic partial nephrectomy. *J Urol*. 2007;177(1):70-74; discussion 74.
2. Jemal A, Siegel R, Ward E, Hao Y, Xu J, Thun MJ. Cancer statistics, 2009. *CA Cancer J Clin*. 2009;59(4):225-249.
3. Clayman RV, Kavoussi LR, Soper NJ, et al. Laparoscopic nephrectomy: initial case report. *J Urol*. 1991;146(2):278-282.
4. Hollingsworth JM, Miller DC, Daignault S, Hollenbeck BK. Rising incidence of small renal masses: a need to reassess treatment effect. *J Natl Cancer Inst*. 2006;98(18):1331-1334.
5. Kane CJ, Mallin K, Ritchey J, Cooperberg MR, Carroll PR. Renal cell cancer stage migration: analysis of the National Cancer Data Base. *Cancer*. 2008;113(1):78-83.
6. Huang WC, Elkin EB, Levey AS, Jang TL, Russo P. Partial nephrectomy versus radical nephrectomy in patients with small renal tumors – is there a difference in mortality and cardiovascular outcomes? *J Urol*. 2009;181(1):55-61; discussion 61–52.
7. Fergany AF, Hafez KS, Novick AC. Long-term results of nephron sparing surgery for localized renal cell carcinoma: 10-year followup. *J Urol*. 2000;163(2):442-445.
8. Lee CT, Katz J, Shi W, Thaler HT, Reuter VE, Russo P. Surgical management of renal tumors 4 cm. or less in a contemporary cohort. *J Urol*. 2000;163(3):730-736.
9. Dash A, Vickers AJ, Schachter LR, Bach AM, Snyder ME, Russo P. Comparison of outcomes in elective partial vs radical nephrectomy for clear cell renal cell carcinoma of 4–7 cm. *BJU Int*. 2006;97(5):939-945.
10. Miller DC, Hollingsworth JM, Hafez KS, Daignault S, Hollenbeck BK. Partial nephrectomy for small renal masses: an emerging quality of care concern? *J Urol*. 2006;175(3): 853-857.
11. Winfield HN, Donovan JF, Godet AS, Clayman RV. Laparoscopic partial nephrectomy: initial case report for benign disease. *J Endourol*. 1993;7(6):521-526.
12. Gill IS, Matin SF, Desai MM, et al. Comparative analysis of laparoscopic versus open partial nephrectomy for renal tumors in 200 patients. *J Urol*. 2003;170(1):64-68.
13. Gill IS, Kavoussi LR, Lane BR, et al. Comparison of 1,800 laparoscopic and open partial nephrectomies for single renal tumors. *J Urol*. 2007;178(1):41-46.
14. Berryhill R Jr, Jhaveri J, Yadav R, et al. Robotic prostatectomy: a review of outcomes compared with laparoscopic and open approaches. *Urology*. 2008;72(1):15-23.
15. Bhayani SB, Das N. Robotic assisted laparoscopic partial nephrectomy for suspected renal cell carcinoma: retrospective review of surgical outcomes of 35 cases. *BMC Surg*. 2008;8:16.
16. Benway BM, Bhayani SB, Rogers CG, et al. Robot assisted partial nephrectomy versus laparoscopic partial nephrectomy for renal tumors: a multi-institutional analysis of perioperative outcomes. *J Urol*. 2009;182(3):866-872.
17. Rogers CG, Singh A, Blatt AM, Linehan WM, Pinto PA. Robotic partial nephrectomy for complex renal tumors: surgical technique. *Eur Urol*. 2008;53(3):514-521.
18. Desai MM, Strzempkowski B, Matin SF, et al. Prospective randomized comparison of transperitoneal versus retroperitoneal laparoscopic radical nephrectomy. *J Urol*. 2005;173(1):38-41.

19. Berglund RK, Gill IS, Babineau D, Desai M, Kaouk JH. A prospective comparison of transperitoneal and retroperitoneal laparoscopic nephrectomy in the extremely obese patient. *BJU Int*. 2007;99(4):871-874.
20. Gill IS, Delworth MG, Munch LC. Laparoscopic retroperitoneal partial nephrectomy. *J Urol*. 1994;152(5 Pt 1):1539-1542.
21. Wright JL, Porter JR. Laparoscopic partial nephrectomy: comparison of transperitoneal and retroperitoneal approaches. *J Urol*. 2005;174(3):841-845.
22. Richstone L, Montag S, Ost M, Reggio E, Permpongkosol S, Kavoussi LR. Laparoscopic partial nephrectomy for hilar tumors: evaluation of short-term oncologic outcome. *Urology*. 2008;71(1):36-40.
23. Rogers CG, Metwalli A, Blatt AM, et al. Robotic partial nephrectomy for renal hilar tumors: a multi-institutional analysis. *J Urol*. 2008;180(6):2353-2356; discussion 2356.
24. Gill IS, Colombo JR Jr, Frank I, Moinzadeh A, Kaouk J, Desai M. Laparoscopic partial nephrectomy for hilar tumors. *J Urol*. 2005;174(3):850-853; discussion 853–854.
25. Gill IS, Rassweiler JJ. Retroperitoneoscopic renal surgery: our approach. *Urology*. 1999;54(4):734-738.
26. Benway BM, Wang AJ, Cabello JM, Bhayani SB. Robotic partial nephrectomy with sliding-clip renorrhaphy: technique and outcomes. *Eur Urol*. 2009;55(3):592-599.
27. Shapiro EY, Hakimi AA, Hyams ES, Cynamon J, Stifelman M, Ghavamian R. Renal artery pseudoaneurysm following laparoscopic partial nephrectomy. *Urology*. 2009;74(4):819-823.
28. Bishoff JT, Allaf ME, Kirkels W, Moore RG, Kavoussi LR, Schroder F. Laparoscopic bowel injury: incidence and clinical presentation. *J Urol*. 1999;161(3):887-890.
29. Borden LS Jr, Kozlowski PM, Porter CR, Corman JM. Mechanical failure rate of da Vinci robotic system. *Can J Urol*. 2007;14(2):3499-3501.

Retroperitoneal Robotic Partial Nephrectomy

7

James R. Porter

Abstract The ability to perform reconstructive surgery with the robotic surgical platform has recently led to the application of robotics to nephron sparing surgery. Because of space limitations and the size of the robot at the patient side, the standard approach to robotic partial nephrectomy (RPN) has been transperitoneal. However, posterior located tumors are difficult to approach transperitoneally, and require the kidney to be completely mobilized and flipped medially. Laparoscopic partial nephrectomy (LPN) has been performed using a retroperitoneal approach and affords the advantages of direct access to the renal hilum, no need for bowel mobilization, and excellent visualization of posteriorly located tumors.

Retroperitoneal robotic partial nephrectomy is performed with the patient in the full flank position with the table flexed to increase the space between the 12th rib and iliac crest. Access to the retroperitoneal space is performed using a balloon dilating device and pneumoretroperitoneum is maintained using a 12-mm Hasson balloon trocar. Three robotic trocars are used with one 12-mm assistant trocar placed in the anterior axillary line. A 0° robotic laparoscopic is routinely used but on occasion the 30° up lens is necessary due to conflict with the iliac crest. The robot is brought in over the patient's head parallel to the spine. The renal artery is exposed to allow a bulldog clamp on the artery. The renal vein is rarely clamped. The renal mass is exposed with the assistance of laparoscopic ultrasound and a 5 mm margin is scored circumferentially around the tumor. The tumor is excised under warm ischemic conditions and care was taken to maintain a clear operative field to allow identification of tumor if encountered. Entrance into the collecting system is easily identified with the 3-D robotic visualization and closed with suture. The renal defect is reconstructed in two layers using the sliding locking clip technique on both the deep layer and the cortical layer.

Retroperitoneal robotic partial nephrectomy was performed successfully in the vast majority of patients. One procedure was converted to LPN due to conflict between the robotic arm and the psoas muscle. Posterior and lateral tumors are ideally suited for the retroperitoneal approach, while anterior and medial tumors are better excised using the transperitoneal technique. The psoas muscle and Gerota's fascia are the major landmarks used to maintain orientation during dissection. Inadvertent entrance into the peritoneal cavity was seen in two cases, but this did not prevent the completion of the procedure by the retroperitoneal approach.

Retroperitoneal robotic partial nephrectomy is a safe and reproducible approach to minimally invasive partial nephrectomy. The retroperitoneal approach is ideally suited to posterior and lateral tumors, eliminating the need to rotate the kidney. The limitations of the retroperitoneal space do not prohibit the use of the robot.

Keywords Kidney cancer • Nephron sparing surgery • Reconstruction • Retroperitoneoscopy • Robotic surgery

J.R. Porter
Surgical Robotics, Department of Urology, Swedish Medical Center, 1101 Madison, Suite 1400, 98104 Seattle, WA, USA
e-mail: porter@swedishurology.com

J.V. Joseph and H.R.H. Patel (eds.), *Retroperitoneal Robotic and Laparoscopic Surgery*,
DOI: 10.1007/978-0-85729-485-2_7, © Springer-Verlag London Limited 2011

Key Points

- The retroperitoneal approach for partial nephrectomy is indicated for posterior or lateral renal masses and in patients who have had previous abdominal surgery.
- The trocar placement for robotic retroperitoneal partial nephrectomy is closer to the iliac crest and more anterior than traditionally described with laparoscopic retroperitoneal surgery.
- The robot is docked over the patient's head, parallel to the spine which is distinction from the transperitoneal approach to robotic renal surgery where the robot is docked perpendicular to the patient's spine.
- The key landmarks for retroperitoneal robotic renal surgery are the psoas muscle posteriorly, the peritoneal reflection anteriorly and Gerota's fascia just above the psoas muscle. It is essential to maintain proper orientation during retroperitoneal robotic surgery to avoid misidentification of vascular structure which could lead to vascular injury.
- It is important to dissect within Gerota's fascia to avoid inadvertent entry into the peritoneal cavity, thereby decreasing the retroperitoneal space.

7.1 Introduction

Nephron sparing surgery is the accepted standard for removal of small renal masses. Originally described using open surgery, partial nephrectomy utilizes temporary vascular occlusion to allow precise removal of the renal mass in a bloodless field and permit accurate reconstruction of the renal defect.[1] Laparoscopic partial nephrectomy (LPN) has gained acceptance as an alternative to open partial nephrectomy with equivalent oncologic outcome and reduced patient morbidity.[2] However, the technical challenge of renal reconstruction under time constraints to minimize warm ischemic injury has made this procedure reproducible only in high volume laparoscopic centers.[3]

With the introduction of robotic technology to surgical procedures, several advantages have been recognized over conventional laparoscopic surgery. These include a magnified 3-D view of the operative field, improved surgeon ergonomics, and enhanced reconstructive capabilities. The wristed technology afforded by robotic instruments allows suturing with more degrees of freedom than laparoscopic instruments, which are limited by the fixed position of laparoscopic trocars. Given the need for accurate and efficient suturing during partial nephrectomy, robotic assisted laparoscopic partial nephrectomy (RALPN) has been performed increasingly with excellent short-term oncologic outcomes and improved warm ischemia times as compared to LPN.[4,5] To date, the majority of RALPN have been performed via a transperitoneal (TP) approach given the spatial requirements of the robotic platform.[6]

The retroperitoneal (RP) approach for minimally invasive surgery has been applied to LPN. We previously identified several advantages of the RP approach over the TP technique for LPN, which include faster operative time, earlier return of oral intake, and shorter length of hospital stay.[7] By accessing the kidney behind the peritoneal cavity, the RP approach avoids bowel manipulation and allows direct exposure to the renal hilum. The RP approach is ideal for posteriorly located tumors, and avoids the need for complete mobilization and rotation of the kidney, which is required when the TP technique is used for posterior tumors. The RP approach is also preferred for patients who have had previous abdominal surgery and avoids the scarring and adhesions that may prohibit access to the kidney transperitoneally. Finally, if bleeding or urine leakage occurs after partial nephrectomy, blood and urine are sequestered within the retroperitoneal cavity decreasing bowel irritation and peritonitis.

Given the reconstructive advantages of robotic surgery over conventional laparoscopy and our experience with RP minimally invasive surgery, we pursued RP-RALPN in an effort to determine the feasibility of this approach and identify any potential advantages.

7.2 Indications and Patient Selection

The usual indications for RALPN are renal masses 4 cm or less in patients with a normally functioning contralateral kidney. Patients with exophytic or polar tumors should be selected early in the experience of the surgeon. With increasing experience tumors greater than 4 cm, central tumors, endophytic tumors, and tumors in solitary kidneys have been treated.[8,9]

The RP approach is ideally suited for posterior or lateral renal masses, but can be applied to anterior masses in patients who have had previous abdominal surgery and pose a risk for intraabdominal scarring and adhesions. Medial masses are best approached by the TP method. Obese patients are more difficult to treat RP due to excessive retroperitoneal fat. However, with experience these patients can be treated with the RP approach. Patients with a BMI over 35 should undergo RALPN by the TP approach.

Contraindications to RALPN include patient with bleeding disorders and anticoagulated patients. Patients who have had previous RP surgery around the kidney represent a relative contraindication to RALPN.

Preparation for RP-RALPN includes evaluation for evidence of possible metastatic renal cell carcinoma with chest imaging and liver function studies. Laboratory studies including coagulation parameters are checked prior to surgery. Blood is typed and crossed for patients despite a low risk of transfusion. Patients routinely do not undergo bowel preparation, and are counseled that they may require conversion to TP-RALPN, conventional LPN or open surgery. They are also informed of the possibility of radical nephrectomy if nephron sparing surgery cannot be performed safely or if an adequate margin of resection cannot be obtained.

7.3 Technique

General anesthesia is required for RP-RALPN and in our experience some patients may experience higher end tidal CO_2 levels with the RP approach due to tracking of insufflated gas within the subcutaneous tissues and greater absorption of CO_2.

Patients are placed in the full flank position for RP-RALPN (Fig. 7.1). The patient is well padded and an axillary roll is placed on the chest wall below the axilla on the contralateral side. The ipsilateral arm is secured on pillows placed on an arm board and the patient is carefully taped to the table. Every effort is made to fully flex the patient to increase the space between the 12th rib and iliac crest. This allows sufficient space between trocars to prevent robotic arm collisions. Early in our experience, ureteral catheters were placed cystoscopically to allow identification of the open collecting system by injecting blue dyed saline. However, with increasing experience and the improved visualization of the robotic view, ureteral catheter placement is no longer necessary.

The retroperitoneal space is created by first making a 12–15 cm incision in the mid-axillary line, 2 cm above the iliac crest. This initial incision is more caudal than other descriptions of retroperitoneal access, which use

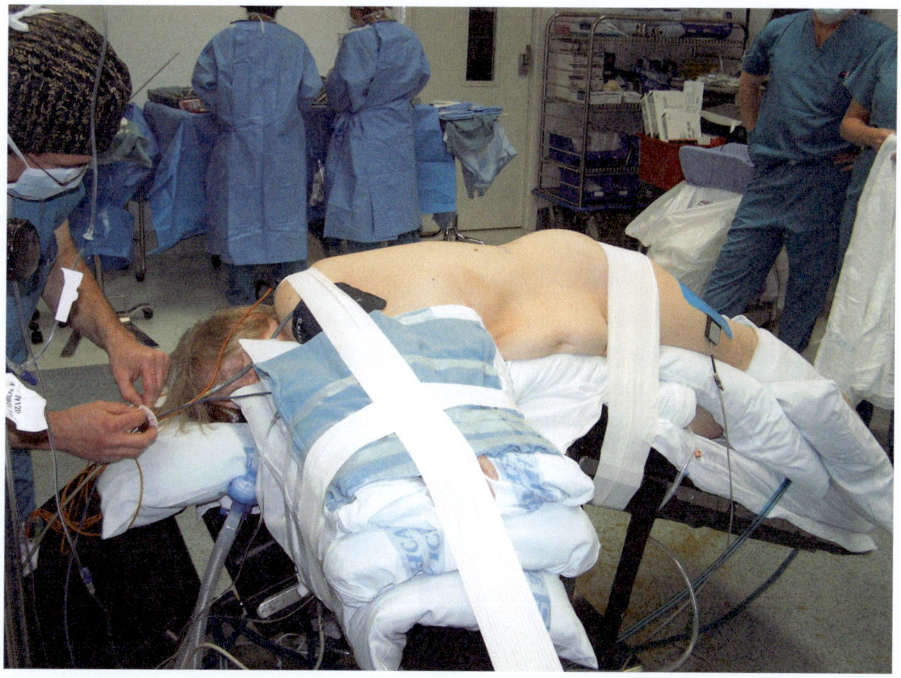

Fig. 7.1 Flank position for retroperitoneal robotic partial nephrectomy

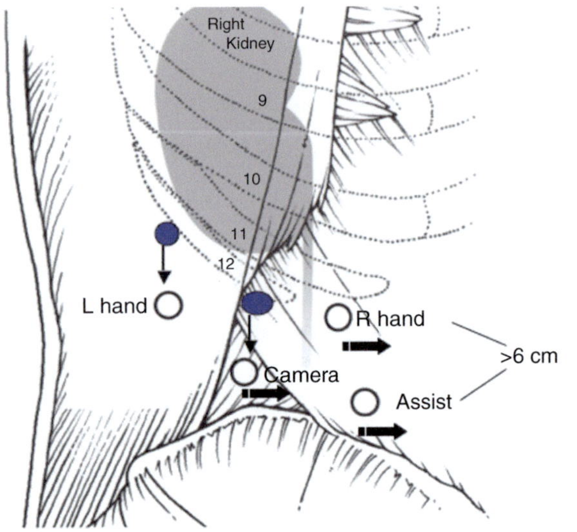

Fig. 7.2 Retroperitoneal robotic port placement on right flank. Note the camera and posterior trocar sites have been placed closer to the iliac crest to allow access to the kidney. The assistant and right hand trocar are placed more anteriorly to gain more space between the robotic arms

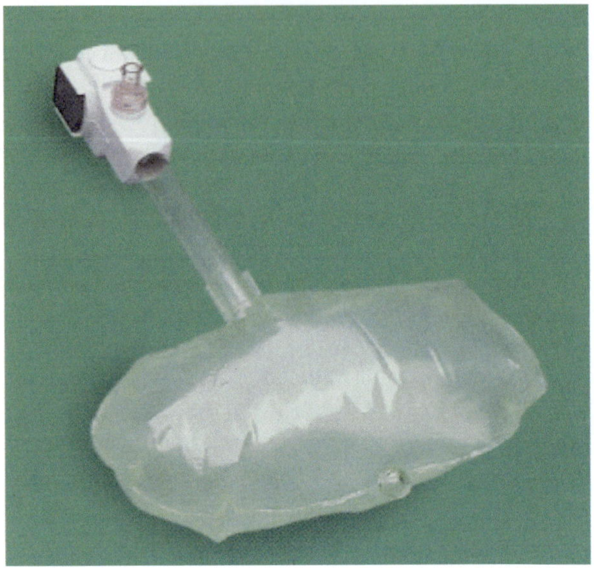

Fig. 7.3 Retroperitoneal balloon dilator (Courtesy Covidien; used with permission)

the tip of the 12th rib as a landmark.[10] We have found the 12th rib incision to be too far cephalad to allow access to the lower pole of the kidney (Fig. 7.2). Once the incision has been created dissection is carried to the external oblique fascia, which is incised with cautery, and dissection is carried down through the oblique muscles with an index finger. The entrance to the retroperitoneal space is obtained after going through the lumbodorsal fascia, which can be entered with a finger in women or a tonsil clamp in men. Once the retroperitoneal space has been entered, it is further developed with an index finger to allow enough room to place the balloon dilator in the retroperitoneum. Landmarks such as the inside of iliac crest and tip of the 12th rib can be palpated to confirm the correct location.

The dilating balloon (Covidien, Mansfield, MA) (Fig. 7.3) is then carefully placed in the retroperitoneum with the aid of the obturator. A 30° laparoscope is placed within the balloon to allow direct visualization of the retroperitoneum during expansion of the balloon. Care should be taken to expand the balloon slowly and to watch for potential thin areas in the peritoneum. Patients who have had previous abdominal surgeries are particularly at risk for developing holes in the peritoneum, which could result in deflation of the retroperitoneal space. Landmarks that are commonly visible during expansion of the balloon include the psoas muscle, the gonadal vessels, the ureter, the vena cava on the right side, and the aortic pulsation on the left. The most important landmark during balloon dilation is the peritoneal reflection anteriorly, which will act as a guide for the placement of the anterior robotic trocar. The balloon is expanded until enough working space is created and to allow the trocars to be placed. As mentioned earlier, care must be taken to not overinflate the balloon, which could result in a small hole in the peritoneum resulting in loss of CO_2 into the peritoneal cavity and compression of the retroperitoneum.

Once the dilating balloon is deflated and removed a 12-mm Hasson balloon trocar (Covidien, Mansfield, MA) (Fig. 7.4) is placed, and secured with the sponge

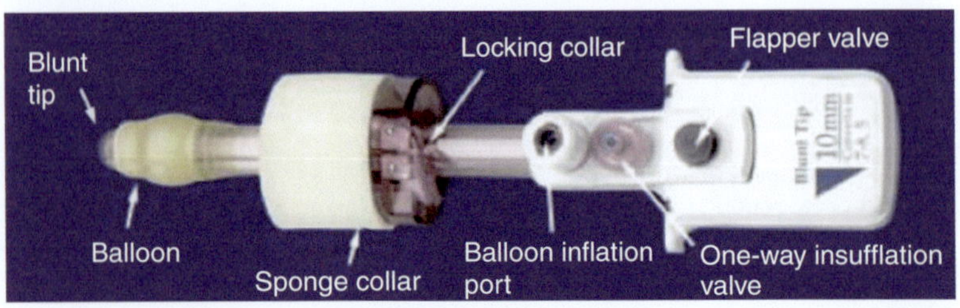

Fig. 7.4 Hasson balloon trocar with locking sponge collar (Courtesy Covidien; used with permission)

collar to prevent loss of CO_2 from the incision. The CO_2 pressure is maintained between 12 and 15 mmHg depending on the patient. We have found some patients will retain CO_2 more readily with the RP approach and may require a higher minute ventilation to maintain a normal end tidal CO_2 level. The remaining trocars are then placed under direct vision using the laparoscope to guide placement.

A four-port configuration is routinely used for RP-RALPN (Fig. 7.5). The spacing between the camera port and the left and right robotic ports is usually 7–8 cm, but can be smaller if necessary. The assistant 12 mm port is placed inferior to the anterior robotic port and should be no closer than 6 cm to avoid conflict with the anterior robotic arm. The anterior robotic port should be placed as close to the peritoneal reflection as possible without going through the peritoneum to avoid CO_2 leak into the peritoneum. The posterior robotic port should be placed far enough above the psoas muscle to avoid conflict with the muscle, which could limit access to the renal hilum. A 0° robotic laparoscope is most commonly used, but on occasion a 30° up lens is needed to avoid camera conflict with the iliac crest.

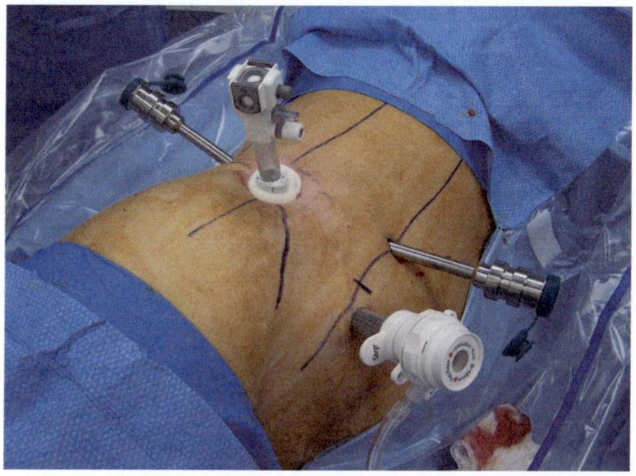

Fig. 7.5 Right sided retroperitoneal trocar configuration with Hasson balloon trocar just above iliac crest and assistant 12 mm port in anterior axillary line

Once the ports are placed the robot is docked by bringing the robot in over the patient's head, parallel to the spine (Fig. 7.6). This is in distinction to the TP approach where the robot is docked over the patient's back. The camera arm is docked to the Hasson balloon port. We routinely use monopolar scissors through the right robotic port, fenestrated bipolar through the left robotic port, and the assistant uses the suction/irrigation device. We prefer the fenestrated bipolar over the Maryland bipolar because it provides atraumatic grasping and retracting. We have found that the da Vinci standard system, the da Vinci S and the da Vinci Si can be used to perform RP-RALPN.

The first step is exposure of the renal hilum and isolation of the renal artery. Enough artery is dissected free to allow two bulldog clamps (Klein Surgical Systems, San Antonio, TX) to be placed on the artery. The vein is isolated but rarely clamped. The vein is clamped if

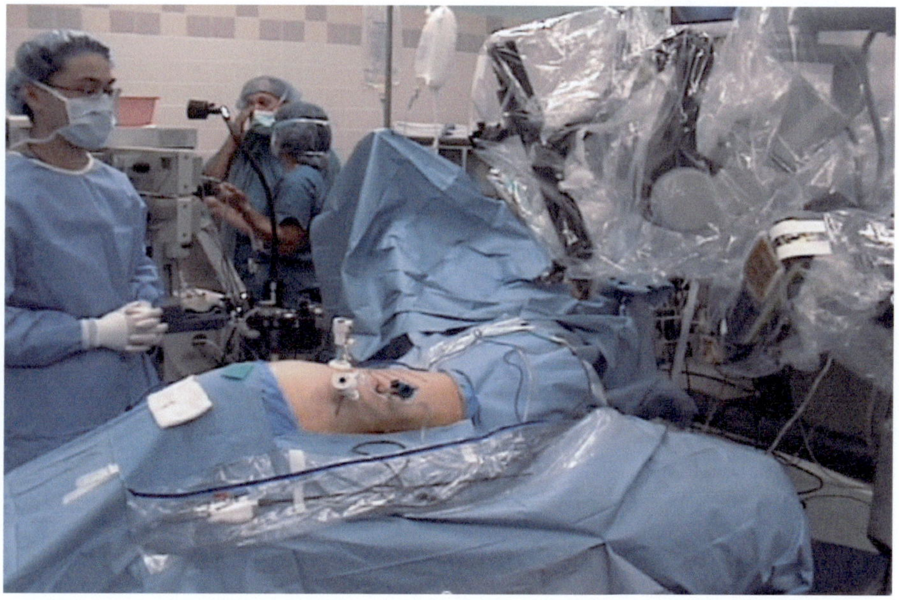

Fig. 7.6 Docking of robot over patient's head parallel to the spine for retroperitoneal robotic partial nephrectomy

the tumor is large or centrally located to avoid excessive venous back bleeding. The renal mass is then exposed by removing the perinephric fat surrounding the tumor. Enough renal parenchyma is exposed to allow a 5–10 mm margin around the tumor and closure of the defect. The perinephric fat is usually left on the surface of the mass, but it can be removed and sent as a separate specimen. Laparoscopic ultrasound is then brought in by the bedside assistant to allow visualization of the tumor and determine the depth of invasion. This will permit the depth of resection to be confirmed which is usually one level below than the depth of the tumor. The margin of resection is then scored around the mass and the tumor is checked a final time with laparoscopic ultrasound.

Prior to clamping the renal artery, 12.5 g of mannitol and 20 mg of furosemide are given intravenously to induce diuresis. Sutures are cut to appropriate length and oxidized cellulose bolsters are made. Every effort is made to limit warm ischemia time by having all necessary supplies prepared before clamps are placed on the artery. The same OR team is maintained throughout warm ischemia time.

Two bulldog clamps are routinely placed on the artery beginning warm ischemia time (Fig. 7.7). We have found one bulldog clamp inadequate for complete occlusion of the artery due to decreasing closing strength with repeated use of the bulldog clamps over time.[11] The renal vein is clamped for hilar tumors or for heminephrectomies. The tumor is excised with cold scissors and cautery is avoided to prevent charring of the normal renal parenchyma and preserve excellent visualization. During excision of the mass, careful attention is paid to distinguish between normal parenchyma and gross tumor and a margin of normal renal tissue is maintained around the tumor (Fig. 7.8). Once the tumor is freed, it is placed in an endoscopic entrapment sac for later removal.

The renal defect is reconstructed by first closing the collecting system, if it is entered, with 4–0 absorbable braided sutures (Fig. 7.9). Individual vessels are oversewn with 4–0 sutures. The base of the defect is oversewn with 3–0 monofilament absorbable suture in a running fashion and secured on the outside of the kidney with locking clips. The renal cortex is then closed using 2–0 absorbable braided suture using the sliding locking clip technique.[12] Depending on the size of the renal defect, an oxidized cellulose bolster may be

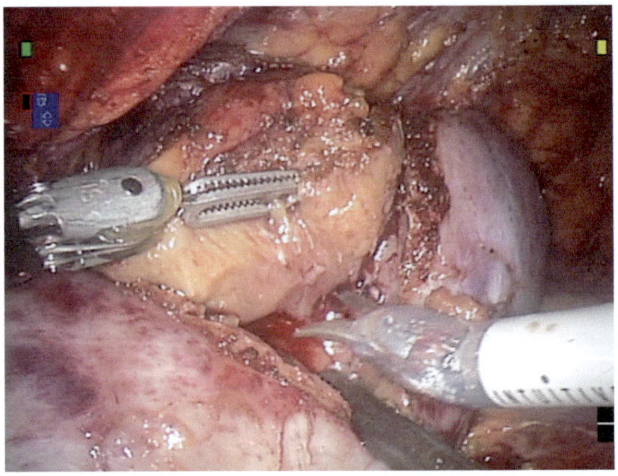

Fig. 7.8 Excision of renal mass during retroperitoneal RALPN

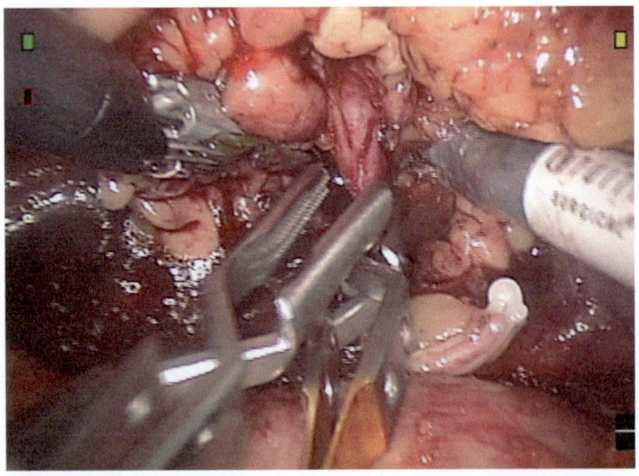

Fig. 7.7 Two bulldog clamps on renal artery

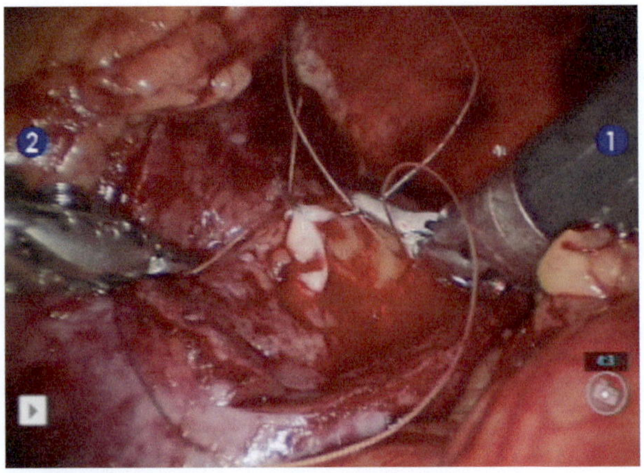

Fig. 7.9 Closure of collecting system during retroperitoneal RALPN

placed in the base of the defect prior to closing the renal cortex.

Once the defect is closed the bulldog clamps are removed ending warm ischemia time. The renal closure is observed and additional 2–0 absorbable sutures are placed and secured with sliding locking clips if needed. The patient's systolic blood pressure is increased until it reaches between 120 and 130 to look for arterial bleeding. A drain is placed and the renal mass is removed and sent to pathology for immediate analysis. The margin is assessed with the pathologist by covering the deep parenchymal margin with ink and serially sectioning the tumor to determine the thickness of the margin.

7.4 Results

Our experience with RP-RALPN began in June 2006 and 47 procedures have been performed. The mean age for the group is 59.6 years (range 36–82). There were 30 males and 17 females with renal masses in 28 right and 19 left kidneys. Mean BMI for the group was 27.5. The mean preoperative size of the renal masses was 2.60 cm, and 95% were found incidentally during radiographic evaluation for other reasons. There were 16 upper, 16 mid, and 15 lower pole masses. Twenty-three were located posteriorly, nine laterally, three medially and one anteriorly. Three masses were complex cysts, while the remainder were solid renal masses. One procedure was performed in a solitary kidney while another was performed in a polycystic kidney.

Mean operative time was 151 min and mean blood loss was 71 cm^3. Mean warm ischemia time was 22.4 min for the group and decreased to 18 min for the last 10 patients. The collecting system was entered and repaired in 17 (36%) patients. The mean hospital stay was 2.3 days.

Pathologic analysis revealed renal cell carcinoma in 35 (74%) patients with clear cell in 18, papillary in 13 and chromophobe in 4. There were 12 benign tumors with oncocytoma in six, angiomyolipoma in four and benign cysts in two patients. Mean postoperative tumor size was 2.69 cm. There were two positive margins. One patient had a 4.7 cm Type I papillary tumor and has been followed for 18 months with no evidence of recurrence. The other positive margin was in a patient with a 4.5 cm clear cell carcinoma. Laparoscopic radical nephrectomy (LRN) was performed 4 months after RP-RALPN and there was evidence of residual carcinoma in the radical nephrectomy specimen.

Complications occurred in 5 (10.6%) patients. The most common complication was delayed bleeding due to arterial pseudoaneurysm formation in the partial nephrectomy resection bed. This was identified in three patients at postoperative day number 3, 4, and 16. All three patients were successfully treated with angioembolization. One of the patients had von Willebrand's disease and required a transfusion during the episode of bleeding. This was the only transfusion in the series. One patient suffered a myocardial infarction based on cardiac enzymes and recovered without difficulty. One patient developed high CO_2 levels during the procedure and, despite increasing minute ventilation, the pneumoretroperitoneum had to be taken down temporarily to allow a normal CO_2 level to be obtained. The procedure was completed after resuming a lower CO_2 pressure. Postoperative chest x-ray revealed a small pneumothorax in the ipsilateral pleural space which resolved without tube thoracostomy. There were no episodes of urine leakage in the series.

7.5 Discussion

The RP approach for laparoscopic renal surgery has been applied to multiple procedures including laparoscopic pyeloplasty, laparoscopic radical nephrectomy (LRN), and laparoscopic partial nephrectomy (LPN).

One of the earliest evaluations of the RP approach was performed by McDougall and Clayman for laparoscopic nephrectomy (LN) for benign conditions.[13] They compared 23 TP-LN to ten patients undergoing the RP technique. The two groups were similar with regard to age, ASA score, and specimen weight. They found no significance difference between the two groups with regard to operative time, hospital stay, and analgesic requirements as measured by morphine equivalents. They did note earlier return of bowel function in the RP group and when the weight of the nephrectomy specimen was 100 cm^3 or less, the RP patients required less narcotic pain medication (11 mg morphine equivalent vs. 28 mg for TP). They concluded that the RP approach was their method of choice for removal of kidneys with benign indications.

Gill and colleagues preformed the only randomized comparison of the TP and RP approaches for patients undergoing LRN.[14] They randomized 102 patients with a renal mass to receive either TP or RP LRN with intact specimen extraction. The two groups were comparable with regard to age, BMI, ASA score, laterality of tumor, and tumor size (mean mass size 5.3 cm TP and 5.0 RP). They found a significantly shorter time to vessel exposure and shorter operative time with the RP approach as compared to the TP technique. However, there was no significant difference with regard to estimated blood loss, hospital stay, complications, or postoperative analgesic requirements. While the RP approach did not result in an anticipated faster discharge from the hospital, the authors noted several advantages of the RP technique and this was the preferred method for LRN at this institution.

The same group reported their experience with LPN via the RP approach in 63 patients and compared it to the TP technique in 100.[15] They used tumor location as the determining factor in choosing the approach with posterior tumors excised with the RP technique and anterior and lateral tumors removed with the TP technique. The two groups were very comparable except for tumor size with the TP approach associated with larger tumors (3.2 vs. 2.5 cm; $p<0.001$). When comparing the two approaches they found the RP technique to result in statistically significant shorter operative time (208 vs. 173 min; $p<0.001$), warm ischemia time (31 vs. 28 min; $p<0.04$), and hospital stay (2.9 vs. 2.2 days; $p<0.01$). Blood loss, analgesic requirements, complications and post-op renal function were without significant difference between the two techniques. Despite the advantages seen with the RP approach, the authors stated they prefer the TP approach for LPN due to the larger working area and superior suturing angles necessary for renal reconstruction.

Kieran retrospectively compared their experience with 27 RP-LPN with 45 TP-LPN.[16] The two groups were similar except that tumor size was smaller (2.1 RP vs. 2.7 cm TP; $p=0.03$) and the RP technique was used more commonly on right kidneys. They found shorter operative time (160 vs. 192 min; $p=0.008$), decreased blood loss (100 vs. 225 cm^3; $p=0.06$), and earlier hospital discharge (1.0 vs. 2.0 days; $p=0.001$) in the RP group as compared to the patients undergoing TP-LPN. They concluded that depending on the patient and anatomic considerations, the RP technique may have advantages over the TP approach and that these differences may become more apparent with surgeon experience and increasing patient number.

Similar to Kiernan's experience we found the RP approach to offer several advantages over the TP technique for LPN. Using tumor location to determine the approach, we compared 19 TP with 32 RP patients. Patients with posterior or lateral tumors underwent RP-LPN while anterior and medial tumors were treated with the TP approach. The RP approach resulted in shorter operative time (3.2 vs. 5.4 h, $p=0.0001$), less blood loss (192 vs. 403 cm^3, $p=0.002$), shorter time to regular diet (1.2 vs. 1.7 days, $p=0.02$), and shorter time to discharge from the hospital (2.3 vs. 3.6, $p=0.0008$). There was no difference in warm ischemia time for the two groups.

The largest RP experience for LPN was reported by Pyo and Grasso in 2008, who reported on 110 patients.[17] They applied the RP approach irrespective of tumor location. Mean tumor size was 2.4 cm. Mean OR time was 199 min, mean blood loss was 260 cm^3, and mean length of stay was 2.6 days. There were no positive margins in the series. With a mean follow-up of 23 months, there was one local recurrence noted 1 year after LPN in a patient with a negative margin of resection. Residual cancer was confirmed at subsequent radical nephrectomy. There were two persistent urine leaks despite placement of double-J stents in almost all patients. They concluded that RP approach offers perioperative outcomes comparable to open and TP LPN, with excellent cancer control and preserved renal function. They also point out the advantage of containing blood and urine outside the peritoneal cavity which decreases patient morbidity.

While the RP technique has been employed for LPN, this approach has not been routinely used for RALPN. Gettman et al. reported the first experience with RALPN in 13 patients and described both the TP and RP techniques in this series.[18] However, there was no indication as to how many patients underwent the RP approach and there were no results reported for the RP patients.

Our results using the RP approach for RALPN represents the largest experience to date. All published reports of RALPN describe the TP approach and these studies emphasize the advantages of robotic technology which include 3-D visualization, increased degrees of freedom of movement, and enhanced reconstructive capabilities.[19,20] However, posterior tumors treated with the TP technique require complete mobilization and medial rotation of the kidney. Based on our experience with LPN, we recognized that the RP approach provided direct access to the renal hilum and posterior tumors. This led to the combination of the robotic surgical platform and the RP approach for posterior and lateral tumors. Of note, we still use the TP approach during RALPN for anterior and medial tumors and feel that the approach for RALPN should be tailored to tumor location.

Our results comparing RP-LPN to RALPN are presented in Table 7.1. The tumor size was slightly smaller in the LPN group reflecting the larger tumor size and more complex tumors that we are now removing with RALPN. This difference was not statistically significant. Despite increasing tumor size and more complex tumors, the operative time, estimated blood loss and warm ischemia time were shorter in the RALPN group. The most noteworthy improvement was the reduction in warm ischemia time which decreased by approximately 10 min. This difference was both statistically and clinically significant and has been identified by other investigators when LPN is compared to RALPN.[21,22] The other finding of note was three pseudoaneurysms in the RALPN group which may reflect the use of the robot for more central and hilar tumors. All pseudoaneurysms were successfully managed with selective angioembolization. There was no difference in length of stay for the two groups.

Table 7.1 Results of retroperitoneal LPN vs. RALPN

	LPN	RALPN	p-value
N	32	47	
Tumor size (cm)	2.38	2.59	0.38
OR time (min)	229	151	0.0004
EBL (cc)	192	71	0.00006
Warm ischemia time (min)	32.9	22.4	0.00005
LOS (days)	2.53	2.29	0.25
Complications	5/32 (15.6%)	5/47 (10.6%)	
Pseudoaneurysm	1	3	
Urine leak	1	0	
Myocardial infarction	0	1	
Clostridium difficile colitis	1	0	
CO_2 retention	0	1	
Acute tubular necrosis	1	0	
Ileus	1	0	

Table 7.2 Results of trans vs. retro RALPN

	Trans	Retro	p-value
N	22	26	
Tumor size (cm)	2.57	2.60	0.91
OR time (min)	210	174	0.035
EBL (cc)	165.9	73.6	0.0009
Warm ischemia time (min)	27.9	25.1	0.30
LOS (days)	3.27	2.50	0.01
Complications	2/22 (9%)	3/26 (11.5%)	
Pseudoaneuryms	0	2	
Myocardial infarction	0	1	
CVA	1	0	
Chylous ascites	1	0	

We perform TP-RALPN for anterior and medial tumors and feel that the surgical approach should be based on tumor location. The two approaches complement each other and we have found medial tumors to be very difficult to remove with the RP technique. A comparison of TP and RP-RALPN is presented in Table 7.2. The two approaches were performed concurrently so there is no learning curve benefit for one technique over the other. Based on our experience, the RP approach resulted in shorter operative time, less blood loss, and shorter length of stay as compared to the TP technique. Warm ischemia time was not significantly different between the two approaches.

7.6 Conclusions

The RP approach for RALPN provides direct access to the renal hilum and posterior located tumors. This technique is ideal for patients who have had previous abdominal surgery avoiding any adhesions that may be present. RP surgery sequesters any urine leakage or blood that may result from partial nephrectomy.

The combination of the RP approach and the advantages of robotic technology have resulted in several advantages over LPN which include decreased blood loss, shorter operating time, and most importantly, decreased warm ischemia time. Compared to the TP approach, RP-RALPN resulted in less blood loss, shorter operative time, and shorter length of stay due to earlier return of bowel function. With experience, the limitations associated with the RP approach can be minimized and adequate space can be created for the da Vinci robot.

References

1. Fergany AF, Hafez KS, Novick AC. Long-term results of nephron sparing surgery for localized renal cell carcinoma: 10-year followup. *J Urol*. 2000;163:442.
2. Gill IS, Matin SF, Desai M, et al. Comparative analysis of laparoscopic versus open partial nephrectomy for renal tumors in 200 patients. *J Urol*. 2003;170:64.
3. Gill IS, Kavoussi LR, Lane BR, et al. Comparison of 1,800 laparoscopic and open partial nephrectomies for single renal tumors. *J Urol*. 2007;178:41-46.
4. Benway BM, Bhayani SB, Rogers CG, et al. Robot assisted partial nephrectomy versus laparoscopic partial nephrectomy for renal tumors: a multi-institutional analysis of perioperative outcomes. *J Urol*. 2009;182:866-872.
5. Gautam G, Benway BM, Bhayani SB, Zorn KC. Robot-assisted partial nephrectomy: current perspectives and future prospects. *Urology*. 2009;74:735-740.
6. Bhayani SB. da Vinci robotic partial nephrectomy for renal cell carcinoma: an atlas of the four-arm technique. *J Robo Surg*. 2008;1:279-285.
7. Wright JL, Porter JR. Laparoscopic partial nephrectomy: comparison of transperitoneal and retroperitoneal approaches. *J Urol*. 2005;174:841-845.
8. Patel MN, Krane LS, Bhandari A, et al. Robotic partial nephrectomy for renal tumors larger than 4 cm. *Eur Urol*. 2009;13:2009.
9. Rogers CG, Metwalli A, Blatt AM. Robotic partial nephrectomy for renal hilar tumors: a multi-institutional analysis. *J Urol*. 2008;180:2353-2356.
10. Gill IS, Delworth MG, Munch LC. Laparoscopic retroperitoneal partial nephrectomy. *J Urol*. 1994;152:1539.
11. Lee HJ, Box GN, Abraham JBA, et al. Laboratory evaluation of laparoscopic vascular clamps using a load-cell device—are all clamps the same? *J Urol*. 2008;180:1267-1272.
12. Benway BM, Wang AJ, Cabello JM, Bhayani SB. Robotic partial nephrectomy with sliding-clip renorrhaphy: technique and outcomes. *Eur Urol*. 2009;55:592-599.
13. McDougall EM, Clayman RV. Laparoscopic nephrectomy for benign disease: comparison of the transperitoneal and retroperitoneal approaches. *J Endourol*. 1996;10:45-49.
14. Desai MM, Strzempkowski B, Gill IS, et al. Prospective randomized comparison of transperitoneal versus retroperitoneal laparoscopic radical nephrectomy. *J Urol*. 2005; 173:38-41.
15. Ng CS, Gill IS, Ramani AP, et al. Transperitoneal versus retroperitoneal laparoscopic partial nephrectomy: patient selection and perioperative outcomes. *J Urol*. 2005; 174:846-849.
16. Kieran K, Montgomery JS, Daignault S, et al. Comparison of intraoperative parameters and perioperative complications of retroperitoneal and transperitoneal approaches to laparoscopic partial nephrectomy: support for a retroperitoneal approach in selected patients. *J Endourol*. 2007;21: 754-759.
17. Pyo P, Chen A, Grasso M. Retroperitoneal laparoscopic partial nephrectomy: surgical experience and outcomes. *J Urol*. 2008;180:1279-1283.
18. Gettman MT, Blute ML, Chow GK, Neururer R, Bartsch G, Peschel R. Robotic-assisted laparoscopic partial nephrectomy: technique and initial clinical experience with daVinci robotic system. *Urology*. 2004;64:914-918.
19. Bhayani SB, Das N. Robotic assisted laparoscopic partial nephrectomy for suspected renal cell carcinoma: retrospective review of surgical outcomes of 35 cases. *BMC Surg*. 2008;24:8-16.
20. Michli EE, Parra RO. Robotic-assisted laparoscopic partial nephrectomy: initial clinical experience. *Urology*. 2009;73: 302-305.
21. Wang AJ, Bhayani SB. Robotic partial nephrectomy versus laparoscopic partial nephrectomy for renal cell carcinoma: single-surgeon analysis of >100 consecutive procedures. *Urology*. 2009;73:306-310.
22. Benway BM, Bhayani SB, Rogers CG, et al. Robot assisted partial nephrectomy versus laparoscopic partial nephrectomy for renal tumors: a multi-institutional analysis of perioperative outcomes. *J Urol*. 2009;182:866-872.

8 Laparoscopic and Robotic Mid and Distal Ureteral Reconstructive Surgery

Alireza Moinzadeh

Abstract Laparoscopic and robot-assisted distal ureteral reconstruction techniques and outcomes are well described. In this chapter, we summarize our surgical technique for reconstruction of non-malignant ureteral strictures. We detail ureteroneocystotomy, psoas hitch, and Boari flap procedures. Preoperative and postoperative considerations are presented.

Keywords Boari flap • Laparoscopy • Psoas hitch • Stricture • Ureter

Key Points

- Appropriate preoperative work up includes retrograde ureteropyelogram, cystogram, anterograde study (if nephrostomy tube is placed), and studies to rule out ureteral malignancy if concern exists (urine cytology, ureteroscopy/biopsy).
- Ureteral dissection minimizing the use of thermal injury to avoid ureteral injury
- Bladder dissection to increase mobility and reduce anastomotic tension if necessary.
- Appropriate bladder flap width during Boari flap (at least 5 cm) to preserve blood supply to the flap
- Watertight, tension free anastomosis over ureteral stent no matter which surgical procedure is undertaken.

A. Moinzadeh
Institute of Urology, Lahey Clinic Medical Center,
41 Mall Road, Burlington 01805, MA, USA
e-mail: moinza00@lahey.org

8.1 Introduction

Lower ureter injuries are frequently the result of iatrogenic injury. The most frequent iatrogenic injuries include ureteroscopy for stone disease and radical hysterectomy.[1] Other abdominal or pelvic surgeries that lead to ureteral injury include distal colectomy[2], vascular procedures,[3] and vaginal procedures including anterior colporrhaphy and hysterectomy. Iatrogenic injuries far outnumber those caused by trauma. Traumatic injuries may include either blunt or penetrating. The injury may be recognized at the time of original iatrogenic insult, or may present at a later date. In this chapter we review the diagnosis, preoperative preparation, and operative steps involved in laparoscopic or robotic distal ureteral reconstruction. Emphasis is placed on ureteroneocystotomy, psoas hitch, and Boari Flap procedures. We have refrained from applying these techniques to cases of lower ureter transitional cell cancer given the potential concern of cancer cell seeding.[4]

8.2 Preoperative Preparation

It is important to have complete radiographic assessment prior to surgery. Cross sectional imaging in the form of computed tomography (CT) scan is commonly available at the time of referral to the surgeon. The radiological study should include delayed images to visualize the collecting system. Inflammatory reaction around the ureter may provide the surgeon with clues regarding the relative difficulty of peri-ureteral dissection planes. Given the potential evolving nature of some benign ureteral strictures, we recommend imaging

J.V. Joseph and H.R.H. Patel (eds.), *Retroperitoneal Robotic and Laparoscopic Surgery*,
DOI: 10.1007/978-0-85729-485-2_8,

within 3 months of the proposed definitive surgery. As such, the propagation of the stricture may be noted allowing for better surgical planning.

If the obstruction is complete and the patient has an existing nephrostomy tube, then to-and-fro imaging including concomitant nephrostogram and retrograde pyelogram is most helpful in precisely defining the length and location of the stricture. Cystogram under general anesthesia at 20 cm height is useful to assess bladder capacity in the event of planned Boari flap or psoas hitch. A 24 or 48 h voiding diary also aids in determining functional bladder capacity. If a filling defect is noted during radiographic ureter studies, or if the clinical scenario warrants, a urine cytology/ureteroscopy is necessary to rule out transitional cell carcinoma. In the event of unilateral compromised renal unit, we obtain a nuclear renal scan to assess differential function. In cases where renal function is less than 20%, nephrectomy rather than reconstruction is recommended.

Preoperative preparation includes one bottle of magnesium citrate starting at 1 pm the day prior to planned surgery. Patient is instructed to only consume clear liquids starting at noon the day prior to surgery. All patients are instructed to withhold any non-steroidals or medications which may induce bleeding for a period of 10 days prior to surgery. Given the likely history of prolonged indwelling ureteral stent or nephrostomy tube, urine culture preoperatively is strongly recommended. We administer organism specific antibiotics prior to surgery to sterilize or decrease urine bacterial counts.

Although any patient who is a candidate for open distal ureteral reconstructive repair is a candidate for robotic or laparoscopic repair, certain caveats are worth mentioning. If the patient has had an attempt at open repair in the past and the surgery has failed, this patient is best approached in open fashion as use of bowel or auto transplant may be necessary. Patients who have had prior cautery balloon or laser incision in an attempt to rectify short strictures present a particularly challenging case. In the author's experience these patients have an increased amount of inflammatory reaction around the site of extravasation. This leads to extremely adherent tissue planes around the ureter akin to surgery for retroperitoneal fibrosis. Surgeons lacking significant minimally invasive experience operating in such an environment may strongly consider performing open surgery.

8.3 Operative Positioning and Trocars

Patients are placed in a position similar to the one used for robotic radical prostatectomy. We prefer the split leg table, with the patient supine. For patients with significant abdominal girth, we place table side extenders so that arms may rest comfortably, without excessive pressure. This is particularly important for distal ureter surgical cases as it is often difficult to predict the exact length of the operation.

After sterile preparation/draping and administration of intravenous broad spectrum antibiotics, a Foley catheter is placed. Although we are facile with both retroperitoneal renal access and extraperitoneal pelvic access,[5] we prefer the transperitoneal approach for ureteral reconstructive surgery. The transperitoneal approach allows the surgeon the option of continued cephalad proximal

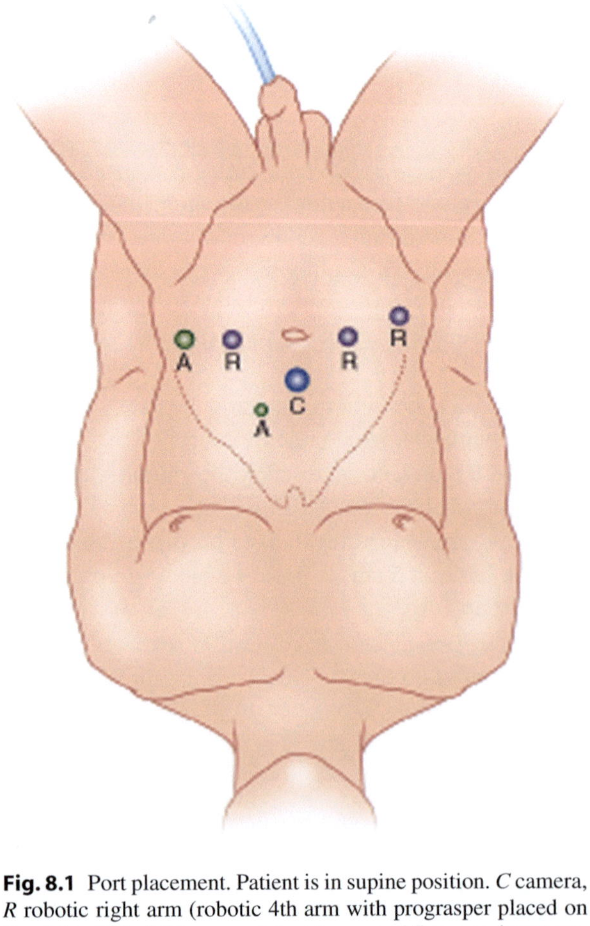

Fig. 8.1 Port placement. Patient is in supine position. *C* camera, *R* robotic right arm (robotic 4th arm with prograsper placed on the right side), *A* 12 mm assistant trocar and 5 mm assistant trocar (optional)

dissection of the ureter when necessary. Trocars for robotic procedures are placed after transperitoneal insulation with Veress needle or open Hasson technique. Trocars are placed slightly more cephalad (about 2-finger breadth) than for other robotic pelvic surgeries (radical prostatectomy or cystectomy) to allow access to the proximal ureter if necessary (Fig. 8.1). We prefer to place the robotic "4th arm" on the patient's right side and have the assistant stand on the patient's left side. This allows for simultaneous movement of two grasping instruments (left hand bipolar/right hand prograsper) when the 4th arm is engaged.

8.4 Dissection of Ureter

For left side ureter dissection, the 4th arm equipped with the prograsp is used to gently retract the sigmoid medially, while scissors and the bipolar are used to reflect the large bowel mesentery. We generally locate the ureter cephalad to the common iliac artery as in most cases the ureter has less inflammatory reaction away from the area of ureteral stricture. Once the ureter is identified and circumferentially dissected, a vessel loop is placed around it. Hem-o-lock clips are placed on the vessel loop ends to prevent migration of the loop during retraction. The loop may then be moved cephalad or caudal on the ureter allowing for a relatively atraumatic retraction of the ureter during the remaining distal dissection (Fig. 8.2). We aim to

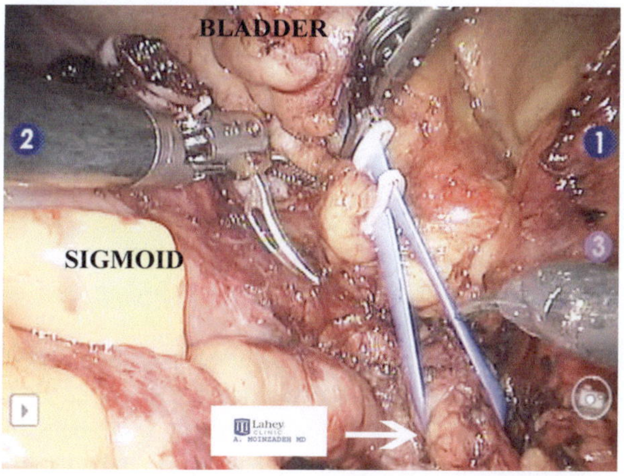

Fig. 8.2 Right ureter dissection (*white arrow*); ureter is lifted up and medial with the 4th arm prograsper using the atraumatic vessel loop

preserve as much peri-ureteral tissue as possible during dissection so as to avoid cautery or de-vascularization injury to the distal ureter.

Distal ureter dissection is carried out to the point of obstruction. The area of stricture is typically appreciated externally given the abundance of reactionary adherent tissue. Some have advocated the use of Fogarty balloons placed cystoscopically, at the outset, to locate the strictured area. We have not found this technique to be necessary. Use of preoperative cross sectional imaging and retrograde ureterogram allows for accurate determination of the strictured area. Proximally the ureter is dissected about 4–5 cm above the point of obstruction. A tagging suture of 4–0 Vicryl is placed anteriorly on the ureter to allow for future retraction and orientation. The ureter is then incised approximately 1 cm above the point of obstruction. Visualization of the lumen integrity confirms the obstructive nature of the ureter. The ureter is spatulated to a healthy appearing widely patent proximal portion. It is not necessary to continue distal dissection of the ureter beyond the area of scar tissue formation. The distal strictured portion of ureter may be extremely adherent to the surrounding structures increasing risk of adjacent organ risk. A portion of the distal stump may be sent for pathologic analysis to confirm lack of transitional cell cancer.

If a ureteral stent has been paced previously, care is taken not to traumatize the stent. We prefer the use 4.8 French × 22–30 cm stent (Boston Scientific, Natick, MA, USA). The variable length of the stent allows mobility within the ureter minimizing the risks of inadvertent stent migration during surgery. Small stent circumference decreases luminal obstruction which may become problematic while suturing the anastomosis.

If a ureteral stent was not placed prior to surgery given complete obstruction, it may be placed after ureter division. We prefer the use of Sensor® wire (Boston Scientific, Natick, MA, USA) as the floppy tip may easily negotiate tortuous anatomy, while the PTFE coating can be handled by the robotic prograsper or needle drivers. Caution must be taken to avoid unnecessary angulation and stress of the PTFE coating with the needle drivers as this may lead to shear effects on the wire with loss of PTFE material. The wire may be introduced into the peritoneum via the assistant 5 mm port to minimize loss of pneumoperitoneum.

8.5 Bladder Dissection

After completion of ureter dissection, the bladder is dropped down in similar fashion to the transperitoneal radical prostatectomy. The space of Retzius is entered. Lateral dissection is carried down dividing the peritoneal window lateral to the obliterated ligament. Care is taken not to traumatize the contralateral ureter during this portion of the dissection. If necessary, division of the vas deferens may be necessary to increase bladder and or ureteral mobility. Preoperative discussion with the young male patient about this issue is warranted. Distal bladder dissection is continued to completely separate the bladder from the pubic bone down to the endopelvic fascia.

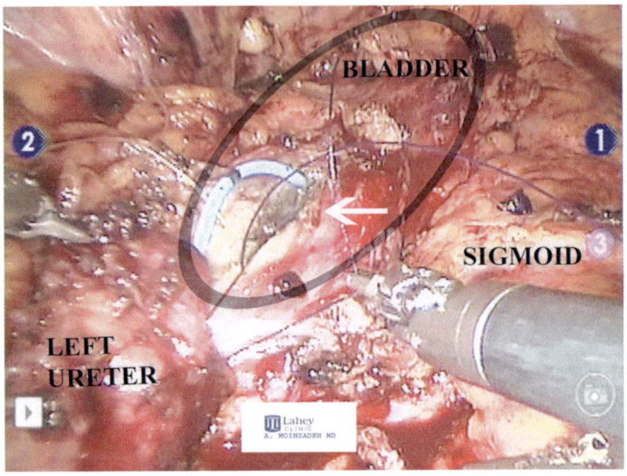

Fig. 8.3 Left sided psoas hitch. The bladder has already been hitched to the left psoas. *White arrow* shows extravesical trough. Blue stent is visualized prior to tying down of placed interrupted sutures between the left ureter and bladder

8.6 Ureteroneocystotomy Versus Psoas Hitch

For all reconstruction techniques, the goals remain the same: tension free mucosa to mucosa anastomosis over a JJ stent. The bladder and ureter may be apposed using graspers to test approximation in tension free fashion. If this is not possible, consideration should be given to creation of a Boari flap (see below). The bladder is filled with sterile irrigation to assess distance between the terminal ureter and the bladder. For the most distal ureter strictures, the ureter may be sewn back to the bladder in an extravesical fashion (ureteroneocystotomy). Ureteroneocystotomy is preferred over other techniques if a tension free water tight anastomosis can be obtained. If necessary, a psoas hitch is performed to aid in decreasing the distance between the bladder and ureter and to relieve tension on the anastomosis. Two permanent sutures are placed near full thickness on the posterior peritoneal dome reflection of the bladder and secured to the psoas fascia or psoas ligament. Care is taken not to damage the genitofemoral nerve during suture placement on the psoas fascia. The exact location of the genitofemoral nerve is typically appreciated. A horizontal incision on the mid bladder which is then closed vertically (Heineke Mikulicz closure) may augment achievable length. Although rarely necessary, one may dissect and ligate the contralateral blood supply to the bladder to achieve additional mobility on the bladder.

The extravesical ureteral reimplantation for both ureteroneocystotomy and psoas hitch is completed in similar fashion. Both may result in a refluxing anastomosis depending on the type of anastomosis completed. The bladder is filled with approximately 200 cc of sterile irrigant. An extravesical trough is created on the bladder surface about 2 cm in length, down to the bladder mucosa. Anastomosis of the spatulated ureter and the bladder is completed with a series of interrupted sutures of 4–0 and 3–0 Vicryl in interrupted fashion (Fig. 8.3). The 3–0 Vicryl serves as an anchor point in the most distal portion of the anastomosis. Two or three sutures are placed prior to tying of the sutures to allow for easier identification of the ureteral/bladder mucosa. Using the Foley catheter, the integrity of the anastomosis is tested by retrograde filling of the bladder with dilute methelene blue irrigation mixture. A Jackson Pratt drain is placed in the perivesical space.

8.7 Boari Flap

When a psoas hitch is inadequate to provide needed length, a bladder flap is constructed. Described in a canine model in 1894 and subsequently in humans in 1947, the Boari Ockerblad flap has proven to be useful for mid to lower ureter obstruction.[6,7] Depending on bladder capacity and elasticity of the bladder, defects as long as 15 cm may be bridged. The laparoscopic technique is now well described.[8,9] Contraindications

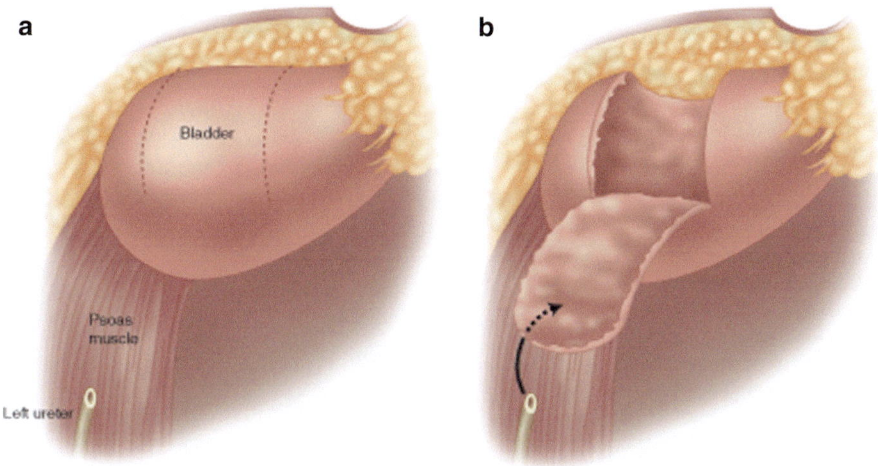

Fig. 8.4 Robotic view of proposed Boari flap. The U-shaped bladder flap (**a**) is angled in the direction of the proposed ureter anastomosis (**b**)

to a flap procedure would include cases of compromised bladder capacity/fibrosis or poor blood supply (pelvic radiation). Formal urodynamic studies may be conducted preoperatively in patients with significant voiding dysfunction.

After dissection of the ureter, bladder, and psoas fascia as described above for the psoas hitch procedure, an anterior bladder flap is created in the direction of the proposed ureteral anastomosis. We have found it useful to place a disposable ruler via the 12 mm trocar into the abdomen to carry rout measurements on the bladder. The proposed bladder flap dissection may then be marked on the bladder using electrocautery. The U-shaped flap is angled in the direction of the ureter so as to increase flap size and relieve tension on the anastomosis (Fig. 8.4). The bladder is filled with enough sterile irrigation (~200 cc) to allow for partial filling. In order to preserve blood supply to the flap, the base is measured to at least 5 cm with a narrowing to about 3 cm at the tip. The flap is sewn to the psoas fascia or psoas ligament as described for the psoas hitch. A submucosal tunnel is created for the anastomosis of the ureter and anastomosis is completed.[9] The submucosal tunnel is really a mucosal/submucosal trough about 1.5 cm in length. The anteriorly spatulated ureter is then laid into the trough and 3–0 or 4–0 Vicryl suture is used in interrupted fashion to anastomose the ureter to the bladder flap (Fig. 8.5). A 4.8 French multi-coil stent is placed over a wire. The bladder flap is then closed over the ureter anteriorly and the flap and bladder defect is closed. The integrity of the anastomosis and bladder defect closure is tested by retrograde filling of the bladder via the Foley catheter. A Jackson-Pratt drain is placed in the perivesical space.

8.8 Postoperative Management

Antibiotics are continued for 7 days postoperatively. At approximately day 7 (ureteroneocystotomy or psoas hitch) and day 10–14 (Boari flap) a cystogram is performed. After confirming no leak, the Foley catheter is removed. Ureteral stent is removed about 4–6 weeks after surgery. Three months after surgery a diuretic renal scan is performed to assess emptying time of the kidney. Alternatively, an intravenous urogram may be performed. Given the high likelihood of reflux, we place a Foley catheter prior the radiographic imaging. Culture specific antibiotics are administered for stent removal if a history of prior urinary tract infections exists.

8.9 Complications

Complications during surgery are primarily related to adjacent organ injury (bowel, blood vessels, etc.). Infectious complications are minimized by checking preoperative urine cultures and continuing appropriate antibiotics during the peri-operative period. Care should be taken during ureter dissection to avoid excess use of thermal injury. This may aid preservation of blood supply to the ureter. For psoas hitch or Boari flap procedures, during placement of the fixation suture on to the psoas muscle, one must avoid genitofemoral nerve entrapment. If bladder spasms occur postoperatively, anticholinergic medications

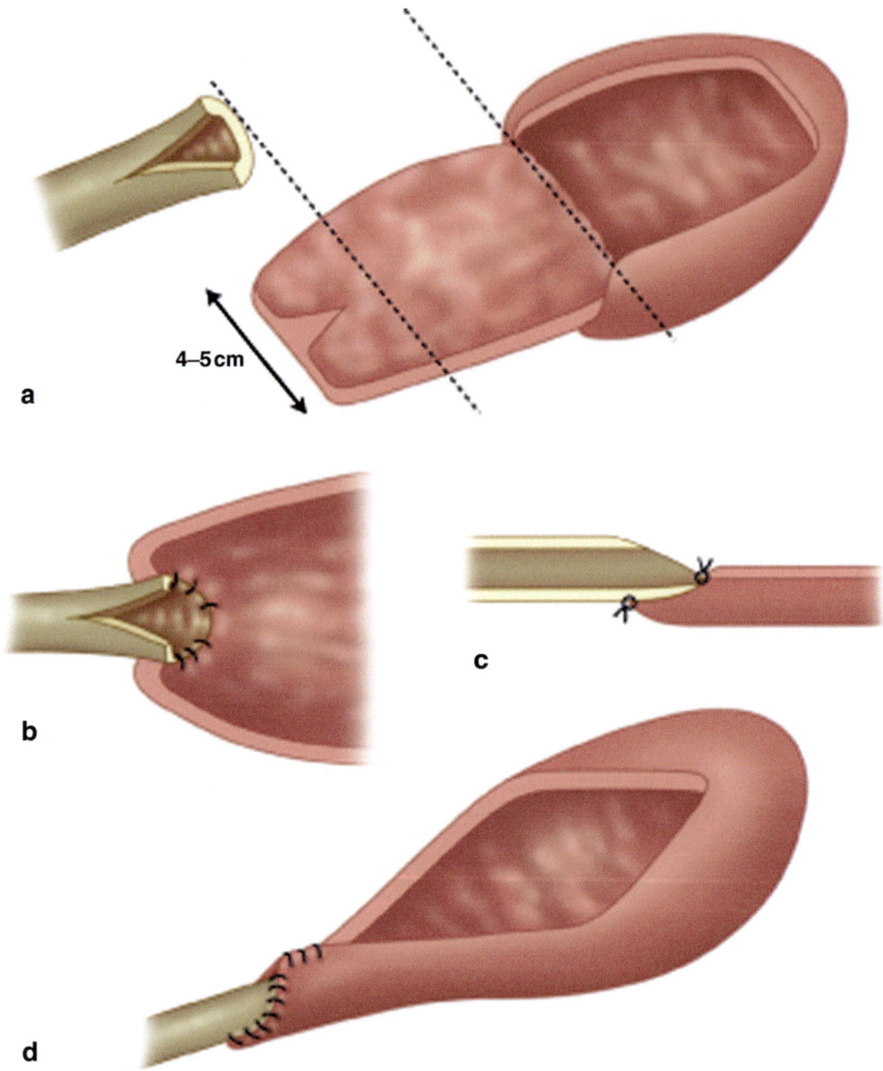

Fig. 8.5 Anastomotic technique of Boari flap. (**a**) Trough created in the submucosa for approximately 1 cm. (**b**) Approximation of spatulated ureter and "troughed" mucosal edge allows for double inverse spatulation. (**c**) Seromuscular sutures used overlap anastomosis with detrusor. (**d**) Interrupted sutures were used to tubularize the flap adjacent to the anastomosis. Tubularization 1–2 cm beyond anastomosis was conducted with running closure

are initiated to minimize disruption of the anastomosis. During bladder mobilization, the contralateral ureter must not be injured. If a refluxing anastomosis is performed, the patient should be aware of potential sequela of temporary renal colic. This "kidney pressure" may occur when the bladder is full or during voiding. Although failure from recurring stricture varies, between 5% and 10% of patients may develop recurrent stenosis. As such continued follow-up during the first 1–2 years is warranted.

8.10 Summary

Laparoscopic or robot-assisted ureteral reconstruction surgical steps are described in detail. Preoperative radiographic work up to assess the length of the ureter is useful in surgical planning and patient discussion. It is paramount to perform a tension free, watertight, anastomosis over a ureteral stent. Minimally invasive surgical options may be the preferable surgical option given the lack of need for a specimen extraction site.

References

1. Hunter RW, McCartney AJ. Ureteric injuries at laparoscopic hysterectomy. *Am J Obstet Gynecol*. 1993;169:752.
2. Graham JW, Goligher JC. The management of accidental injuries and deliberate resections of the ureter during excision of the rectum. *Br J Surg*. 1954;42:151.
3. Spirnak JP, Hampel N, Resnick MI. Ureteral injuries complicating vascular surgery: is repair indicated? *J Urol*. 1989;141:13.
4. Moinzadeh A. Re: Robotic distal ureterectomy with reimplantation in malignancy: technical nuances. *Can J Urol*. 2009;16:4676. discussion 4676.
5. Kaouk JH, Hafron J, Parekattil S, et al. Is retroperitoneal approach feasible for robotic dismembered pyeloplasty: initial experience and long-term results. *J Endourol*. 2008; 22:2153.
6. Boari A, Casati E. Contributo *sperimentale alla plastica* dell'urretere [A *contribution* to the experimental plastic surgery of ureter]. *Atti Accad Sci Med Nat Ferrar*. 1894;68:149.
7. Ockerblad N. Reimplantation of ureter into the bladder by flap method. *J Urol*. 1947;57(5):845-7.
8. Fugita OE, Dinlenc C, Kavoussi L. The laparoscopic Boari flap. *J Urol*. 2001;166:51.
9. Simmons MN, Gill IS, Fergany AF, Kaouk JH, Desai MM. Technical modifications to laparoscopic Boari flap. *Urology*. 2007;69:175.

9 Robot-Assisted Laparoscopic Nephroureterectomy

Sijo J. Parekattil, Hany N. Atalah, and Li-Ming Su

Abstract Laparoscopic nephroureterectomy is a well-established surgical treatment option for patients with transitional cell carcinoma of the upper urinary tract and has well-published data supporting an advantage in decreased patient morbidity compared to open techniques with similar oncologic outcomes. With the recent addition of the da Vinci Surgical System (Intuitive Surgical Inc., Sunnyvale, CA), robot-assisted laparoscopic nephroureterectomy (RLNUx) may provide additional technical advantages to the surgeon to further improve upon the outcomes noted with the conventional laparoscopic technique. This chapter provides a detailed description of the RLNUx technique, its indications, contraindications, preoperative preparation, operative steps, and complications.

Keywords Laparoscopy • Nephroureterectomy • Robotic surgery • Transitional cell carcinoma

Key Points

- For single robot docking for the entire procedure, the robot must be brought in from the caudal position to allow for both renal hilar dissection and distal ureteral and bladder cuff excision.
- Creation of a psoas window below the ureter and above the gonadal vein for right-sided cases (below gonadal vein for left-sided cases) allows for superior traction of the kidney to access the renal hilum.
- During a right-sided procedure, the renal artery and/or vein are ligated using the vascular stapler with care taken to visualize the vena cava inferiorly and superiorly to prevent any inadvertent caval injury.
- The ipsilateral medial umbilical ligament is dissected and then ligated to allow the ipsilateral side of the bladder to be mobilized, thus providing optimal visualization of the ureterovesical junction.
- Once the ureter and bladder cuff are freed, a hemoclip may be placed across the ureter to prevent any urine and possible tumor spillage. The anterior retraction with the stay stitch and drainage of the bladder with the Foley help to prevent any urine or potential tumor spillage from the bladder.

9.1 Introduction

Approximately 5–10% of all renal malignancies are transitional cell carcinomas.[1] Radical nephroureterectomy (NUx) with formal bladder cuff excision was

S.J. Parekattil (✉)
Department of Urology, University of Florida,
1600 Archer Road, Gainesville, FL 32610, USA
e-mail: sijo.parekattil@winterhavenhospital.org

DOI: 10.1007/978-0-85729-485-2_9,

first proposed in 1933 by Kimball and Ferris[2] and remains the standard of care. Laparoscopic nephroureterectomy (LNUx) was first described by Clayman et al. in 1991.[3,4] Although initially a tedious procedure, with greater experience and surgical modifications, this technique has become the new standard of care at many institutions worldwide with increasing evidence supporting equivalent oncologic outcomes and a faster convalescence as compared to open surgery.[5-17]

More recently, robot-assisted laparoscopic radical nephroureterectomy (RLNUx) has been presented as an alternative to LNUx with potential advantages including improved surgeon efficiency and suturing, ergonomics, ease of bladder reconstruction after bladder cuff excision in addition to equivalent oncologic efficacy as compared to LNUx.[18-22] This chapter is dedicated to the detailed description of the RLNUx technique: indications, contraindications, preoperative preparation, operative steps, and complications.

9.2 Indications and Contraindications

RLNUx is classically performed as a treatment option for transitional cell carcinoma of the renal pelvis and/or ureter. In this situation, complete excision of the entire urothelium of the affected kidney, ureter, and bladder cuff is required in order to minimize local tumor recurrence. This procedure may also be utilized in certain congenital or acquired conditions where the patient has an atrophic or non-functional renal unit. In cases of renal atrophy associated with high-grade vesicoureteral reflux, if surgical removal of the renal unit is warranted on the grounds of flank pain and/or recurrent infection, complete excision of the ureter is necessary in addition to the kidney in order to prevent reflux of urine into a retained ureteral stump resulting in persistent symptoms. Patients with a duplicated renal collecting system and a non-functional moiety may also be candidates for RLNUx.

RLNUx may be contraindicated in patients with severe cardiopulmonary compromise or those with uncorrectable bleeding disorders. One relative contraindication is in those patients with locally advanced transitional cell carcinoma where there is preoperative radiographic evidence of local extension of disease into surrounding structures or lymph node involvement. The use of an open technique in these unique circumstances may be prudent. However, there is mounting evidence that such patients may do poorly whatever surgical approach is used, and may benefit from multi-disciplinary approaches to treatment incorporating neoadjuvant or adjuvant chemotherapy.[23] Although patients with prior extensive abdominal surgery or morbid obesity may be technically more challenging, these are not absolute contraindications to RLNUx and are dependent upon the skill and experience of the surgeon.

9.3 Preoperative Preparation

Patients are instructed to avoid any aspirin, ibuprophen-containing products, blood thinners or Vitamin E for 1 week before surgery to minimize the risk of operative or postoperative bleeding. A mechanical bowel prep is given to the patient the day before surgery (one bottle magnesium citrate) and the patient is instructed to adhere to a clear liquid diet up until midnight the day before surgery.

9.4 Operative Steps for Robot-Assisted Laparoscopic Nephroureterectomy

9.4.1 *Patient Positioning*

An orogastric tube is placed in the patient at the beginning of the case. The patient is positioned in a modified lateral decubitus position at a 45° angle to reveal the side that is being approached (transperitoneal approach). The bed is flexed to approximately 30°–40° with the break of the bed lined up to the superior margin of the iliac crest. The dependent leg is flexed to a 90° angle at the knee and supported at the ankle and knee with gel or foam padding. Pillows are placed between the legs to support the non-dependent leg, which is aligned straight on top of the pillows.

The dependent arm is supported by foam padding and either tucked at the patient's side or placed on top of an arm board that is angled cephalad to allow room for the robotic arms and assistant during the procedure. A rolled up foam support cushion is placed in the axilla to prevent any brachial nerve injuries (there is no need for axillary support if the flexion of the bed is less than 40°). An additional rolled up foam support is

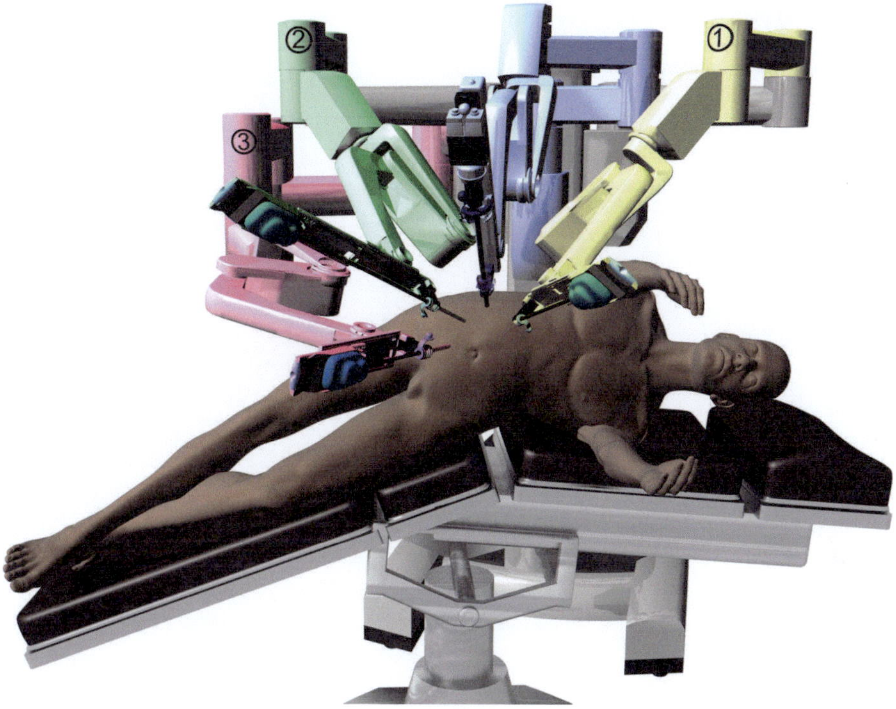

Fig. 9.1 Patient and robot positioning for right-sided robot-assisted laparoscopic nephroureterectomy

placed over the supraclavicular area between the neck of the patient and the shoulder. Two pillows are placed on top of the dependent arm to support the non-dependent arm, which is also aligned in an outward and cranial fashion to expose the abdomen fully. It is important that the two arms are kept in a comfortable yet low profile position as possible as placing too much padding between the arms may result in elevation of the non-dependent arm causing direct contact with the robotic arms during the operation. Towels are placed on the upper torso and hips. Two-inch cloth tape is used to secure the patient to the operative table by wrapping the patient at the upper torso and hips to the bed. The patient's abdomen is then prepped and draped in the standard fashion. A Foley catheter is inserted in the sterile field so that Methylene blue-tainted saline can be inserted into the bladder during the bladder cuff excision portion of the surgery. Figure 9.1 illustrates the patient positioning with the robotic surgical platform.

9.4.2 Port Placement

Figures 9.2 and 9.3 illustrate the port placement for RLNUx that allows for a single docking position of the robot for a right-sided case. For right-sided cases, an additional 5 mm laparoscopic port may be placed if desired at the subcostal margin near the xiphoid process to place a locking non-traumatic laparoscopic grasper that is used as a liver retractor. This port should be placed left to the midline to avoid the falciform ligament, to allow better retraction of the liver. For right-sided cases, the fourth robotic arm is brought in cephalad (above the right robotic arm).

For left-sided cases, the port placement mirrors that for right-sided case, however the additional 5 mm assistant port is generally not necessary for retraction of the spleen. Release of the spleno-renal ligament leads to adequate visualization of the kidney without the need for any additional retraction of the spleen. For left-sided cases, the fourth robotic arm is brought in cephalad (above the left robotic arm).

Initially, the nephrectomy portion of the case is completed using the port configuration shown in Fig. 9.2. In order to maintain a single robotic docking position for the entire case, the distal ureter with bladder cuff excision is performed using the port configuration shown in Fig. 9.3 by making the following port adjustments:

1. The left robotic arm port is piggy-backed into the 12 mm assistant port,
2. A new 12 mm port is placed at the previous left robotic port site in order to create new assistant port, and

Fig. 9.2 Port placement for right-sided robot-assisted laparoscopic nephroureterectomy – nephrectomy portion

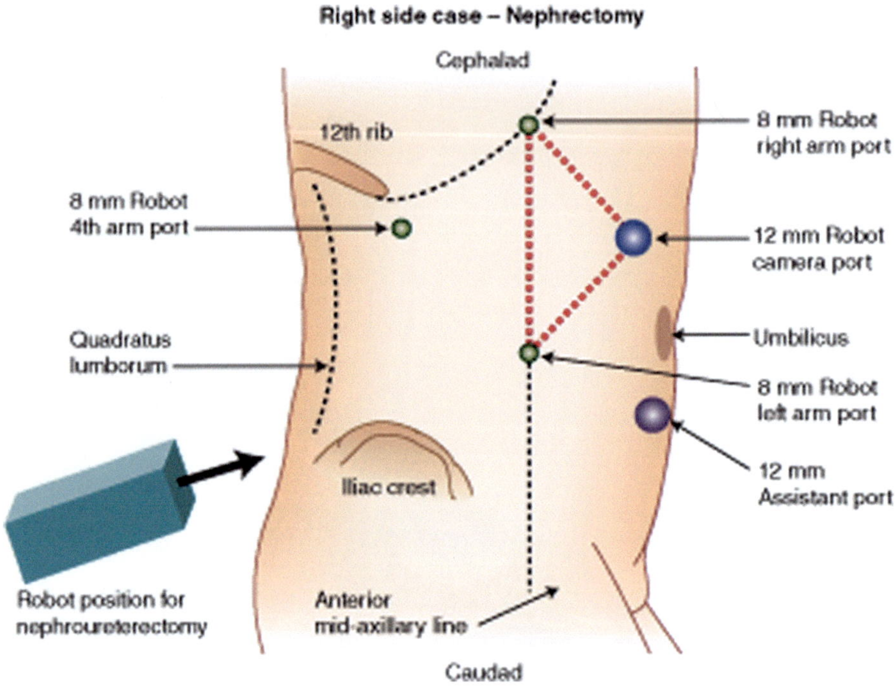

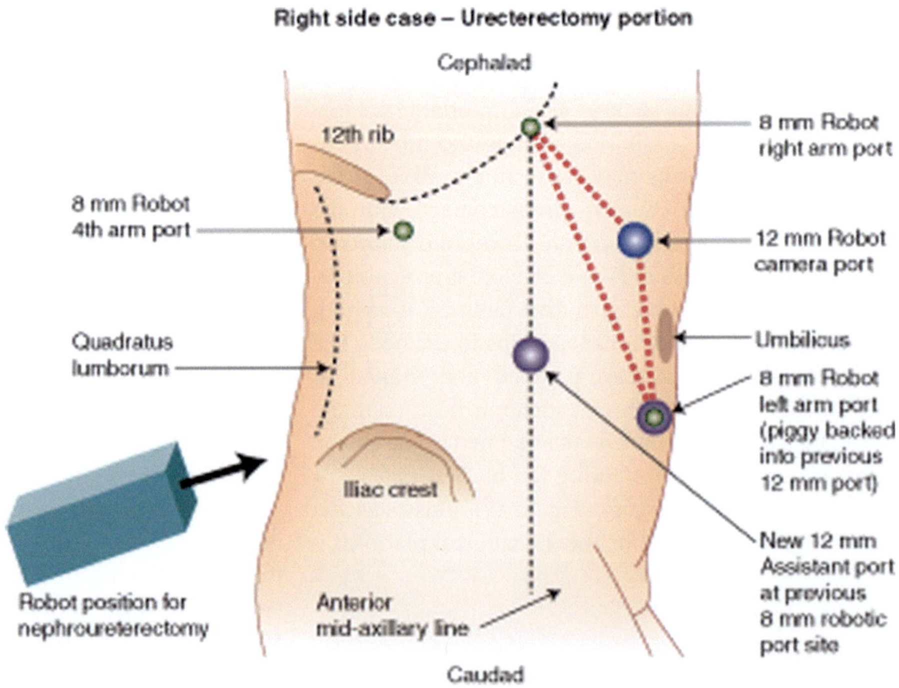

Fig. 9.3 Port placement for right-sided robot-assisted laparoscopic nephroureterectomy – ureterectomy and bladder cuff portion

3. The fourth robotic arm may be used as the surgeon's right arm or an additional retraction tool to reach the lower pelvis for bladder cuff excision and bladder closure.

This modification of ports allows for a single docking position for the robot during the entire case. Use of single robotic docking approach has been shown to be beneficial in decreasing operative duration.[19] Alternatively, a two docking approach may be used with the robot initially docked at a 45° angle entering from the head of the operating table to address the nephrectomy portion of the operation. The robot is then redocked entering from the foot of the table to address the ureterectomy and bladder cuff.

9.4.3 Surgical Assistant

For robot-assisted laparoscopic procedures, it is imperative to have a skilled surgical assistant at the bedside, since the primary surgeon will be located at the robotic console for the majority of the procedure. The assistant provides necessary counter traction, suctioning of fluids, clip and stapler application. The assistant is also responsible for readjustment of the robotic arms to prevent any external mechanical clashing between arms. The single docking approach requires a well-trained surgical assistant to perform the subtle port adjustments mentioned above especially when the distal ureter and bladder cuff are tackled.

9.4.4 Approach to the Kidney

The robotic curved monopolar scissors are used in the right robotic arm, the curved bipolar or Prograsp forceps are used in the left robotic arm and a Prograsp forceps may be used in the fourth robotic arm (use of the fourth arm is based on surgeon preference). The ascending colon is reflected medially by sharply incising along the white line of Toldt in an athermal fashion. Once the colon is fully reflected medially, the inferior portion of the renal moiety is dissected in order to visualize the ureter and gonadal vein. A hemoclip is placed across the ureter at this point (without ligation) to prevent any tumor cells from migrating down the ureter during manipulation of the kidney. The gonadal vein may be clipped and ligated to prevent any traction injury to the inferior vena cava. A window to the psoas muscle is created above the gonadal vein and under the ureter (for left-sided cases, the window would be created under both the ureter and gonadal vein). This window is utilized as a traction point with the left robotic arm to lift the kidney anteriorly in order to access and facilitate dissection of the renal hilum. If the fourth robotic arm is used, it can serve to elevate the kidney instead of the left arm.

The hilum is now carefully approached with gentle blunt dissection. Care must be taken to avoid the duodenum medially and any accessory crossing renal arteries or lumbar vessels. A monopolar hook electrocautery may be used in the right robotic arm at this point for fine dissection of the perivascular tissues as shown in Fig. 9.4. The assistant provides critical medial traction of the duodenum and vena cava for exposure of the renal hilum.

Once the renal hilum is carefully dissected, and the renal artery and vein are well visualized, the renal artery may be clipped or stapled as per surgeon preference. A 2–3 cm proximal segment of renal artery should be dissected free to allow ease of placement of hemoclips or a linear stapling device. Proximal dissection of the renal

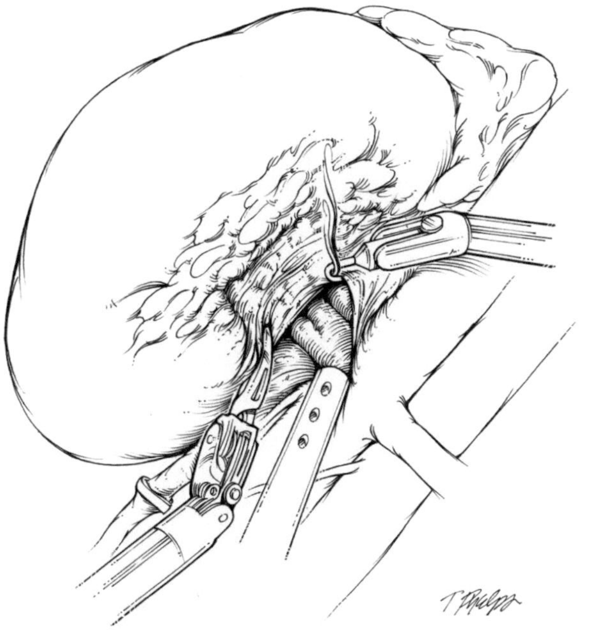

Fig. 9.4 Robot-assisted renal hilar dissection (© Li-Ming Su, University of Florida; used with permission)

artery should be performed before it branches into segmental arteries for ease of ligation. Once the artery is ligated, the renal vein is ligated using a linear stapling device with care taken to visualize the vena cava inferiorly and superiorly to prevent any inadvertent caval injury.

Once the renal hilum is freed, the upper pole attachments of the kidney may be divided and released using a vascular stapler, harmonic scalpel, monopolar hook electrocautery, or LigaSure device (Valleylab, Colorado). Usually, an adrenal sparing approach is utilized unless direct extension of the tumor is radiographically evident. However, if there is suspicion of adrenal involvement, the adrenal is removed en block with the renal specimen. During preservation of the adrenal gland, bleeding may be encountered while separating the upper pole of the kidney from the adrenal gland. As such, this dissection should be performed carefully with any of the above four hemostatic techniques previously mentioned. Biosealants such as Floseal™(Baxter, Illinois) or Surgicel™(Ethicon, North Carolina) may be applied to the adrenal bed if there is any concern for residual minor venous bleeding. Finally, the lateral attachments of the kidney are divided thus completely freeing the kidney and its surrounding perirenal fat from its attachments.

If perihilar adenopathy is encountered, a limited retroperitoneal lymph node dissection may be performed along the border of the great vessels for staging purposes.

9.4.5 Approach to the Distal Ureter and Bladder Cuff

For this portion of the case, a few port adjustments are made as previously described in the port placement section. Attention is now focused in dissecting out the distal ureter. Following division of the gonadal vessels as they course toward the inguinal ring, the ureter is dissected from the pelvic brim down toward the bladder. In the male patient, the vas deferens is divided and in the female the round ligament to allow for exposure and dissection of the distal ureter. The ipsilateral medial umbilical ligament is divided to allow the bladder to be mobilized medially. The ipsilateral superior vesical artery may be sacrificed (if needed) to further mobilize the lateral portion of the bladder providing optimal exposure of the ureterovesical junction. The fourth robotic arm (Prograsp forceps) may be used to retract the ureter anteriorly and medially to aid in its dissection if needed.

The bladder is filled with approximately 300 mL of indigo carmine-stained saline or water to demonstrate the bladder outline. The peritoneal layer covering the bladder and the distal ureter is dissected to reveal the uretero-vesicle junction noted by the splaying of the mucosa and surrounding muscle fibers as the ureter enters into the bladder. An extravesical approach is utilized to incise the detrusor muscle 2 cm around the ureterovesical junction as shown in Fig. 9.5. The incision is carried down until the bluish mucosa of the bladder is identified. Care must be taken so as to not perforate the mucosa prior to draining the bladder via the Foley. A 0-vicryl stay stitch may now be placed at the distal edge of the bladder cuff and held anteriorly with the fourth robotic arm. The bladder cuff is now carefully incised using the curved monopolar scissors in the right robotic arm with care taken to obtain a clear margin around the ureteral orifice. Once the ureter and bladder cuff are completely freed, a hemoclip may be placed across the terminal end of the ureter to prevent any urine and possible tumor spillage. By applying anterior retraction on the bladder with the stay stitch and draining the

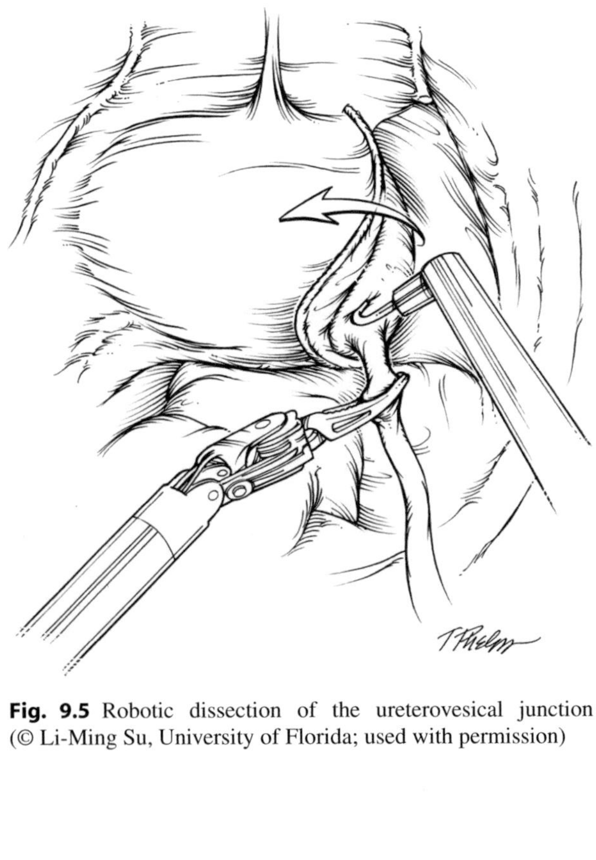

Fig. 9.5 Robotic dissection of the ureterovesical junction (© Li-Ming Su, University of Florida; used with permission)

bladder prior to cystotomy, urine and potential tumor spillage from the bladder is minimized. A laparoscopic entrapment sac is introduced through the 12 mm assistant port by the surgical assistant and the renal specimen, ureter and bladder cuff is carefully entrapped to be later extracted intact at the end of the operation.

9.4.6 Bladder Closure

The bladder is now closed in two layers using 2-0 polyglactin sutures on a SH or UR6 needle in a running continuous fashion. Once the bladder closure is completed, the integrity of the closure is tested by filling the bladder with approximately 100–200 mL of saline (may use Methylene blue-tainted fluid if desired). The specimen bag is now removed by enlarging the new 12 mm assistant port into a 3–4 cm muscle splitting Gibson incision or through an infraumbilical incision. Upon removal of the specimen, the Gibson incision is closed using 0-Vicryl or 0-PDS running suture at the fascial level. All the ports are removed under laparoscopic view. The port sites and extraction site are closed using 4-0 Monocryl running subcuticular stitches. A closed suction pelvic drain is left at the end of the operation, exiting the port site used by the fourth robotic arm.

9.5 Postoperative Management

Patients are admitted to the hospital and are usually discharged on postoperative day 1 or 2. Emphasis is placed on early mobilization and an aggressive bowel regimen including stool softeners, milk of magnesia, and simethicone. Patients are discharged home with the Foley catheter and follow up in the office for Foley catheter removal in 1–2 weeks. The pelvic drain is removed prior to discharge if the output remains low.

9.6 Complications

The published data on RLNUx currently consists of a number of small case series without a comprehensive review of complications. However, based on publications of large series of LNUx, the minor complication rate ranges from 6% to 40% and the major complication rate ranges from 6% to 24%.[24] However, several studies have shown that LNUx results in less blood loss, less postoperative pain, faster oral intake, and more rapid recovery for patients as compared to open surgery.[25]

9.6.1 Port Site Tumor Recurrences

Transitional cell carcinoma has a tendency for local implantation.[26] There are three reported cases of port site recurrences in patients who underwent LNUx in the literature.[27,28] Although very rare, this complication is quite serious and has grave consequences. This emphasizes the need for careful manipulation and prevention of spillage during these procedures. To date there are no reported cases of port site recurrences in patients who have undergone RLNUx, however, as mentioned the series are small with short-term follow up.

9.7 Conclusions

Robot-assisted laparoscopic nephroureterectomy is an alternative minimally invasive technique which offers improved visualization and ergonomics as compared to traditional laparoscopic surgery. This procedure is an alternative especially for individuals with limited skills and training in advanced laparoscopic techniques such as suturing. RLNUx is a challenging procedure that requires a dedicated robotic team and a skilled bedside assistant. Further studies are needed to assess and define its role amongst other competing techniques.

References

1. ACS: Detailed Guide of Kidney Cancers 2009. American Cancer Society, 2009.
2. Kimball F, Ferris HV. Papillomatous tumor of the renal pelvis associated with similar tumors of the ureter and bladder: a review of the literature and report of two cases. *J Urol.* 1933;31:257.
3. Kerbl K, Clayman RV, McDougall EM, Urban DA, Gill I, Kavoussi LR. Laparoscopic nephroureterectomy: evaluation of first clinical series. *Eur Urol.* 1993;23(4):431-436.

4. Clayman RV, Kavoussi LR, Figenshau RS, Chandhoke PS, Albala DM. Laparoscopic nephroureterectomy: initial clinical case report. *J Laparoendosc Surg*. 1991;1(6):343-349.
5. Berger A, Fergany A. Laparoscopic nephroureteroectomy: oncologic outcomes and management of distal ureter; review of the literature. *Adv Urol.* 2009: 826725.
6. Busby JE, Brown GA, Matin SF. Comparing lymphadenectomy during radical nephroureterectomy: open versus laparoscopic. *Urology*. 2008;71(3):413-416.
7. Berger A, Haber GP, Kamoi K, et al. Laparoscopic radical nephroureterectomy for upper tract transitional cell carcinoma: oncological outcomes at 7 years. *J Urol.* 2008;180(3): 849-854; discussion 854.
8. Colombo JR Jr, Haber GP, Jelovsek JE, et al. Complications of laparoscopic surgery for urological cancer: a single institution analysis. *J Urol*. 2007;178(3 Pt 1):786-791.
9. Busby JE, Matin SF. Laparoscopic radical nephroureterectomy for transitional cell carcinoma: where are we in 2007? *Curr Opin Urol*. 2007;17(2):83-87.
10. Matin SF, Gill IS. Recurrence and survival following laparoscopic radical nephroureterectomy with various forms of bladder cuff control. *J Urol*. 2005;173(2):395-400.
11. Kawauchi A, Fujito A, Ukimura O, Yoneda K, Mizutani Y, Miki T. Hand assisted retroperitoneoscopic nephroureterectomy: comparison with the open procedure. *J Urol.* 2003;169(3):890-894; discussion 894.
12. Matsui Y, Ohara H, Ichioka K, et al. Retroperitoneoscopy-assisted total nephroureterectomy for upper urinary tract transitional cell carcinoma. *Urology*. 2002;60(6):1010-1015.
13. Stifelman MD, Hyman MJ, Shichman S, Sosa RE. Hand-assisted laparoscopic nephroureterectomy versus open nephroureterectomy for the treatment of transitional-cell carcinoma of the upper urinary tract. *J Endourol*. 2001;15(4):391-395; discussion 397.
14. Shalhav AL, Dunn MD, Portis AJ, Elbahnasy AM, McDougall EM, Clayman RV. Laparoscopic nephroureterectomy for upper tract transitional cell cancer: the Washington University experience. *J Urol*. 2000;163(4):1100-1104.
15. McNeill SA, Chrisofos M, Tolley DA. The long-term outcome after laparoscopic nephroureterectomy: a comparison with open nephroureterectomy. *BJU Int*. 2000;86(6):619-623.
16. Gill IS, Sung GT, Hobart MG, et al. Laparoscopic radical nephroureterectomy for upper tract transitional cell carcinoma: the Cleveland Clinic experience. *J Urol*. 2000;164(5):1513-1522.
17. Dunn MD, Shalhav AL, McDougall EM, Clayman RV. Laparoscopic nephrectomy and nephroureterectomy for renal and upper tract transitional cell cancer. *Semin Laparosc Surg*. 2000;7(3):200-210.
18. Rogers CG, Laungani R, Bhandari A, et al. Maximizing console surgeon independence during robot-assisted renal surgery by using the Fourth Arm and TilePro. *J Endourol*. 2009;23(1):115-121.
19. Park SY, Jeong W, Ham WS, Kim WT, Rha KH. Initial experience of robotic nephroureterectomy: a hybrid-port technique. *BJU Int*. 2009;104:1718-1721.
20. Park SY, Jeong W, Choi YD, Chung BH, Hong SJ, Rha KH. Yonsei experience in robotic urologic surgery-application in various urological procedures. *Yonsei Med J*. 2008;49(6):897-900.
21. Eun D, Bhandari A, Boris R, Rogers C, Bhandari M, Menon M. Concurrent upper and lower urinary tract robotic surgery: strategies for success. *BJU Int*. 2007;100(5): 1121-1125.
22. Rose K, Khan S, Godbole H, Olsburgh J, Dasgupta P. Robotic assisted retroperitoneoscopic nephroureterectomy – first experience and the hybrid port technique. *Int J Clin Pract*. 2006;60(1):12-14.
23. Margulis V, Shariat SF, Matin SF, et al. Outcomes of radical nephroureterectomy: a series from the Upper Tract Urothelial Carcinoma Collaboration. *Cancer*. 2009;115(6): 1224-1233.
24. Hyams ES, Kanofsky JA, Stifelman MD. Laparoscopic Doppler technology: applications in laparoscopic pyeloplasty and radical and partial nephrectomy. *Urology*. 2008;71(5):952-956.
25. Matin SF. Laparoscopic radical nephroureterectomy: current status. In: Gill IS, ed. *Textbook of Laparoscopic Surgery*. New York: Informa Healthcare; 2006:573-585.
26. Pearlstone DB, Feig BW, Mansfield PF. Port site recurrences after laparoscopy for malignant disease. *Semin Surg Oncol*. 1999;16(4):307-312.
27. Matsui Y, Ohara H, Ichioka K, Terada N, Yoshimura K, Terai A. Abdominal wall metastasis after retroperitoneoscopic assisted total nephroureterectomy for renal pelvic cancer. *J Urol*. 2004;171(2 Pt 1):793.
28. Ong AM, Bhayani SB, Pavlovich CP. Trocar site recurrence after laparoscopic nephroureterectomy. *J Urol*. 2003;170 (4 Pt 1):1301.

Laparoscopic Pelvic Lymphadenectomy in Prostate Cancer

10

Evangelos Liatsikos, Minh Do, Panagiotis Kallidonis, Iason Kyriazis, Alan McNeil, Roman Ganzer, and Jens-Uwe Stolzenburg

Abstract Pelvic lymphadenectomy (PLA) for the time being appears to be the most reliable staging method for localized prostate cancer (PCa), retrieving information concerning lymph node (LN) invasion that is important for the initiation of adjuvant therapy. LN metastasis is associated with poor prognosis and consequently there is a trend to perform PLA in all patients with respectable probability to harbor LN metastasis. The importance of PLA for prostate cancer (PCa) outcome is unclear. Laparoscopic PLA is a surgical operation carried out in an operative field adjacent to many important and vulnerable structures and is associated with an increased risk for surgical complications. Thus, expert surgical skills and a meticulous knowledge of pelvic anatomy are required in order for this challenging procedure to be carried out with effectiveness and reasonable risk to the patient.

Keywords Extended lymphadenectomy • Laparoscopic • Pelvic lymphadenectomy • Prostate cancer

J.-U. Stolzenburg (✉)
Department of Urology, University of Leipzig, Leipzig, Germany
e-mail: stolj@medizin.uni-leipzig.de

Key Points

- The role of PLA in PCa outcome is still under debate.
- The percent of invaded LNs detected is proportional to the number of LNs that have been dissected.
- PLA is associated with significant incidence of complications that rises with increase of the number of dissected LNs.
- In patients with PSA<10, biopsy Gleason sum<7 and in T1c or T2 clinical stage, the incidence of exclusively nonobturator LN invasion is very limited and a standard PLA should be offered.
- At the end of a PLA using the extraperitoneal approach, bilateral fenestration of the peritoneum reduces the incidence of lymphocele at the levels of the transperitoneal approach.

10.1 Introduction

Pelvic lymphadenectomy (PLA) is the surgical procedure through which resection of the lymph nodes (LNs) of the pelvis is taking place. PLA usually takes place before a radical prostatectomy but the performance afterwards or separately is also possible. An eightfold decrease in the incidence of LN invasion as diagnosed by PLA has been observed over the last 20 years. This can be explained by the widespread use of prostate-specific-antigen (PSA) screening

J.V. Joseph and H.R.H. Patel (eds.), *Retroperitoneal Robotic and Laparoscopic Surgery*,
DOI: 10.1007/978-0-85729-485-2_10, © Springer-Verlag London Limited 2011

and prostate cancer (PCa) awareness in the community, which have caused a downward shift in the pathologic stage of PCa at diagnosis. However, LN metastases are reported in 6% of patients with newly diagnosed PCa and in about 11% of patients undergoing radical prostatectomy.[1] Currently, PLA seems to be the most reliable staging method for localized prostate cancer, since the alternative routinely used screening methods such as computed tomography (CT) and magnetic resonance imaging (MRI) of the pelvis have insufficient sensitivity. Thus, these techniques are inadequate to replace PLA.[2] Several newly introduced techniques such as positron emission tomography (PET) scan, MRI using intravenous lymphotropic superparamagnetic nanoparticles, and sentinel LN mapping using radioisotopes have demonstrated promising results in terms of sensitivity and specificity on LN invasion detection.[3] However, further clinical evaluation is deemed necessary for the routine use in clinical practice of these techniques. PLA remains the gold standard method of LN evaluation in case of PCa.

Several controversies exist in the field of PLA. First, the effect of PLA on the outcome of the malignant disease and its effect on the prognosis are currently under debate. Examination of large series of patients with varied risk of LN metastasis has failed to prove that PLA influences significantly the biochemical relapse free survival of the disease. Nevertheless, each of the performed studies suffers from severe limitations and randomized studies are not yet available. As a result, no strict conclusions can be drawn.[2,4] Moreover, PCa is a disease characterized by slow progression and current evidence supports that even in cases of detected LN invasion long-term survival is not definitely prohibited. In an investigation of 10,261 men who underwent prostatectomy, 507 were found positive for LN invasion. The 5- and 10-year rates of biochemical free survival were reported to be 69% and 56%, respectively, and the 5- and 10-year rates of cancer-specific survival were reported to be 94% and 86%.[5] On the contrary, locoregional LN resection is considered as a therapeutic procedure in other malignancies such as breast or bladder cancer and the proper performance offers tumor spreading reduction and improvement of prognosis.[3] In PCa, even the most extensive LN dissection is inefficient to retrieve all LNs draining the prostate. As a result, the potential to extract all spreading cancer cells with the combination of radical prostatectomy and extensive LN resection is questionable. Thus, the therapeutic role of PLA is still under debate and PLA should be performed only for staging purposes.

Another controversy regarding PLA is the extent of LN excision that should be performed. It is generally acceptable that the incidence of invaded LNs grows as the extent of PLA increases.[6] The more extended the PLA is, the higher the possibility of detecting LN invasion. The removal of more than ten LNs is related to more than double incidence of LN metastasis in comparison to more limited lymphadenectomy retrieving less than ten LNs (10.3% versus 4.6%). In fact, extended PLA has been observed to retrieve three times more LNs in comparison to standard PLA.[4,7] The above trend could be attributed to the significant portion of LN metastases (19–42%) that occur at LN groups outside the resection template of limited PLA and consequently the limited procedure would underestimate the incidence of LN metastases in these cases.[1,8,9] As a result, several investigators consider extended PLA as treatment of choice and perform the procedure in all cases. Nevertheless, PLA is associated with a high incidence of complications that rises in accordance to the anatomical extent of the procedure. Therefore, an approach combining low morbidity and complication rate with a representative LN sampling should be introduced. Briganti et al. in an accurate nomogram (up to 80% accuracy) presented data demonstrating that not all patients with PCa should undergo an extensive LN dissection. For example, patients with PSA<10 ng/dl, biopsy Gleason sum<7, and clinical stage T1c or T2 have a very limited (1–1.5% accordingly) possibility to harbor nonobturator LN metastases.[1,5] As a result, in the latter group, which represents the majority of PCa patients, a limited to obturator fossa PLA would predict with high accuracy LN invasion and extended PLA would be avoided.

A final point of controversy is the exact anatomic field of LN dissection included in the variety of LN dissection approaches. In general, three approaches for PLA have been described in relation to the anatomical extent of the procedure: the limited, the extended, and the standard or modified PLA. Nevertheless, there is no consensus regarding the exact LN groups excised in each of the above PLA approaches. Some investigators characterize the extent of PLA according to the number of extracted LNs. Consequently, any PLA that resects more than ten LNs is considered as extended.[9] Yet, the mean number of LNs retrieved from the obturator fossa is 9.[1] According to the above-mentioned classification, any additional LN group dissected would characterize the procedure as extended PLA, a fact argued by the authors who use the LN groups dissected as the criterion to characterize the different kinds of PLA. PLA literature becomes even more complicated by the fact that LN groups dissected in case of extended PLA are not common in all studies (some investigators include presacral LNs, other external iliac, etc.) while on the other hand particular LN groups can be interpreted differently. For example, the LNs laying in the internal surface of external iliac vessels are described either as obturator or as external iliac LNs, while the LNs lying medially to internal iliac vessels are being described either as internal iliac, either as presacral LNs. The variability of extracted LNs and the confusion in LN terminology have rendered multi-institutional retrospective studies of large series of cases very difficult.

In this chapter, an attempt is made to clarify the above-mentioned controversies, to describe in detail the indications of LN dissection, the anatomical boundaries of the different LN dissection approaches, and the surgical approach that should be followed in each case.

10.2 Indications

The indication of PLA followed by the majority of urologists worldwide is a PSA greater than 10 ng/mL and a Gleason score of 7 or higher with/without the presence of palpable tumor.[9,10] This group of patients sustains a reasonable possibility to harbor LN metastases enough to overcome the risk of PLA complications.[11] However, many authors have adopted PLA as a routine procedure preceding radical prostatectomy in all patients, given the excellent long-term outcome of the approach even when LN invasion is detected.[12] Today, nomograms are used to stratify the risk of harboring LN metastases according to clinical parameters such as PSA, clinical stage, and Gleason biopsy score.[1,4,5,9] Using these nomograms, the clinician can select the proper candidates for PLA and decide the extent of LN resection based on evidence. For example, patients with Gleason score of 6 or less and with a PSA<10 ng/mL have a very small possibility of having LN metastases and consequently PLA is not warranted.[13] Enlargement of pelvic LNs as seen by imaging techniques can be considered as a relative indication.

The importance of PLA for the determination of the presence of metastatic disease in pelvic LNs of PCa patients is questioned in the literature by several investigators. These investigators propose that the down-staging of PCa due to the wide use of PSA screening and the establishment of predictive nomograms could render the performance of PLA as an unnecessary intervention.[11,14] In addition, several physicians base their decision to perform PLA on nomograms designed for the limited PLA and the application of these nomograms in cases of extended PLA is questionable.[11]

Our experience indicates that currently predictive nomograms and noninvasive screening techniques do predict the possibility of LNs harboring PCa, but fail to predict accurately if LNs of a particular patient are actually invaded. Consequently, we still perform the procedure in all patients with a reasonable possibility to harbor LN metastases. Growing experience and multicenter retrospective analyses are expected to reinforce the predictive accuracy of nomograms and, with the evolution of screening techniques, may lead to the abandonment of the procedure in the future.

10.3 Contraindications

Despite the fact that a limited number of authors have proposed otherwise,[7] PLA offers no therapeutic benefit in cases of metastatic prostate cancer. Consequently, evidence of metastasis (regardless of the organ) is considered a strict contraindication of the procedure. Additional absolute contraindications for the performance of laparoscopy are uncorrectable coagulopathy, severe cardiopulmonary disease, intestinal obstruction, generalized peritonitis, abdominal wall infection, massive hemoperitoneum, and malignant ascites.[14] Moreover, previous extraperitoneal or transperitoneal mesh placement for inguinal hernia repair are also contraindications since the adhesions induced by the aforementioned procedures do not allow the excision of LNs. Open hernia repair does not represent a problem for PLA. Relative contraindications for laparoscopic procedure include extensive prior abdominal or pelvic surgery, pelvic fibrosis, morbid obesity, organomegaly, ascites, pregnancy, diaphragmatic hernia, and the presence of iliac or aortic aneurysm. Relative contraindications are related to either adhesion formation or anatomical problems that could represent a significant challenge intraoperatively. Nevertheless, the majority of patients presenting relative contraindications could be laparoscopically managed by careful assessment of the patient and sufficient laparoscopic experience.[15]

10.4 Preoperative Evaluation

Meticulous preoperative evaluation of candidates for possible laparoscopic surgery includes past history, physical examination, and assessment of any concomitant medical conditions, which are initial steps for the successful performance of PLA. Age- and health-related laboratory studies are necessary. Blood cell count, biochemical and coagulation profile, as well as urinalysis and urine culture should be evaluated. An assessment of perioperative risk by a cardiologist, particularly in patients with a cardiac history and an electrocardiogram (ECG) should be routinely performed. According to the cardiac history of the patient, additional cardiological investigations should take place when necessary. Severe cardiac arrhythmias represent significant risk for the myocardium due to the pneumoperitoneum-induced hypercapnia and concomitant acidosis.

Chest and abdominal radiograph should also be performed in all cases. Since pneumoperitoneum influences negatively the respiratory function of the patient, pulmonary investigation by an expert is necessary in the presence of a concomitant respiratory pathology. Patients with chronic obstructive pulmonary disease should be further evaluated with blood gases and pulmonary function tests according to the recommendation of the expert physician.

10.5 Preoperative Preparation

Preoperative bowel preparation usually is necessary for the decompression of the bowel and takes place the day before surgery. Clear liquid diet and laxative suppositories or tablets are sufficient. Mechanical and antibiotic preparation of the bowel is appropriate for cases that could be related to dense abdominal adhesions. Determination of patient blood type is usually enough and blood transfusion should not necessarily be planned for the performance of laparoscopic PLA since the procedure is associated with minimal intraoperative blood loss. When the procedure takes place along with a laparoscopic radical prostatectomy, the preparation does not change due to the low blood loss and transfusion requirement of laparoscopic radical prostatectomy. The informed consent of the patient regarding the risks and complications of laparoscopic PLA should always be obtained and the possibility for conversion to open surgery should also be discussed.[14,15]

10.6 Patient Positioning and Draping

The placement of the patient on the operative table requires special care. The patient should be appropriately secured to avoid sliding off the table when in the Trendelenburg position. PLA is performed with the patient in supine position with the arms secured at the sides. Tape and security belts across the chest and thighs provide stable and safe positioning. Compression stockings should always be used for antiembolic prophylaxis. The use of an active warming system is sometimes necessary in order to avoid hypothermia. Preparation and draping should include the full extent of the abdominal wall from nipples to pubis. Skin preparation and sterilization should take place with special consideration for possible conversion to open surgery. If radical prostatectomy follows PLA, the genitalia should also be prepared and draped in order to maintain sterile conditions of the urethral catheter during the prostatectomy. Nasogastric tube and Foley catheter are placed for stomach and bladder decompression, respectively. The above measures reduce the risk for perforation of these organs.

10.7 Operative Steps

Preoperative patient assessment and patient preparation is identical in all approaches for PLA. The steps of the operation are dependent on the extent of lymphadenectomy performed and current literature has not concluded regarding the exact anatomical boundaries of lymphadenectomy. Thus, the following anatomic definition will be adopted throughout the text:

- Limited lymphadenectomy: excision of LNs of the obturator fossa and along external iliac vein (anterior and medial surface).
- Standard lymphadenectomy: excision of LN groups in the obturator fossa, medially and laterally of the external iliac artery/vein up to the bifurcation of the common iliac vessels as well as along the internal iliac artery (Fig. 10.1).

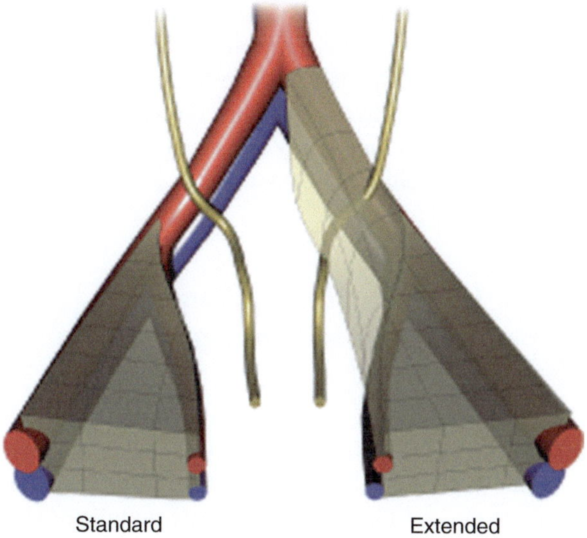

Fig. 10.1 Graphical presentation of the superior level of lymph node (LN) dissection performed in the case of standard and extended pelvic lymphadenectomy

- Extended lymphadenectomy: excision of LN groups at the obturator fossa, medially and laterally to external iliac artery/vein, LNs lateral and medial to internal iliac vessels (similarly to the standard lymphadenectomy). In addition, excision of LNs up to the level of the bifurcation of the aorta is also performed (Fig. 10.1).

In addition, the transperitoneal and extraperitoneal techniques of PLA have several differences and will be described separately. In case of the transperitoneal approach, the standard lymphadenectomy will be described in detail and the differences between the latter with limited and extensive PLA will be given.

10.8 Transperitoneal Approach

10.8.1 Operating Room and Patient Set Up

The patient should be placed supine in a 20–30° Trendelenburg position. The operating surgeon stands on the side opposite to the site of operating LN group, with the assistant standing on the ipsilateral side. The patient should also be rolled slightly towards the operating surgeon. A urinary catheter should be placed in order to ensure an evacuated urinary bladder.

10.8.2 Trocar Placement

In total, four or five trocars should be placed. The following landmarks are used for trocar placement:

- Umbilicus: 10–12 mm trocar
- Left lower quadrant of abdominal wall, 2 cm medial to the anterior superior iliac spine: 5-mm trocar
- Right lower quadrant of abdominal wall, 2 cm medial to the anterior superior iliac spine: 5-mm trocar
- Right lateral border of the rectus muscle, approximately 2 cm lower than umbilicus: 5-mm trocar
- Left lateral border of the rectus muscle, approximately 2 cm lower than umbilicus: 5-mm trocar
- Halfway between the umbilicus and the pubic bone in the midline: 5-mm trocar

The PLA with or without concomitant laparoscopic radical prostatectomy requires the insertion of trocars at the first five aforementioned sites. PLA alone can also be performed with the use of four trocars located at the umbilicus, lower abdominal wall quadrants, and midline. If the use of an additional trocar is deemed necessary intraoperatively, the insertion of a trocar on the lateral rectus muscle border is performed according to the preference of the surgeon.

For the placement of the umbilical trocar and creation of pneumoperitoneum, two techniques have been proposed. The introduction using Veress needle or by mini-laparotomy is possible. According to the first, the Veress needle is inserted at the lower border of the umbilicus. Care should be taken to avoid organ or bowel injury. The Trendelenburg position of the patient facilitates insertion and limits the risk of organ injury. The inserted needle should be aspirated to check for blood or bowel content. The correct placement of the needle could be checked by the injection of saline into the abdominal cavity. The saline should pass through the needle without resistance. Insufflation follows and the pneumoperitoneum is established primarily at 20 mmHg and then lowered to 12–15 mmHg after port positioning. The edges of the wound are stabilized with towel clips and the initial trocar (12-mm trocar) is inserted through the umbilicus with 70° caudal direction. The insertion of the trocar in the peritoneal cavity is proved by the escape of gas from the open sidearm of the trocar or with the use of laparoscopic camera.

Alternatively, the introduction of the umbilical trocar through a mini-laparotomy is taking place. A semicircular incision is made on the lower edge or slightly below of the umbilicus. The underlining fascia and peritoneum are incised (transverse incision 2–3 cm). Sutures are placed on the posterior fascia and the 12-mm trocar is inserted (Hasson cannula). The trocar should be inserted with the blunt tip protruding in order to avoid organ injury. The pneumoperitoneum is established primarily at 20 mmHg and then lowered to 12–15 mmHg after port positioning.

The other trocars are introduced under visual guidance from the laparoscope. The final two (trocars 3 and 4) should perforate the abdominal wall lateral to the epigastric vessels.

In case of radical prostatectomy following PLA, trocar number and placement should follow the requirements of prostatectomy. Consequently, five trocars should be used, in the designated positions. In case of patients with a small pelvis, some urologists place the umbilical trocar laterally to the umbilicus as a way to increase their working space.

10.8.3 Exposure and Identification of Operative Field

The operative field is covered by the intestinal loops. The 30° Trendelenburg position and the slight lateral rotation towards the surgeon are usually enough to uncover the pelvic wall, causing the intestinal loops to move up towards the upper half of the abdominal cavity. However, in case of left PLA, the sigmoid colon is found to be attached to the parietal layer of the peritoneum. Dissection of the white line of Toldt to release the sigmoid colon is suggested. On the right side, the cecum and appendix may need to be freed from their lower attachments. In some cases, mobilization of right ascending colon or left descending colon is also necessary. At this point, it has to be emphasized that excessive coagulation of the colon should be avoided, given that it could lead to secondary perforation due to coagulative necrosis.

When the pelvic floor is uncovered, the following landmarks should be identified prior to surgical intervention: the obliterated umbilical ligament medially, the testicular vessels passing through the internal inguinal ring and the vas deferens laterally. The peritoneal fold covering the external iliac vessels (artery and vein) is directly visible while the vessels are pulsating underneath. In thin patients, the ureter crossing over the common iliac artery can usually be identified medial to the umbilical ligament.

10.8.4 Incision of the Peritoneum and Vas Deferens Ligation

In the transperitoneal laparoscopic PLA, the approach towards the pelvic LNs requires an opening of the peritoneum. A peritoneal incision parallel to the external iliac vessels and lateral to the medial umbilical ligament is made with the use of ultrasonic scissors. The incision follows an anterior–posterior direction. Identification of the artery can be made through its pulsation that is notable upon inspection. The incision is extended high over the pubic bone and downwards just medial to the pulsating internal iliac artery, back toward the bifurcation of the common iliac artery where the ureter is located. A large incision is advised in order to ease the dissection of the superior part of the LN group. Special care should be taken not to damage the iliac vessels and the crossing ureter. Then, identification of the vas deferens takes place, as it runs transversally through the anterior part of the peritoneal incision. In obese patients, the identification of the vas deferens can be difficult due to the presence of fatty tissue. It is important to distinguish between vas deferens and the adjacent ureter. Traction on the spermatic cord that mobilizes the vas deferens facilitates the distinction between these two structures. Vas deferens is then clipped or coagulated and divided. The internal segment of the divided vas is retracted medially to reveal the underlying LN dissection area. The external iliac vein should appear during this traction within the anterior part of the incision.

In case of radical prostatectomy following PLA, the above-described bilateral peritoneal incision parallel to external iliac vessels can be omitted. In the latter case, the inverted U-shaped transverse incision of the parietal peritoneum superior to the dome of the bladder, performed for the access to the prostate, can be expanded laterally. Then the surgeon, grasping the pelvic lip of the peritoneal incision can dissect the parietal peritoneum from the underlying tissues revealing the LN dissection area.

10.8.5 Lymph Node Group Dissection

10.8.5.1 Standard Lymphadenectomy

The anatomic limits of the standard pelvic lymphadenectomy are as follows:

- Laterally: internal surface of the external iliac vein and the ilio-psoas muscle
- Medially: the umbilical ligament
- Caudally: the pectineal ligament
- Anteriorly: the iliopubic branch of the pelvis
- Cephaladly: the confluence of the external iliac vein and the internal iliac vein

Each LN group should be excised en bloc. The following order of excision borders should be followed: external, internal, inferior, posterior, and finally superior limit of the LN group.

External Limit

The internal border of the external iliac vein is dissected medially and underneath the vein until the underlying ilio-psoas muscle has been revealed. Retraction of LN group medially facilitates the dissection (Fig. 10.2a, b). The obturator nerve lies in the bottom of this area and the dissection should carefully take place in order to prevent its injury (Fig. 10.2c, d). The following landmarks verify that this part of excision has been done properly: the pectineal ligament caudally and the obturator nerve posteriorly.

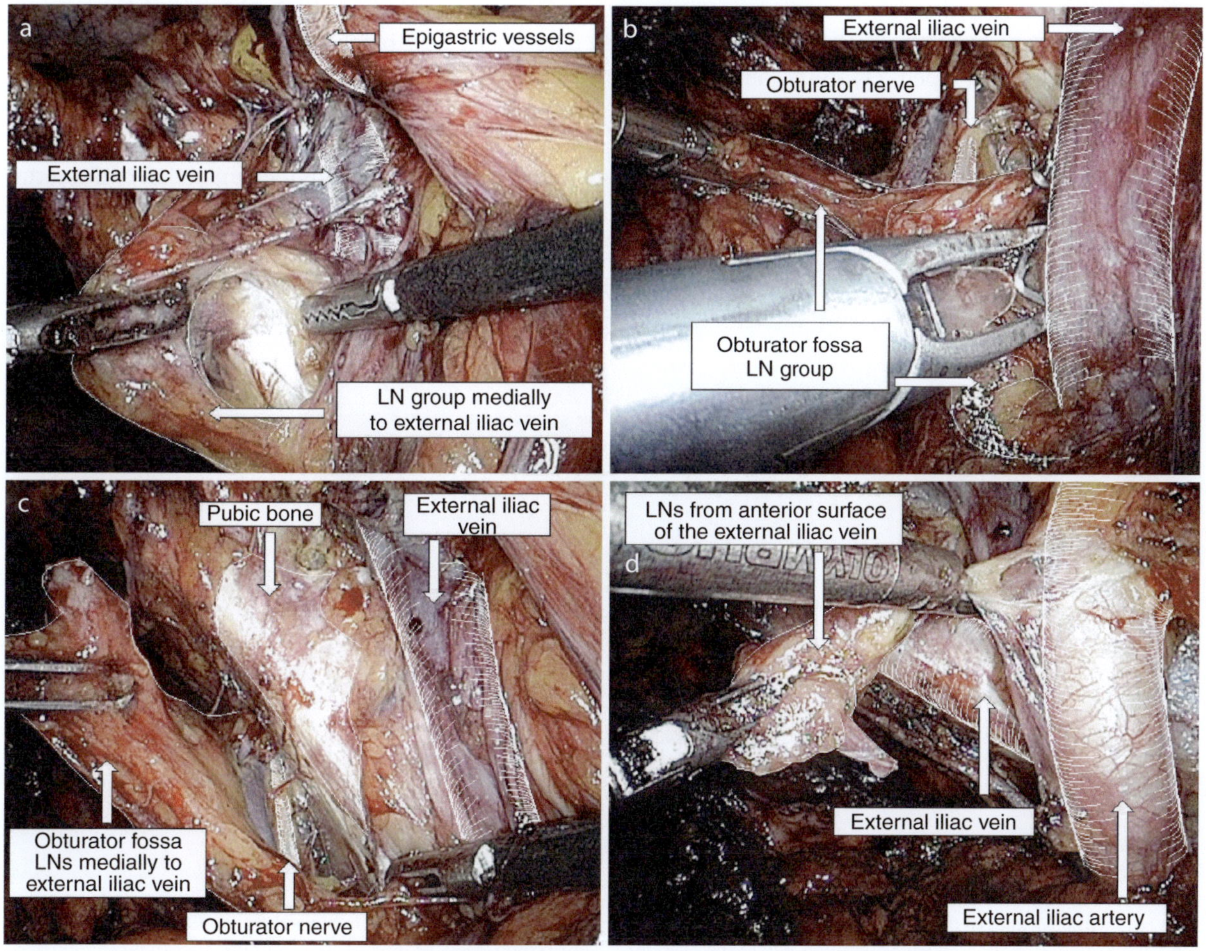

Fig. 10.2 (**a**) Retraction of the medial to the external iliac vein lymph node group. (**b**) Application of clips on lymphatic vessels. (**c**) Coagulation of lymphatic vessels. (**d**) Final excision of lymph node group at the site of the obturator fossa. The underlying obturator nerve is exposed

Internal Limit

The preperitoneal space is located between the anterior surface of the internal edge of the peritoneal incision and the LN group. Deep preparation of the preperitoneal space follows with direction laterally to the umbilical ligament and caudally towards the pelvic floor. Retraction of both LN group laterally and vas deferens internal segment medially facilitates this part of the dissection. The umbilical ligament forms the lower medial limit of the lymphadenectomy.

Inferior Limit

Inferiorly, the pectineal ligament defines the inferior boundary of the dissection. LN group is attached to the underlying tissue through a varying number of lymphatics. In order to free the LN group, the lymphatics should be clipped carefully and divided, revealing the pectineal ligament. Other investigators prefer the use of coagulation in order to ligate the lymphatics and to avoid postoperative lymph extravasation. Noncontrolled division of the lymphatic vessels will result in lymphocele formation. The underlying obturator vessels located underneath the excision area may be injured resulting in excessive bleeding. Obturator artery and any protruding vessels should be clipped and divided.

Posterior Limit

The obturator nerve defines the posterior lower limit of dissection and special care should be taken to avoid injury. Macroscopically, it can be mistaken for the obturator artery and eventually be ligated. Many authors suggest electrical stimulation as a way to distinguish between these two structures.

Superior Limit

For the termination of the excision, the confluence between the external iliac artery and the internal iliac artery is exposed (Fig. 10.3a, b). The LN group is being excised en block, using clips. The descending preparation of the internal iliac artery follows and the excision of LNs surrounding the latter vessel. In the case of extended lymphadenectomy, the dissection continues cephalad towards the bifurcation of the aorta. Care should be taken to avoid injuring structures such as the ureter. During the limited PLA, the excision at the level of the confluence of the common iliac artery

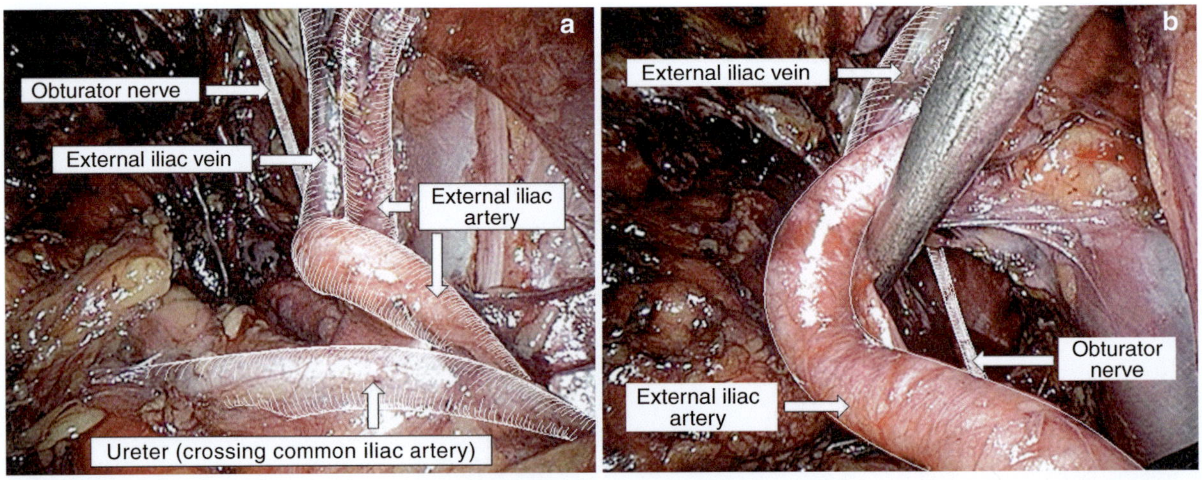

Fig. 10.3 (**a**) Exposure of the external iliac artery and vein up to the level of common iliac artery bifurcation where the crossing ureter is located. (**b**) Retraction of the external iliac artery and exposure of the obturator fossa as well as nerve. The lymphatic tissue of the site has been excised. (**c, d**) Complete excision of the lymph node groups of the obturator fossa and the external iliac vessels, bilaterally

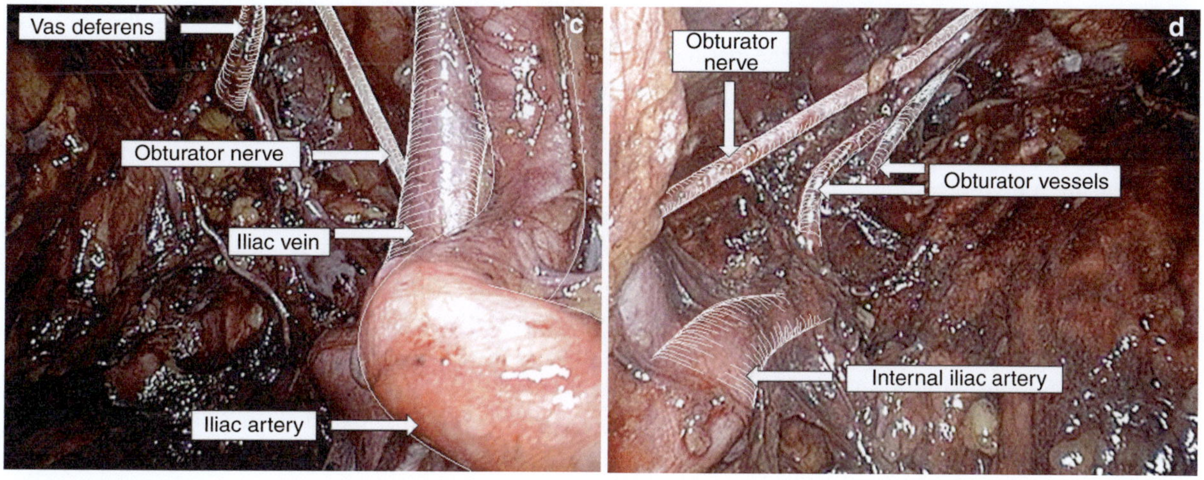

Fig. 10.3 (continued)

does not take place; the dissection is terminated when the LN group located at the site of the obturator fossa and external iliac vein is removed.

10.8.5.2 Contralateral Lymphadenectomy

The specimen is placed in the pelvis until the contralateral PLA is performed or is extracted through a 12-mm trocar (if possible). Contralateral lymphadenectomy is performed in a symmetrical fashion following the steps described previously (Fig. 10.3c, d).

10.8.5.3 End of the Procedure

Hemostasis should be checked at the end of the procedure and performed when necessary using a bipolar grasper. Hemostatic material could be placed at the dissection site. Peritoneum should be left open as a way to prevent lymphocele. Finally, the extracted specimens should be placed in an extraction bag (i.e., Endo-Bag) and retrieved through the umbilical port. Left and right LN groups should be marked differently in order to be discriminated in the histological examination. A drain is not usually necessary. However, some authors tend to place two drains, one in each side of dissection, as a way to reduce the incidence of lymphocele formation. Trocars are then removed under direct vision, with the optical trocar to be removed last. Careful inspection at trocar sites is imperative since injury of the epigastric vessels is a significant cause of postoperative bleeding.[16] In the umbilical port, the muscle aponeurosis is approximated using absorbable sutures and the skin is closed in all five trocar wounds using sutures or staples.

10.9 Extraperitoneal Approach

10.9.1 Patient Set Up

In extraperitoneal approach, patient setup remains the same as in the transperitoneal approach. However, the steep Trendelenburg position is not required, because the lower part of the peritoneum will hold intestinal loops outside the operative field. In case of peritoneal lesion, a cephalad operative table gradient can be applied to pull peritoneum with its contents towards the upper half of abdominal cavity.

10.9.2 Trocar Placement

In the extraperitoneal approach, trocars are placed in the same landmarks as in the transperitoneal approach. However, the umbilical trocar's insertion is differentiated. Using an open technique, the anterior fascia of rectus abdominis muscle is incised, careful dissection of the muscle layer follows and without peritoneal fenestration, an opening in the preperitoneal space is created. Blunt dissection of the preperitoneal connective tissue that connects the posterior surface of abdominal muscles with the anterior surface of the peritoneum is performed caudally until the pubic bone is reached (if possible). The umbilical trocar is inserted and a working space in the preperitoneal retropubic space is formed using a high-pressure balloon dilator. During the preparation of the preperitoneal space with the balloon dilator, the endoscopic camera is inserted and anatomical landmarks such as the epigastric vessels are visualized. The insertion of a Hassan trocar follows. The trocar is stabilized on the anterior fascia of the rectus abdominis with two absorbable sutures and gas insufflations are initiated. Then, the second trocar is inserted between the first port and the pubic bone. An instrument is introduced through the second trocar. Under visual guidance, insertion of the right and left lateral trocars takes place. The trocars should enter the abdominal wall lateral to the epigastric vessels.

10.9.3 Exposure and Identification of Operative Field

In the extraperitoneal approach, the vas deferens and the umbilical ligaments are adherent to the peritoneum, thus they are retracted cephalad upon the creation of the working space. The following landmarks should be identified prior to any surgical intervention:

- The pectineal ligament
- The external iliac vein and artery
- The vas deferens
- The epigastric vessels
- The site of the obturator fossa

In obese patients, external iliac vessels can be found covered by a fat layer. Using blunt gentle dissection of the fatty tissue, the vessels can be identified. The palpation of external iliac artery can be used as a landmark for the above maneuver.

10.9.4 Lymph Node Group Dissection

The extraperitoneal approach does not allow the performance of extended lymphadenectomy as described previously. Standard dissection can be performed with excision of LN groups at the site of external and internal iliac arteries while not including the common iliac artery LNs. The anatomical boundaries of the LN group dissection are similar to the transperitoneal approach. In case of extraperitoneal approach, vas deferens does not have to be ligated since it is retracted by the peritoneum cephalad. Instead of vas deferens, the umbilical ligament can serve as a structure facilitating medial retraction. The latter maneuver is performed by the assistant using a grasper. The LNs are located just medial to the external iliac vein. The procedure will now follow the same route as in the transperitoneal approach, excising the borders of LN group in the same sequence: the external, internal, inferior, posterior, and finally the superior limit of LN group.

10.9.5 Termination of the Procedure

Termination of extraperitoneal approach follows the same steps as with the transperitoneal approach. Nevertheless, after careful hemostasis bilateral peritoneal fenestration should be performed. The extraperitoneal approach is associated with a higher incidence of postoperative lymphocele due to lack of space to host any leaking lymph from the dissected lymphatics. Symptomatic lymphoceles represent a significant postoperative complication of the extraperitoneal approach (up to 3.8%). Fenestration of the peritoneum diminishes the aforementioned disadvantage of extraperitoneal approach.[17]

10.10 Postoperative Management

Postoperative antibiotics are not usually indicated except for cases of bowel perforation or other complications. The urinary catheter should be left in place usually for 1 day. Concomitant laparoscopic radical prostatectomy requires additional catheterization period. When drains are placed, they should be clamped on the first postoperative day and unclamped the same evening. If the outflow of lymph fluid is insignificant, the drain can be removed since the prolonged presence of drain induces the production of lymph fluid. Food should be restricted until the return of bowel function. Light food is usually allowed on postoperative day 1 and subcutaneous administration of low molecular weight heparin (LMWH) for 10 days is recommended as a prevention measure for deep vein thrombosis. The patient is discharged on postoperative day 1 or 2 depending on the return of both preoperative general condition of the patient and bowel function.

In our institutions, the catheter is removed on first postoperative day in case of pelvic lymphadenectomy and on the fifth postoperative day in cases of concomitant laparoscopic/endoscopic radical prostatectomy. Liquid diet is allowed on the first evening after the operation. LMWH is administered as described earlier. Ultrasonographic examination takes place on the day of discharge in order to detect any lymphocele formation.

10.11 Complications

Complications associated with laparoscopic pelvic lymphadenectomy can be categorized into three categories: complications associated with any laparoscopic surgery, complications associated with the surgery of the pelvic floor, and finally complications associated with the dissection of the lymphatics.

10.11.1 General Laparoscopic Surgery

Complications associated with any laparoscopic surgery include hypercapnia and acidosis and hypoxemia due to CO_2 pneumoperitoneum and steep Trendelenburg position that do not allow proper expansion of the diaphragm. The anesthesiologist should be familiar with the appropriate setup for laparoscopy in order to avoid the above-mentioned complications.[18] Moreover, gas embolism during Veress needle insertion and subcutaneous emphysema at the site of trocar insertion are possible but very rare complications. Significant cause of postoperative morbidity is injury of vessels and/or organ injury during trocar placement. The insertion of trocars under visual control and the use of trocars with blunt obturator are methods to avoid injury. Postoperative bleeding from the epigastric vessels represents one of the most common bleeding complications in our experience with laparoscopic radical prostatectomy and pelvic lymphadenectomies.[19] Bleeding complications frequently require re-intervention and consequently represent significant cause of postoperative morbidity. Rare but significant complications are the postoperative infection and hernia formation at the sites of trocar placement.

10.11.2 Pelvic Floor Surgery

Associated with the surgery of the pelvic floor are the injuries of vessels related to LN dissection (mainly the external iliac vessels). In case of vein injury, bleeding can be controlled by tamponnade or selective suturing.[16] The injury of the external iliac artery is a devastating complication since a large lesion and significant bleeding could compromise visibility of the operative field. A confident laparoscopist could manage the complication by selective suturing. Otherwise, open conversion should take place. Obturator nerve injury can be identified postoperatively as transient or permanent (in case of nerve ligation) neuropraxia. We have observed 0.2% of obturator nerve apraxia in our series of more than 940 PLAs.[17] For any obturator vein bleeding, vein ligation and clip appliance is suggested for bleeding control. Additional complications are ureteral injury as well as urinary bladder and bowel perforation. The ureteral injury occurs more easily in transperitoneal approach cases, since the ureter can be mistaken for vas deferens and ligated. Our experience with the extraperitoneal approach does not include any ureteral injury due to PLA, since the ureter is usually adherent and retracted upwards with the peritoneum away from the operative field. In addition, we have never encountered any urinary bladder or bowel perforation. These complications could take place during dissection or trocar insertion. Careful dissection and direct visual control trocar insertion are adequate for complication prevention.[16]

10.11.3 Dissection of the Lymphatics

The main complication related to the dissection of the lymphatics is the creation of lymphocele, which is reported to be more frequent in the case of the extraperitoneal approach. The incidence of symptomatic lymphoceles with the extraperitoneal approach was observed to be 3.8% of the PLA cases.[19] Nevertheless, the fenestration of peritoneum at the end of the procedure significantly reduces lymphocele formation. In fact, the incidence of lymphocele in the latter case appears to be equal in both trans- and extraperitoneal approach.[17] Moreover, edema of lower extremities and deep vein thrombosis has been reported to occur in a frequency related to the extent of LN dissection. The more LNs dissected the higher incidence of these complications.[9]

10.12 Advantages and Pitfalls of the Technique

The main advantage of transperitoneal approach is the presence of a preexisting working place that allows an easy trocar placement and a large operative field. Moreover, it is suitable for the extended LN dissection allowing access to the cephalad LN groups, around aorta and common iliac vessels. The access of LNs through the peritoneal cavity provides communication of the dissected area with the wide space of peritoneal cavity which drains any postoperative lymph extravasation. Thus, the risk of lymphocele formation is reduced. Nevertheless, the presence of intraperitoneal organs in the operative field is related to an increased risk of organ injury, such as bowel perforation. Moreover, the transperitoneal approach might require the aforementioned colon mobilization from the parietal layer of the peritoneum which increases the risk of colon perforation due to the use of coagulation. In case of a prior intra-abdominal surgery, the operative field could be significantly altered due to the presence of adhesions. The latter phenomenon adds challenging difficulties to the procedure. During the performance of transperitoneal PLA, the ureter can be mistaken for vas deferens and ligated resulting in significant postoperative morbidity.[13]

The main advantages of extraperitoneal approach are the lack of interference from intraperitoneal organs that minimizes the risk of bowel injury and the ease to be performed in case of the presence of intraperitoneal adhesions. However, the extraperitoneal approach provides the potential to perform only standard lymphadenectomy including the LNs of external and internal iliac vessels but not those of common iliac vessels. In addition, the benefit of the extended dissection at the level of the common iliac vessels is not clearly proven. An extended PLA is not feasible by the extraperitoneal approach due to the peritoneum and its content protrusion towards the upper half of the abdominal cavity. As a result, the pelvic vessels from the level of the bifurcation of common iliac vessels and above are not accessible. In addition, lymphocele formation is reported to be higher with the extraperitoneal approach. In our department, fenestration of peritoneum at the end of the procedure diminishes the incidence of lymphocele formation to the level of the transperitoneal approach despite the use of extraperitoneal approach.[17]

10.13 Summary

In summary, transperitoneal and extraperitoneal laparoscopic PLA have been proven feasible, safe, and effective and can be regarded as the gold standard surgical approach of LN evaluation in case of PCa. Large retrospective studies using data derived from the growing multicenter experience in PLA are expected to increase the potential of predictive nomograms in the near future and limit PLA application only to patients that will be most benefited, since high concomitant morbidity has to be balanced against the possible therapeutic effects of the procedure. Moreover, the evolution of noninvasive or minimal invasive LN screening techniques is expected to replace PLA as soon as several drawbacks such as the cost-effectiveness and the accuracy of prediction are addressed.

References

1. Briganti A, Chun FK, Salonia A, et al. A nomogram for staging of exclusive nonobturator lymph node metastases in men with localized prostate cancer. *Eur Urol*. 2007;51:112-120.
2. Sivalingam S, Oxley J, Probert JL, et al. Role of pelvic lymphadenectomy in prostate cancer management. *Urology*. 2007;69(2):203-209.
3. Liatsikos E, Kallidonis P, Stolzenburg JU. Management of lymph nodes in early prostate cancer. *Minerva Urol Nefrol*. 2008;60(1):41-49.
4. Briganti A, Blute ML, Eastham JH, et al. Pelvic lymph node dissection in prostate cancer. *Eur Urol*. 2009;55(6):1251-1265.
5. Prostate Cancer. AUA 2007 Highlights. http://cme.medscape.com/viewarticle/559037. Accessed May 7, 2007.
6. Briganti A, Chun FK, Salonia A, et al. Validation of a nomogram predicting the probability of lymph node invasion based on the extent of pelvic lymphadenectomy in patients with clinically localized prostate cancer. *BJU Int*. 2006;98:788-793.

7. Studer UE, Collette L. Morbidity from pelvic lymphadenectomy in men undergoing radical prostatectomy. *Eur Urol.* 2006;50:887-892.
8. Briganti A, Chun FK, Salonia A, et al. Validation of a nomogram predicting the probability of lymph node invasion among patients undergoing radical prostatectomy and an extended pelvic lymphadenectomy. *Eur Urol.* 2006;49:1019-1027.
9. Heidenreich A, Bolla M, Joniau S, et al. Guidelines on prostate cancer. *Eur Urol.* 2008;53(1):68-80.
10. Graefen M. Editorial comment on: is pelvic lymph node dissection necessary in patients with a serum PSA < 10 ng/ml undergoing radical prostatectomy for prostate cancer? *Eur Urol.* 2006;50:272-279.
11. Winfield HN, Cadeddu JA. Laparoscopic pelvic lymph node dissection. In: *Campbell's Urology.* 8th ed. Philadelphia: Saunders; 2002:3687-3690.
12. Borley N, Fabrin K, Sriprasad S, Mondaini N, et al. Laparoscopic pelvic lymph node dissection allows significantly more accurate staging in "high-risk" prostate cancer compared to MRI or CT. Scand J *Urol Nephrol.* 2003;37(5): 382-6.
13. Liatsikos E, Rabenalt R, Burchardt M, et al. Prevention and management of perioperative complications in laparoscopic and endoscopic radical prostatectomy. *World J Urol.* 2006;24(6):668-675.
14. Stolzenburg JU, Wasserscheid J, Rabenalt R, et al. Reduction in incidence of lymphocele following extraperitoneal radical prostatectomy and pelvic lymph node dissection by bilateral peritoneal fenestration. *World J Urol.* 2008;26(6):581-586.
15. Stolzenburg JU, Aedtner B, Olthoff D, Foenig F, et al. Anaesthetic considerations for endoscopic extraperitoneal and laparoscopic extraperitoneal radical prostatectomy. *BJU Int.* 2006;98:508-513.
16. Stolzenburg JU, Rabenalt R, Do M, et al. Endoscopic extraperitoneal radical prostatectomy: the University of Leipzig experience of 2000 cases. *J Endourol.* 2008;22(10): 2319-2325.
17. Mattei A, Fuechsel FG, Bhatta Dhar N, et al. The template of the primary lymphatic landing sites of the prostate should be revisited: results of a multimodality mapping study. *Eur Urol.* 2008;53:118-125.
18. Heidenreich A, Ohlmann CH, Polyakov S. Anatomical extent of pelvic lymphadenectomy in patients undergoing radical prostatectomy. *Eur Urol.* 2007;52:29-37.
19. Schumacher MC, Burkhard FC, Thalmann GN, et al. Is pelvic lymph node dissection necessary in patients with a serum PSA <10 ng/ml undergoing radical prostatectomy for prostate cancer? *Eur Urol.* 2006;50:272-279.

Laparoscopic Simple Prostatectomy

11

Xavier Cathelineau, Rafael E. Sanchez-Salas, Eric Barret,
Francois Rozet, Marc Galiano, and Guy Vallancien

Abstract Open prostatectomy is a long accepted method of treating patients with large hyperplasic glands. New therapeutic options have demonstrated efficiency and safety for high volume benign prostatic hyperplasia (BPH). Minimally invasive laparoscopic and endourological treatments have reproduced similar results to open simple prostatectomy with some clinical advantages. Results indicate that laparoscopic simple prostatectomy is a viable option for the surgical treatment of BPH. Available clinical series evidence that in patients with BPH and formal surgical indication, surgery could be safely and properly performed by a laparoscopic technique. Publications concerning laparoscopic simple prostatectomy (LSP) or laparoscopic adenomectomy are mostly based on non experimental studies, such as comparative studies, correlation studies and case reports. The studies underpinning this current chapter were identified through a systematic research using PubMed. There are no randomized or high levels of evidence studies available for LSP. Our objective is to present the available experience in laparoscopic simple prostatectomy which, in our view, is a reproducible, effective procedure for removal of large prostatic adenomas with overall low perioperative morbidity.

Keywords Adenomectomy • Benign prostatic hyperplasia • Extraperitoneal approach • Laparoscopy • Laparoscopic simple prostatectomy • Minimally invasive surgery

X. Cathelineau (✉)
Department of Urology, Institut Montsouris,
42 Bd. Jourdan, Paris 75014, France
e-mail: xavier.cathelineau@imm.fr

Key Points

- LSP is a safe and feasible procedure for BPH surgical treatment. The laparoscopic version of the operation requires previous minimally invasive experience.
- The hybrid technique combines the benefits of minimally invasive surgery and digital enucleation of the adenoma.
- The learning curve of LSP is about 50 cases when assessing incidence of complications.
- The novel minimally invasive techniques, NOTES-LESS and robotic surgery will sure play a role in future development of adenoma's surgical approach.
- Open adenomectomy remains the surgical gold standard for the treatment of high volume prostatic adenomas.

11.1 Benign Prostatic Hyperplasia Surgical Treatment: The Rationale for LSP

Benign prostatic hyperplasia (BPH) is a very common benign disease in men; lower urinary tract symptoms (LUTS) are referred by 30% of men older than 65 years.[1] Currently, transurethral resection of the prostate (TURP) remains the gold standard for the surgical treatment of benign prostate hyperplasia for adenomas with volume larger than 30 cc. There is a group of 10% of the patients who do not benefit from TURP, and its major limitation is related to prostate volume and shape which determines a prolonged operative time for resection and may

J.V. Joseph and H.R.H. Patel (eds.), *Retroperitoneal Robotic and Laparoscopic Surgery*,
DOI: 10.1007/978-0-85729-485-2_11,

have an impact on treatment modality. Comorbidities such as urolithiasis, bladder diverticula, inguinal hernia and hip anquilosis might also limit the use of TURP.[2-7] Meanwhile, a group of novel minimally invasive techniques have emerged for the surgical treatment of BPH.[8-10] Among these, Holmium laser has been shown to be superior to other therapeutic options.[11]

Open simple prostatectomy (OSP) has the advantage of complete enucleation of high volume adenomas not amenable to TURP or other minimally invasive management options. Even with all the vascular control techniques, it remains a morbid surgical procedure with significant blood loss and hospital stay.[12,13] Experience with OSP is extensive, with the largest published series of open prostatectomy at 1,800 patients.[14] While fewer OSPs are performed in the western countries due to emerging therapies such as laser prostatectomy, the functional outcomes offered by OSP are comparable to those of TURP,[15] and these results could be achieved by a laparoscopic version of the procedure. The surgical development of laparoscopy brought back an interest in simple prostatectomy as an option for the surgical treatment of BPH. The laparoscopic experience gained with the treatment of prostate carcinoma enhanced the surgical possibilities of performing a simple prostatectomy.[16,17] Several authors[18-21] have reported the advantages for the patients treated in series of laparoscopic simple prostatectomy, which are those claimed for any laparoscopic procedure (lower blood loss, less pain, and shorter convalescence). We present our experience and the role of laparoscopy for simple prostatectomy.

11.2 Surgical Technique for LSP

Both intraperitoneal and extraperitoneal laparoscopic surgical techniques as well as transcapsular (Millin) and transvesical techniques have been reported. In our institution, although we initially explored the feasibility of a transvesical approach, we now perform a hybrid of open and laparoscopic principle approaches, which include:

- A transcapsular incision close to the bladder neck, which avoids potential bleeding from the midportion of the prostate;
- A plane of enucleation completed by inserting the finger through a suprapubic port site; and
- A finger in the rectum assisting the suprapubic finger dissection.

Vascular control can be achieved by suturing, as performed in the classic Millin procedure. We reliably use laparoscopic bipolar energy forceps.

11.2.1 Millin Hybrid Technique

Preoperative prophylactic antibiotics and antithrombotic therapy are administered. Patient under general anesthesia is positioned in a slight Trendelenburg position with legs abducted 30°. An infraumbilical incision is made and an extraperitoneal space is created by the use of finger and balloon dissection.

Four ports are used: two 10-mm ports and two 5-mm ports. One 10-mm port is placed infraumbilically for the camera and the other 10-mm port is placed in the midline between the umbilicus and the pubic bone. The two 5-mm ports are placed on the left and right sides, halfway between the umbilicus and the anterior superior iliac spine (Fig. 11.1).

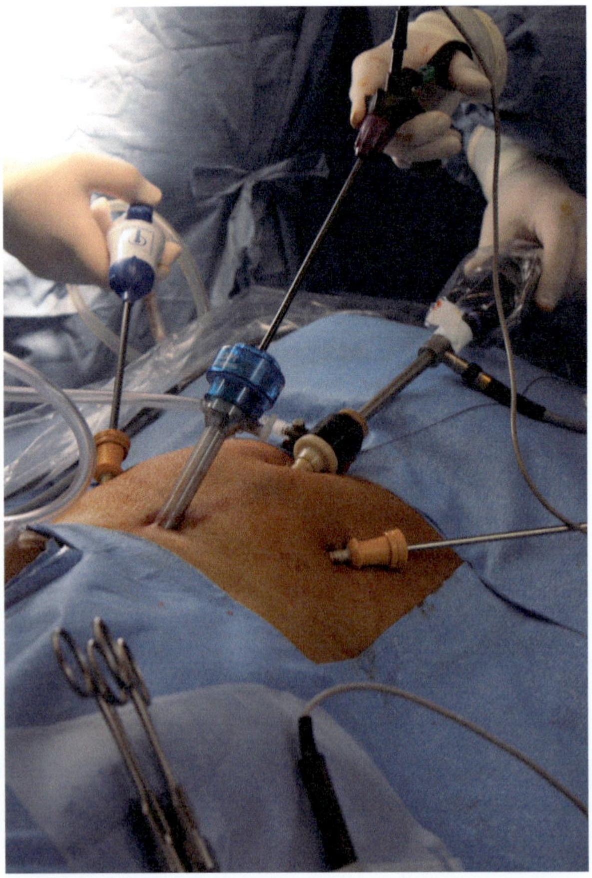

Fig. 11.1 Trocar positioning for LSP. Montsouris technique

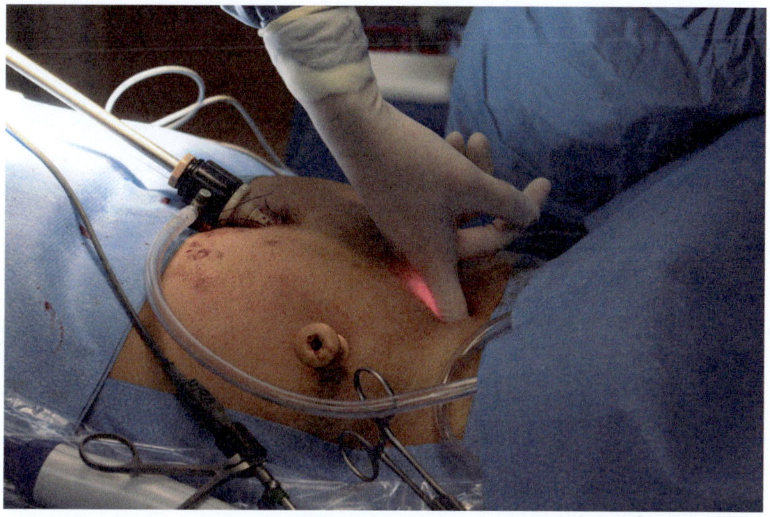

Fig. 11.2 Hybrid technique for LSP. Manual enucleation of the adenoma

Pneumoextraperitoneum is created at 12 mmHg, and after the anterior surface of the prostate is clear of fatty tissue, the prostatic capsule is incised transversely close to the bladder neck. Bipolar electrocautery is used to perform the enucleation of the adenoma. The suprapubic 10-mm port is removed at this point of the procedure, and the right index finger of the operator is inserted through this site to perform a manual enucleation of the adenomatous tissue (Fig. 11.2). The left index finger inserted in the rectum concurrently assists in elevating the prostate toward the anterior abdominal wall. Careful attention is paid to the apex of the prostate in order to maintain the integrity of the urethral sphincter.

Once the adenoma is separated from the capsule, a specimen retrieval bag is used to remove it through the infraumbilical incision. The camera port is replaced and any residual bleeding is controlled with the use of bipolar clamps. Trigonization is performed by reapproximating the posterior prostatic urethra using two stitches of polyglactin 3–0 at 5- and 7-o'clock positions. A 22 F three-way Foley catheter is placed under direct vision, and prostatic capsule is closed using 0-polyglactin. A closed suction drain is placed in the space of Retzius, the ports are closed and catheter connected to bladder irrigation.

11.2.2 Transvesical Technique

For the transvesical technique we use a technique with five ports as described for our radical prostatectomy approach. Once an extraperitoneal space is created, a longitudinal incision is performed in the anterior aspect of the bladder and extended toward the prostatic capsule using scissors and bipolar coagulation. Stay sutures are placed at the edges of the bladder incision and fixed to Cooper's ligament on each side. The bladder neck is circumscribed, remaining anterior to the ureteral orifices. The anterior and posterior planes between the adenoma and prostatic capsule are developed using blunt and sharp dissection. Once the plane between the prostatic capsule and adenoma is achieved, laparoscopic shears and bipolar forceps are deployed to enucleate the specimen completely. Counter traction on the capsule with a toothed grasper helped to facilitate exposure of the appropriate plane. Capsular hemostasis was achieved using bipolar cautery. A catheter is inserted into the bladder and the incision is closed using a running suture.

11.3 Institut Montsouris Experience in LSP

From January 2003 through January 2008, 101 consecutive patients underwent adenomectomy by an extraperitoneal laparoscopic transcapsular (Millin) approach at our institution. Medical therapy was initially attempted and had failed in all patients. Mean operative time was 95 min (62–128) with a mean total catheter time of 5.2 days (3–8) and a mean hospital stay of 6.3 days (4–8). The most common complication was hemorrhage, occurring in 27 (28.1%) patients. No urinary tract infections have been observed in these patients. We have verified in our setting that LSP offers advantages over its open counterpart in terms of shorter catheter time, shorter length of hospital stay, and fewer urinary tract infections.[22]

Although we have proved the feasibility of LSP in our setting, we kept in mind that our group holds an important experience in laparoscopic radical prostatectomy that eases the path toward other minimally invasive procedures. As LSP remains a potential surgical tool for BPH, our consideration was the following: How many cases do we need to become expert surgeons in this technique? This remains a controversial question that we still need to address in every urological minimal access surgery procedure. The arrival of laparoscopy and, later, the robotic interface has emphasized the importance of the "learning curve." In fact, laparoscopic series brought with them a tremendous enthusiasm in terms of validation of the technique and therefore extensive work in the procedure's learning curve.

To assess the process of obtaining proficiency in LSP we examined the outcomes from our first 101 LSP cases by dividing patients into one of two groups: Group 1, cases 1–50; Group 2, cases 51–101. There was no difference between the groups in terms of age, prostate volume, uroflow, IPSS score, or postvoid residual. There was a significant decrease in operative time between the two groups (107±28.6 min vs. 84±33.1 min; $p<0.001$). No significant difference was observed regarding mean blood loss (325 mL vs. 400 mL; $p=0.275$). Although minor complications were more numerous in the last 51 cases, major complications tended to decrease with time ($p=0.014$). The duration of bladder catheter tends to decrease after the 50th case ($p<0.001$). We have not only verified that LSP is safe with comparable outcomes to those published for open prostatectomy series but also that operative time can be effectively reduced with practice and we estimate the learning curve for this procedure to be 50 cases.[23]

11.4 LSP: Origins and Evolution

Laparoscopic simple prostatectomy is a viable option for the surgical treatment of BPH. Present clinical evidence shows that in patients with BPH and a formal surgical indication, surgery could be safely and properly performed by a laparoscopic technique (Table 11.1).[19,21,22,24-29]

As blood loss represents an issue, some authors have considered vascular control a crucial step in the operation. In their rationale, laparoscopy should mimic open techniques in the endoscopic environment and therefore time must be taken in vascular control as open surgeons have previously described for the simple prostatectomy.[5,12,24]

Mariano et al.[18] reported the first laparoscopic simple prostatectomy with vascular control for a 120 g adenoma with a blood loss of 800 cc and an operative time of over 3 h. The prostatic capsule and bladder neck were opened in the midline, and the adenoma was

Table 11.1 Series of laparoscopic simple prostatectomy

Series	# Patient	Approach	Catheter (days)	OR time (min)	EBL (mL)	Conversion	Complication (%)	Prost. vol. (g)
Van Veltoven et al.[19]	18	Millin	3	145	192	No	27.7	47.6
Rey et al.[26]	5	Millin/hybrid open-lap	–	95	–	No	–	>60
Sotelo et al.[21]	17	Transp. extrap	6.3	156	516	No	19	72
Mariano et al.[25]	60	Transp.	4.6	138	330	No	6.6	144.5
Porpiglia et al.[29]	20	Extrap.	6.3	127.2	411.6	No	5	94.2
Castillo et al.[24]	59	Extrap.	4.2	123	415.3	No	7.4	112
Baumert et al.[28]	30	Millin/transves.	4	115	367	No	–	–
Zhou et al.[27]	45	Millin	–	105	–	No	7	>60
McCullough et al.[22]	96	Millin/hybrid open-lap	5.2	95	350	No	28	111

dissected with harmonic scalpel and blunt dissection. The adenoma was removed and morcellated. Bladder neck hemostasis was accomplished with sutures at the 5- and 7-o'clock positions; bladder neck mucosa was then advanced to the prostatic fossa. In 2006 Mariano et al.[25] reported a series of 60 patients treated with their laparoscopic simple prostatectomy technique. The average prostate weight in this series was 144 g. They reported a mean operative time was 138 min. and a mean blood loss of 330 mL. No patient required transfusions or conversion to open surgery. Post operative complications included a case of septicemia and prolonged ileus. Retrograde ejaculation was verified in all patients after 6 months of follow-up. Functional results for this series were adequate: potency was preserved in all patients with preoperatively active sexual performance and no urinary incontinence was reported. The study by Mariano et al. is very interesting as it provides information not only on the technical details of LSP, but also on the quality of life issues of the operation.[25]

Van Velthoven et al.[19] presented 18 laparoscopic simple prostatectomies in which vascular control of lateral pedicles was also performed. In this series, mean operative time was 145 min and mean blood loss was 192 cc. They reported a mean specimen weight of 47.6 g. This feasibility study represents the first comprehensive approach for this surgical technique, and it has the value of being a multicenter study.

Rey et al.[26] published their experience in LSP in a short series of five patients in whom adenoma volume was higher than 60 g. The median operative time was 95 min. These authors performed a finger-assisted technique in three of their patients and a full laparoscopic approach in the other two. They report no use of opioid analgesia in the postoperative period.[26]

Sotelo et al.[21] reported a series of 17 laparoscopic simple prostatectomies with a mean operative time of 156 min, mean blood loss of 516 cc, and mean specimen volume of 72 g. These authors described the evolution of their technique, using different technical maneuvers to minimize intraoperative hemorrhage, including suture ligation of the dorsal vein complex after incising the endopelvic fascia and extravesical suture ligation of the lateral prostate pedicles. In their experience, none of those maneuvers reliably provided a bloodless field. Sotelo and colleagues stated that perhaps performing a capsulotomy directly over the anterior surface of the prostate gland transgressed the subcapsular venous plexus and consequently increased blood loss. They finally opted for an incision of the bladder neck just proximal to the prostatovesical junction and the creation of a posterior and posterolateral subcapsular plane that was then developed circumferentially. The latter technical modification was, in their experience, effective for decreasing blood loss. "It is important to maintain a thick prostate capsule, thus, minimizing violation of the subcapsular venous plexus."[21] At the IMM, we agree with this statement provided by the authors. In our experience, the finger assistance avoids an extensive capsular dissection which probably prevents excessive bleeding. Once the adenoma is dissected free from the capsule, an augmented field of vision allows selective hemostasis; the latter avoids deployment of lateral sutures at the posterolateral aspect of the prostate which could have an impact on potency. These authors have recently updated their experience in 71 patients treated with their technique with the average specimen weight of the excised prostate in this series equal to 84.86% of the gland weight estimated on preoperative transrectal ultrasound.[30]

Castillo et al.[24] presented a series of LSP with mean operative time and mean blood loss comparable with those in previous series; however, their mean specimen weight was higher (95.2 g, 40–150). They operated a total of 59 patients with median age of 65 years with extraperitoneal laparoscopic adenomectomy. All patients had a history of lower urinary tract symptoms (LUTS) and benign prostatic hyperplasia (BPH). Median International Prostate Symptom Score (IPSS) was 20. Their laparoscopic surgical technique included vascular control of dorsal venous complex and lateral bladder pedicles, cervicoscapular incision, and subsequent adenomectomy. All 59 adenomas were excised entirely by laparoscopy with no conversion to open surgery. Median operative time was 123 min with a median blood loss of 415 mL. Four patients (14.8%) in this series required blood transfusion. Two (7.4%) patients presented perioperative complications.

Median hospital stay and catheter time were 3.5 and 4.2 days respectively. They believe that the feasibility of laparoscopic simple prostatectomy for higher-volume adenomas depends on the implementation of a detailed vascular control as stated in the report by Rehman et al.[31] in their initial LSP. More recently Zhou et al.[27] assessed the feasibility of extraperitoneal laparoscopic prostatectomy in China. They performed LSP in 45 patients with prostatic weight more than 60 g. Surgical technique included: hemostatic control of lateral venous vesicoprostatic pedicles and transversal anterior incision of the prostate capsule for prostatic adenomectomy. The average prostate resected weight was 78.2 g with a mean operative time of 105.4 min. No conversion to open prostatectomy was necessary. Three were transfused. Follow-up of their series showed that after a 6-month period, 40 patients had improvement on objective urinary symptoms (mean IPSS score decreased from 25.5 to 6.2 and maximum urine flow [Qmax] Increased from 6.1 to 18.7 mL/s) and any patient presented with urinary incontinence.

This work provides early objective follow-up information which is necessary to validate the outcomes of the procedure.

It would be of utmost importance to establish an objective comparison between open and laparoscopic simple prostatectomy, but a prospective randomized trial to compare these two techniques is unlikely to occur when there is a wider spectrum of minimally invasive procedures for the treatment of BPH, and comparison efforts at this point tend to look at the efficacy of techniques such as holmium laser enucleation of the prostate (HoLEP).[11,32]

Our group has recently reported a comparative study of 280 patients who underwent simple prostatectomy at our institution. Patients underwent either an extraperitoneal laparoscopic (96 patients, 34.3%) or open transvesical (184 patients, 65.7%) prostatectomy.

These patients, for whom medical therapy had failed, were selected for simple prostatectomy by the standardized indications for this procedure. No specific selection criteria were deployed for patient recruitment to either laparoscopic or open groups. This is the largest group of patients undergoing LSP by either intra- or extraperitoneal approaches. The laparoscopic group had longer operative time (95 min vs. 54 min) but a shorter hospitalization period (6.3 days vs. 7.7 days) and shorter catheterization (5.2 days vs. 6.4 days). A limitation of our analysis was that the open group results were influenced by the presence of opening the bladder during the procedure. Because different techniques were deployed for open and laparoscopic techniques, objective comparisons are difficult to make. Interestingly, our series showed a higher rate of urinary tract infection (UTI) and urosepsis in the open surgery group. Eighteen patients of this group showed a culture-documented diagnosis of UTI. On the other hand we have not observed urinary infections in our patients treated by laparoscopy.

Baumert et al.[28] have also presented an interesting comparative study between laparoscopic and open simple prostatectomy that showed advantages in terms of lower blood loss (mean 367 cc), irrigation requirement, catheterization period, and hospital stay in the laparoscopy arm. They reported a mean specimen weight of 74 g and 81 g for their Millin and transvesical groups, respectively. Laparoscopic operative time was longer when compared to the open arm. The operative technique for LSP was changed during the study from a Millin-type procedure to a transvesical prostatic approach because enucleation of the adenoma was found to be difficult through a capsular incision, particularly with large glands or when a large median prostatic lobe was present. Removing concomitant bladder stones was described as easier with the transvesical prostatic approach. Extension of the bladder incision to the anterior aspect of the prostatic surgical capsule improved visualization during enucleation of the adenoma and hemostasis. There was no significant difference in the perioperative variables between the two laparoscopic techniques to suggest that one might be superior to the other. Porpiglia et al.[29] have also presented a non-randomized prospective comparative trial of transcapsular extraperitoneal adenomectomy (Millin) versus open surgery. They compared two groups of 20 patients each and concluded that both techniques were comparable, showing the laparoscopic group advantages in terms of perioperative blood loss.

11.5 LSP: Emerging Techniques

11.5.1 Robotic Simple Prostatectomy

With the arrival of robotic surgery and its improved benefits when compared to laparoscopy in terms of enhanced ergonomics and more dexterous instruments, several groups have developed and presented their techniques for robotic simple prostatectomy (Table 11.2)[33-38]. Recently Sotelo et al.[33] first reported applying the robotic interface to perform simple prostatectomy in seven cases, performed via a transperitoneal approach. Their average operative time was 205 min with a significant blood loss. Average hospital stay was 1.4 days and mean catheterization period was 7 days. Mean specimen weight on pathological examination was 50.48 g.

Table 11.2 Series of emerging techniques for laparoscopic simple prostatectomy

Series	# Patient	Approach	Catheter (days)	OR time (min)	EBL (mL)	Conversion	Complication (%)	Prost. vol. (g)
Sotelo et al.[33]	7	Transp robot	7	205	381	No	14	50
Yuh et al.[34]	3	Robot		211	558	No	No	300
John et al.[35]	13	Robot hybrid technique	6	210 Hybrid: 140	500 Hybrid: 250	No	No	82
Sotelo et al.[36,38]	21	Single port Transumbilical :1 Transvesical: 20	7	91	337	No	10	57
Desai et al.[37]	3	Single port	4	200	500	No	33	>90

Transfusion was necessary in one patient and no complications were observed. They verified considerable improvement from baseline IPSS score (preoperative vs. postoperative 22 vs. 7.25) and Qmax (preoperative vs. postoperative 17.75 vs. 55.5 mL/min). This minimally invasive approach also allowed the enucleation of adenoma without the need for special devices due to the advantages provided by the EndoWrist® of the robotic instrument. It also facilitates hemostatic control, resulting in less intraoperative blood loss. Interestingly, these researchers incorporated hemostatic control into their robotic technique. A previous report from the same group, on laparoscopic simple prostatectomy, did not feature hemostatic stitches in their surgical technique.[21]

Yuh et al.[34] also reported on the feasibility of robot-assisted retropubic prostatectomy. They treated three patients with important benign prostatic enlargement and bothersome lower urinary tract symptoms. Two of these patients had urinary retention. Their technique was a simple prostatectomy through a robot-assisted retropubic (Millin) approach. Average preoperative transrectal ultrasound estimated prostate volume exceeded 300 cc and a mean prostate-specific antigen (PSA) of 25.1. Estimated blood loss averaged 558 mL and mean operative time was 211 min. There were no perioperative complications. Mean hospital stay was 1.3 days and one patient required blood transfusion. As these authors state in their report, the extraction of a gigantic adenoma implies longer operative times and incision enlargement which could offset some of the advantages of the minimally invasive method.

John et al.[35] performed robot-assisted preperitoneal prostate adenomectomy for large benign adenomas. They operated 13 consecutive patients with a median age of 70 years where open adenomectomy was indicated. The total operative time was 210 min with a mean blood loss of 500 mL. No open conversion or transfusions were necessary. These authors deployed a similar hybrid technique to the one used at our institution, with single-finger assistance which they claimed improved the total operative time to 140 min and lowered blood loss to 250 mL. Mean specimen weight was 82 g. The indwelling catheters were removed after 6 days (range 3–15) and at a median follow-up of 13 months, patients showed a median flow rate of 23 mL/s without any postvoid residual urine.

Robotic LSP training as part of mainstream surgical training will be hard to accomplish. The main problems revolve around the inconsistencies of standard technique for LSP. Although, the important elements of robotic surgery actually enhance basic laparoscopic techniques and the prostate has been shown to be an organ where this new technology has a niche, in our opinion the robotic LSP harbors a prolonged operative time and the robotic interface itself remains expensive for this procedure when compared to other minimally invasive options.

11.5.2 NOTES-LESS Simple Prostatectomy

Natural orifice translumenal endoscopic surgery (NOTES) involves the intentional penetration of hollow viscera with an endoscope in order to access the abdominal cavity and perform an intraabdominal operation.[39] In 2002,

Gettman reported the first experience with NOTES, performing transvaginal nephrectomies in pigs.[40] Closely related to NOTES, laparo-endoscopic single-site surgery (LESS) describes minimally access surgical procedures that are performed through a single incision/location.[41] Rane et al. published the first true LESS experience in abstract form in 2007, performing a transumbilical laparoscopic nephrectomy.[42] Currently, the application of NOTES-LESS have been expanding in the clinical setting and several experiences have been published.

Sotelo et al.[30] presented their initial report on NOTES-LESS simple prostatectomy. They operated on a 67-year-old man who presented with acute urinary retention requiring catheterization. A transrectal ultrasound verified and adenoma volume of 110 mL. A LESS intraperitoneal simple prostatectomy was performed using a single multilumen port (R-port) inserted through a solitary 2.5-cm infraumbilical incision. Standard laparoscopic ultrasonic shears and needle drivers, articulating scissors, and specifically designed bent grasping instruments were used for dissection and suturing. No extraumbilical skin incisions were made. Total operative time was 120 min and estimated blood loss was 200 mL. No intra- or postoperative complications occurred. Hospital stay was 2 days and the catheter was removed at seventh postoperative day. Specimen weight was 95 g and revealed benign prostatic hyperplasia. At 3 months follow-up, the patient was completely continent and voiding spontaneously with a Q(max.) of 85 mL/s. This initial report opened the possibilities for NOTES-LESS approach in LSP, as it demonstrated technical feasibility and described a detailed surgical technique. Desai et al.[37] presented their initial report of a novel single-port transvesical enucleation of the prostate in three patients with large-volume benign prostatic hyperplasia. They performed a single-port transvesical enucleation of the prostates with volume higher than 90 mL. The R-port device was introduced percutaneously into the bladder through a 2.5-cm incision under cystoscopic guidance. After establishing pneumovesicum, the adenoma was enucleated in its entirety, transvesically under laparoscopic visualization using standard and articulating laparoscopic instrumentation. The mean operative time for the series was 3.3 h with a mean blood loss of 500 cc. One patient experienced a bowel injury occurred during port insertion; the injury was recognized and repaired intraoperatively and evolved uneventfully. The urethral Foley catheter was removed on day 4, and all patients were voiding spontaneously with a minimal postvoid residual volume and full continence. A transvesical approach represents an interesting proposal to explore in the future as it expands the limits of minimally access surgery.

Sotelo et al.[38] have also presented their initial experience in LESS simple prostatectomy surgery, through multichannel port, articulated instruments, and standard instruments adapted by others for the procedures. They performed both transumbilical simple prostatectomy (PSTU: 1) and transvesical (PSTV: 20). The mean operative time was 91 min with a mean estimated blood loss of 337 cc. Two patients presented hematuria as postoperative complication and underwent endoscopic exploration with satisfactory evolution. This series of 20 cases represents an interesting experience, and it is expected that these authors will follow with publications pertaining to evolution of their technique and results.

NOTES-LESS may represent a new step forward in reducing the morbidity and speeding the recovery from urologic procedures. However, there is much to be done before these techniques become standard in the urologic armamentarium.

11.6 LSP: Disadvantages

LSP includes an increased operative time when compared with any other surgical treatment for BPH. This procedure has a long learning curve and laparoscopic competency is mandatory. Most authors have presented their results on a small number of patients. Clearly this procedure is still in development, with the optimal approach not yet defined and an interesting group of emerging laparoscopic techniques presented as novel options for LSP.

It is important to remember that medical therapy and the novel minimally invasive surgical procedures for BPH remain very expensive and non-reachable worldwide. There are certain environments around the world where open prostatectomy remains the unique therapeutic tool,[19] and we might consider that the laparoscopic version could represent a good option for surgery. Still, there is a wide therapeutic armamentarium for BPH that would make the laparoscopic approach hard to accept by the medical community, as it still has drawbacks in terms of operative time and costs. Open surgery remains the standard treatment for high-volume adenomas.

11.7 Conclusions

LSP is an effective procedure for removal of large prostatic adenomas. In our experience this surgical technique has proved to be doable and reproducible. Although it seems to have less perioperative morbidity, its challenging learning curve needs to be addressed. Novel techniques for LSP need to be explored, standardized, and supported with larger clinical series.

Acknowledgements To former IMM fellows Drs. Jamison Jaffe, Shawn Soon, Casey McCullough, and Flavio Heldwein, who actively contributed to LSP experience at our institution.

Disclaimer

Financial disclosures: None

All authors have made a significant contribution to the findings and methods in the chapter. All authors have read and approved the final draft. There is no financial or commercial interest on this chapter.

References

1. Oelke M, Alivitazos G, Emberton M. Guidelines on benign prostatic hyperplasia. *Eur Urol.* 2004;46:547-554.
2. Tubaro A, Simon C, Ahmad H, et al. A prospective study of the safety and efficacy of suprapubic transvesical prostatectomy in patients with benign prostatic hyperplasia. *J Urol.* 2001;166:172.
3. Luttwak Z, Lask D, Abarbanel J, et al. Transvesical prostatectomy in elderly patients. *J Urol.* 1997;157:2210.
4. Koshiba K, Egawa S, Ohori M, et al. Does transurethral of the prostate pose a risk to life? 22-year outcome. *J Urol.* 1995;153:1506.
5. Sandhu JS, Te AE. Open prostatectomy. *Atlas Urol Clin.* 2002;10:17.
6. Shaheen A, Quinlan D. Feasibility of open simple prostatectomy with early vascular control. *BJU Int.* 2003;93:349.
7. Lam SJ, Volpe MA, Kaplan SA. Transurethral resection and incisión of the prostate. *Atlas Urol Clin.* 2002;10:27.
8. Moody J, Lingerman JE. Holmium laser enucleation for prostate adenoma greater than 100gr.: comparison to open prostatectomy. *J Urol.* 2001;165:459.
9. Hoffman RM, MacDonald R, Slaton JW, et al. Laser prostatectomy versus transurethral resection for treating benign prostatic obstruction: a systematic review. *J Urol.* 2003;169:210.
10. Rainer K, Karin L. Transurethral holmium laser enucleation versus transvesical open enucleation for prostate adenoma greater than 100gr.: a randomised prospective trial of 120 patients. *J Urol.* 2002;168:1465.
11. Tan H, Gilling PJ, Kenneth KM, et al. A randomized trial comparing holmium laser enucleation of the prostate with transurethral resection of the prostate for the treatment of bladder outlet obstruction secondary to benign prostatic hyperplasia in large glands (40 to 200 grams). *J Urol.* 2003; 170:1270.
12. Walsh PC, Osterling JE. Improved hemostasis during simple retropubic prostatectomy. *J Urol.* 1990;143:1203.
13. Amen-Palma JA, Artega RB. Hemostatic technique: extracapsular prostatic adenomectomy. *J Urol.* 2001;166:1364.
14. Serreta V, Morgia G, Fondacaro L, et al. Open prostatectomy for benign prostatic enlargement in southern Europe in the late 1990's: a contemporary series of 1800 interventions. *Urology.* 2002;60:623.
15. Varkarakis I, Kyriakakis Z, Delis A, et al. Long term results of open transvesical prostatectomy from a contemporary series of patients. *Urology.* 2004;64:306.
16. Guillonneau B, El-Fettouh H, Baumert H, et al. Laparoscopic radical prostatectomy: oncological evaluation after 1000 case at Montsouris institute. *J Urol.* 2003;169:1261.
17. Cathelineau X, Cahill D, Rozet F, et al. Transperitoneal or extraperitoneal approach for laparoscopic radical prostatectomy: a false debate over a real challenger. *J Urol.* 2004; 171:714.
18. Mariano MB, Graziottin TM, Tefilli MV. Laparoscopic prostatectomy with vascular control for benign prostatic hyperplasia. *J Urol.* 2002;167:2582.
19. Van Velthoven R, Peltier A, Laguna MP, Piechaud T. Laparoscopic extraperitoneal adenomectomy (Millin): pilot study on feasibility. *Eur Urol.* 2004;45:103.
20. Blew BD, Fazio LM, Pace K, D'A Honey RJ. Laparoscopic simple prostatectomy. *Can J Urol.* 2005;12(6):2891-2894.
21. Sotelo R, Spaliviero M, Garcia-Seguí A, et al. Laparoscopic retropubic simple prostatectomy. *J Urol.* 2005;173:757.
22. McCullough TC, Heldwein FL, Soon SJ, et al. Laparoscopic versus open simple prostatectomy: an evaluation of morbidity. *J Endourol.* 2009;23(1):129-133.
23. Yun HK, Kwon JB, Cho SR, Kim JS. Early Experience with Laparoscopic Retropubic Simple Prostatectomy in Patients with Voluminous Benign Prostatic Hyperplasia (BPH). *Korean J Urol.* 2010 May;51(5):323-9.
24. Castillo O, Degiovanni D, Sanchez-Salas R, et al. Laparoscopic simple prostatectomy with precise vascular control: going back to basics. *Urology.* 2007;70(3 suppl):70.
25. Mariano MB, Tefilli MV, Graziottin TM, et al. Laparoscopic prostatectomy for benign prostatic hyperplasia – a six-year experience. *Eur Urol.* 2006;49(1):127-131.
26. Rey D, Ducarme G, Hoepffner JL, Staerman F. Laparoscopic adenectomy: a novel technique for managing benign prostatic hyperplasia. *BJU Int.* 2005;95(4):676-678.
27. Zhou LY, Xiao J, Chen H, et al. Extraperitoneal laparoscopic adenomectomy for benign prostatic hyperplasia. *World J Urol.* 2009;27(3):385-387.
28. Baumert H, Ballaro A, Dugardin F, Kaisary AV. Laparoscopic versus open simple prostatectomy: a comparative study. *J Urol.* 2006;175:1691-1694.
29. Porpiglia F, Terrone C, Renard J, Grande S. Transcapsular adenomectomy (Millin): a comparative study, extraperitoneal laparoscopy versus open surgery. *Eur Urol.* 2006;49:120-126.
30. Sotelo RJ, Garcia AJ, Carmona O, Banda E. Laparoscopic simple prostatectomy. Experience in 71 cases. *J Urol.* 2007; 177(suppl):578. abstract 1738.
31. Rehman J, Khan SA, Sukkarieh T, et al. Extraperitoneal laparoscopic prostatectomy (adenomectomy) for obstructing

benign prostatic hyperplasia: transvesical and transcapsular (Millin) techniques. *J Endourol*. 2005;19:491-496.
32. Moody JA, Lingeman JE. Holmium laser enucleation for prostate adenoma greater than 100 gm: comparison to open prostatectomy. *J Urol*. 2001;165:459.
33. Sotelo RJ, Clavijo R, Carmona O, et al. Robotic simple prostatectomy. *J Urol*. 2008;179:513-515.
34. Yuh B, Laungani R, Perlmutter A, et al. Robot-assisted Millin's retropubic prostatectomy: case series. *Can J Urol*. 2008;15(3):4101-4105.
35. John H, Bucher C, Engel N, et al. Preperitoneal robotic prostate adenomectomy. *Urology*. 2009;73(4):811-815.
36. Sotelo RJ, Astigueta JC, Desai MM, et al. Laparoendoscopic single-site surgery simple prostatectomy: initial report. *Urology*. 2009;74(3):626-630.
37. Desai MM, Aron M, Canes D, et al. Single-port transvesical simple prostatectomy: initial clinical report. *Urology*. 2008; 72(5):960-965.
38. Sotelo R, Astigueta JC, Carmona O, et al. Laparoendoscopic single site (LESS). *Actas Urol Esp*. 2009;33(2): 172-181.
39. Pearl JP, Ponsky JL. Natural orifice translumenal endoscopic surgery: a critical review. *J Gastrointest Surg*. 2008;12(7): 1293-1300.
40. Gettman MT, Lotan Y, Napper CA, et al. Transvaginal laparoscopic nephrectomy: development and feasibility in the porcine model. *Urology*. 2002;59(3):446-450.
41. Box G, Averch T, Cadeddu J, et al. Nomenclature of natural orifice translumenal endoscopic surgery (NOTES) and laparoendoscopic single-site surgery (LESS) procedures in urology. *J Endourol*. 2008;22(11):2575-2581.
42. Rané A, Rao P. Single-port-access nephrectomy and other laparoscopic urologic procedures using a novel laparoscopic port (R-port). *Urology*. 2008 Aug;72(2): 260-3;

Extraperitoneal Laparoscopic Radical Prostatectomy

12

Sarah P. Psutka and Douglas M. Dahl

Abstract Several trends emerged in recent years to create the possibility of performing complex minimally invasive surgery for prostate cancer. Radical prostatectomy is an operation in which surgical control of cancer and preservation of vulnerable bodily functions require great precision and experience. Only through the development of advanced videoscopic equipment, refined surgical tools, and pioneering surgical techniques has it been possible to achieve excellent outcomes for prostate cancer patients with minimally invasive surgery. In this chapter, the state of the art of laparoscopic radical prostatectomy (LRP) via an extraperitoneal approach will be reviewed. This chapter will detail the considerations for patient selection and preoperative preparation, choice of instruments, surgical technique, and postoperative management for extraperitoneal laparoscopic radical prostatectomy (eLRP). Complications and pitfalls of the techniques will be highlighted based on personal experience with this operation in over 1,300 patients and from the published literature.

Keywords Anastamosis • Complications • Extraperitoneal approach • Laparoscopy • Prior hernia repair • Prostate cancer • Radical prostatectomy

S.P. Psutka (✉)
Department of Urology, Massachusetts General Hospital, GRB 110255 Fruit Street, Boston 02114, MA, USA
e-mail: spsutka@partners.org

Key Points

- Important technical aspects of the eLRP
  - The creation of a preperitoneal space
  - Antegrade dissection of the prostate
- Return to preoperative urinary and sexual function following eLRP requires meticulous handling of tissues intraoperatively, and avoidance of electrocautery during dissection of the neurovascular bundles. We favor the use of harmonic scalpel and do not employ electrocautery at any time.
- Preoperative evaluation of patients is essential for choosing the appropriate patient for eLRP. We find that any patient with a history of surgical intervention in the space of Retzius (e.g. laparoscopic inguinal hernia repair with mesh) is contraindicated to undergo the extraperitoneal approach, but it offers significant advantages in terms of treating patients who have had multiple intraabdominal procedures or a history of intraabdominal pathology, obesity.
- Pathological and intraoperative variables are similar between the tLRP and eLRP, with minimal blood loss, short hospitalization, and similar pathological outcomes including surgical margins, and biochemical recurrence.
- The eLRP is associated with decreased risk of intraperitoneal injuries during laparoscopic access, and is reported to result in decreased rates of ileus and postoperative pain. Complications such as lymphocele, anastomotic urinary leak, and postoperative hemorrhage are confined to the preperitoneal space, which may facilitate diagnosis and management.

J.V. Joseph and H.R.H. Patel (eds.), *Retroperitoneal Robotic and Laparoscopic Surgery*,
DOI: 10.1007/978-0-85729-485-2_12, © Springer-Verlag London Limited 2011

12.1 Introduction

The rapid increase in the incidence of prostate cancer coincided with rapid advances in minimally invasive surgical techniques. The use of laparoscopic technique in surgery was first described in the early twentieth century.[1] With laparoscopy it became possible to greatly reduce the morbidity of abdominal surgery. In the early 1990s, laparoscopic cholecystectomy began to be the standard of care for treatment of gallbladder disease. The average patient was saved a morbid abdominal incision and hospital stay was significantly reduced. Because laparoscopic cholecystectomy is a fairly simple extirpative operation for benign disease and requires no reconstructive surgery, it was successfully accomplished with the relatively rudimentary videoscopic equipment available in the early years of laparoscopy. Image resolution and light intensity have substantially improved since then. The instruments of that era consisted of a small range of graspers, dissectors, and simple electrocautery devices. As surgeons became more comfortable with this relatively simple procedure, more refined instruments and powerful videoscopic devices were developed, allowing progressively more complex procedures to be attempted.

The difficulty for urologists in mastering laparoscopic techniques was that there was no technically simple, common procedure to afford the urologic surgeon a base of skills to advance to more complex procedures. Early pioneers into minimally invasive procedures in urologic surgery were successful in accomplishing radical nephrectomy, a complex extirpative procedure, but one that did not require any reconstructive surgical complement. Prostate cancer staging with laparoscopic pelvic lymphadenectomy was popular for a brief time, but was fraught with a high incidence of iliac vessel injury. Improved cross-sectional imaging, stage migration of earlier detection of prostate cancer, and accurate predictive algorithms such as the Partin tables meant that staging pelvic lymphadenectomy is now rarely indicated. It was not until 1997 that the first report of successful laparoscopic transperitoneal radical prostatectomy (tLRP) was published in a series of nine patients.[2]

Radical prostatectomy became a very common procedure for urologists in the 1990s. The incidence of early prostate cancer increased markedly with the introduction of PSA screening on a widespread basis. The first significant publication of a reproducible technique for laparoscopic radical prostatectomy (LRP) appeared in 2001.[3] It was this publication that sparked the worldwide interest in this technique. Pioneers of the laparoscopic approach to radical prostatectomy soon gained significant experience and made important refinements.[4]

During the rapid adoption and evolution of laparoscopic abdominal surgery, the feasibility of minimally invasive techniques applied to a wide range of urologic operations was demonstrated. The open retropubic radical prostatectomy held the firm ground as the gold standard for the treatment of healthy men with early stage prostate cancer. Minimally invasive techniques had a formidable task to prove that they were able to achieve the same high standards of safety and efficacy while reducing surgical morbidity. Radical prostatectomy is an operation where subtle differences in tissue handling may have a profound impact on the patient's health and quality of life. Combining both meticulous dissection to achieve successful cancer extirpation and complex reconstruction to achieve good bodily function, the laparoscopic radical prostatectomy is a highly challenging procedure. A consensus of experts in laparoscopic urologic surgery rated laparoscopic radical prostatectomy 'extremely difficult', the highest standard for complexity.[5]

This chapter will present the distillation of the wealth of lessons learned in less than a decade during which the extraperitoneal laparoscopic radical prostatectomy (eLRP) has become an important option in the surgical management of prostate cancer.

12.2 Indications and Contraindications

12.2.1 Oncologic Considerations

Laparoscopic radical prostatectomy is suitable for all patients in whom a surgical extirpation of the prostate is likely to offer a reasonable chance for cancer control. For the surgeon who is just learning the techniques of laparoscopic radical prostatectomy, the ideal candidate patient will have a clinical stage T1c or possibly T2a tumor with a Gleason score of 3 + 3. The patient should have a very small likelihood of harboring metastatic disease and therefore will not require staging lymphadenectomy. With the benefit of experience we currently offer this approach to patients even with high stage and high Gleason score, patients who have localized cancer recurrence following radiation therapy, and patients on experimental neoadjuvant chemotherapy protocols. In our series evaluating 1,000 consecutive men undergoing radical prostatectomy, there were no differences in positive margin rate between RRP and LRP in any Gleason grade or T stage, supporting the contention that LRP can provide oncologic control equal to an open approach.[6, 7]

12.2.2 Patient Comorbidities

A broad range of medical conditions may impact the decision to offer a patient radical prostatectomy. Unstable coronary artery syndromes, bleeding diatheses, and poor functional status may pose an unacceptable risk of complications for considering any surgery. Many common medical situations may inform the surgical approach.

Obesity may pose substantial difficulty for performance of RRP. We have found that obese patients remain candidates for LRP by experienced laparoscopists and this may be the preferred approach in this patient population. Brown et al. reported a series of 151 consecutive cases in which 97 nonobese patients were compared to 54 obese patients (35 patients with BMI 30–34.9, 14 with BMI 35–39.9, and 5 with BMI > 40), with the findings that although obesity significantly increased operative time (208 ± 43 vs. 192 ± 34 min, $p = 0.02$), it did not significantly impact the other intraoperative and postoperative surgical parameters they evaluated, including postoperative hemoglobin decrease, length of stay, positive margin rate, anastomotic leakage, biochemical recurrence, early postoperative urinary continence and erectile function.[8] In severely obese patients, we have anecdotally noted an increased incidence of bladder neck stenosis because of significant difficulty with performing the anastomosis given the distance to the deep pelvis and limitations with available equipments.

Though we have not studied it extensively, it is our observation that the extraperitoneal approach is particularly preferable to a transperitoneal laparoscopic or robotic approach in severely obese patients both physiologically and technically. eLRP requires a substantially less exaggerated Trendelenburg position than tLRP. The Trendelenburg position can significantly compromise functional residual capacity of the lungs of the obese patient and predispose them to pulmonary and cardiac complications.[9-11] With steep inclines, the patient's abdominal panniculus can weigh so heavily on his chest that mechanical ventilation is severely compromised. The more neutral positioning of the eLRP is likewise optimal for patients who are elderly or with limited pulmonary reserve as it avoids the steep Trendelenburg positioning. We have successfully completed eLRP in men in whom a transperitoneal robotic approach had been abandoned early in the case due to pulmonary complications from steep Trendelenburg position.

Laparoscopic surgery may be more complicated in patients who have undergone prior abdominal and pelvic surgery. LRP remains feasible and safe for most patients in the hands of experienced surgeons.[4, 12, 13] The extraperitoneal approach offers the additional advantage of avoiding entry into the peritoneum in those patients with a history of prior complicated abdominal surgeries such as appendectomy and colectomy. We have successfully performed eLRP in patients with complicated intraperitoneal surgical histories including colovesical fistula repair, penetrating trauma, and sigmoid colectomy.[9]

Initial reports of aborted open radical prostatectomy or LRP in the setting of prior laparoscopic mesh inguinal hernia repair secondary to an obliterated space of Retzius and the inability to penetrate or mobilize the mesh stapled to the pelvic sidewalls has also been reported.[14, 15] We and others have also demonstrated the safety of performing eLRP in patients with prior laparoscopic mesh inguinal and umbilical herniorrhaphy[16] via an extraperitoneal approach, however, the operation is made markedly more complicated when the retroperitoneum has previously been breached. Therefore, we consider prior laparoscopic extraperitoneal surgery to be a relative contraindication for eLRP. In this situation, it is recommended to take a transperitoneal approach. We have also seen patients in whom a RRP was abandoned after bleeding complications in dissecting the dorsal vein complex. tLRP was successful in these men.

Patients with larger prostates (>90 g) can safely be extirpated via a laparoscopic approach. Rodriguez et al. reported that while larger prostates were associated with increased time to Foley catheter removal (mean 3 days), increased blood loss (56 cc), and slightly prolonged LOS (9 h), there was no increase in blood loss, operative time, time to JP drain removal, risk of transfusion, or positive margin status.[9]

Relative contraindications for this procedure are largely determined by the surgeon's experience. As noted above, with increased experience, more challenging cases, such as patients with prior pelvic surgery or higher body mass index can be safely attempted. In general, we consider absolute contraindications to the extraperitoneal approach to include prior violation of the space of Retzius, such as in prior laparoscopic inguinal mesh herniorrhaphy, as above, abdominal wall infection, uncorrected coagulopathy, and significant systemic disease which would otherwise preclude the patient from undergoing general anesthesia.

Any active or prior inflammatory process of the extraperitoneal space or periprostatic fibrosis will greatly increase the technical difficulty of this procedure. We and others have successfully performed this procedure in patients with prior recto-vesical fistula, in the setting of prior acute or chronic prostatitis, following repeated transrectal biopsies, salvage following androgen deprivation therapy, brachytherapy, or external beam radiation therapy; however, these procedures should only be attempted in the more advanced stages of laparoscopic training.

12.3 Operative Technique and Considerations

12.3.1 Preoperative Preparation

The day prior to surgery, all patients take a clear liquid diet. In the afternoon, 150 mg of magnesium citrate is self-administered orally for bowel preparation followed by an overnight fast. Upon arrival to the operating room they receive a dose of antibiotics, generally Cefazolin (unless a documented allergy exists). We do not use perioperative heparin or anticoagulation, but all patients have compression stockings and pneumatic compression boots placed and activated prior to induction of anesthesia.

12.3.2 Patient Positioning

The patient is positioned in the supine position with the arms supinated and tucked to the patient's body. All bony prominences are padded. The legs are slightly abducted with a pillow behind the legs and the ankles padded, permitting a digital rectal examination prior to the procedure to confirm findings and identify new areas of concern. The patient lies on a vacuum beanbag and is secured in this position by conforming the beanbag to the body and securing it with 6-in. elastic tape from the shoulders to the contralateral side of the bed across the chest. The beanbag holds the patient securely to the bed and therefore allows the bed to be put in Trendelenburg without risk of slipping off the bed (Fig. 12.1a). The patient's anterior abdomen below the costal margin and perineum are prepared and draped in

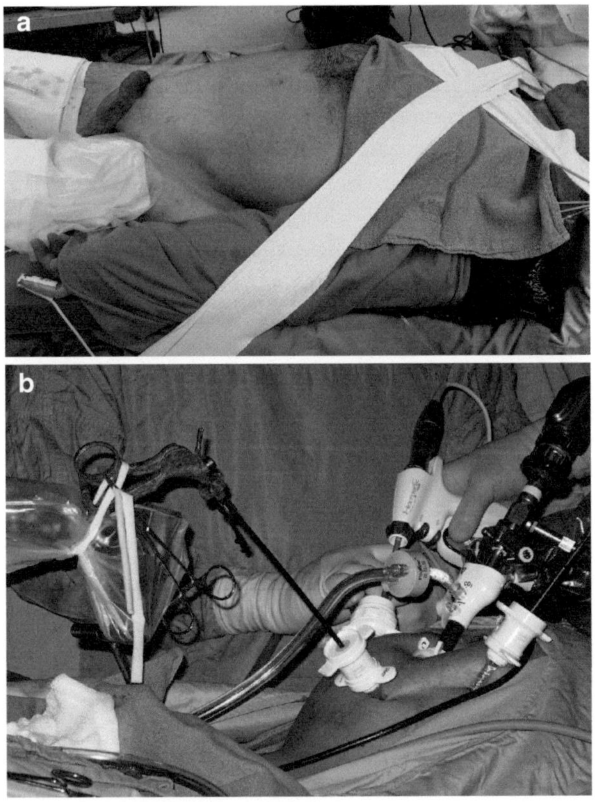

Fig. 12.1 (**a**) Patient positioning prior to extraperitoneal laparoscopic radical prostatectomy. Patients are positioned on a vacuum bean bag with the shoulder extensions draped over the shoulders and padded prior to deflation. Care is taken to avoid hyperextension of the shoulders to avoid injury to the brachial plexus. Tape is crossed over the torso to secure the patient to avoid injury when the table is positioned in steep Trendelenburg. (**b**) Setup of trocars and assistant arms. The AESOP robot is positioned to the left of the assistant and holds the camera in the infraumbilical port. The Civco arm is positioned to the right of the assistant and can secure both the urethral sounds as well as an additional grasper through an optional 5-mm working port in the superpubic region which can be helpful for retraction of the bladder anteriorly

the standard sterile manner. A Foley catheter is inserted on the sterile field and the bladder is drained. An orogastric tube is inserted by the anesthesia team.

We use a voice-activated AESOP robot (Computer Motion Inc., Bethesda, California) to control the laparoscopic camera. The robot arm is positioned superiorly on the right-hand side of the bed with the camera attachment just superior to the infraumbilical port where the camera will be secured and the robotic arm is set parallel to the patient's sternum (Fig. 12.1b).

Trans-urethral metal sounds are extensively used to assist in defining the bladder neck, retracting the prostate anteriorly during the posterior base dissection, obtaining hemostasis, and in defining the urethra. An adjustable laparoscopic instrument holder (Civco, Iowa) is invaluable in holding the sounds allowing stable retraction of the prostate during dissection. The arm is placed on the right-hand side of the operating table, next to the patient's upper leg. Additionally, anterior bladder neck retraction can be accomplished by securing a ratcheted grasper through a 5-mm suprapubic port to the Civco arm, which is useful during the antegrade dissection of the prostate posteriorly or in cases where the peritoneum is unintentionally violated.

The operative team consists of the surgeon, who stands on the patient's left, and an assistant, who stands on the patient's right between the robot and the Civco arm. The scrub nurse or technician stands to the left of the surgeon.

12.3.3 Operative Steps

12.3.3.1 Extraperitoneal Access

A 3-cm vertical incision is made 1 cm inferior to the umbilicus and the subcutaneous tissue is bluntly dissected down to the anterior rectus fascia. The fascia is then incised 1–2 cm lateral to the midline with a long-handled scalpel to create a 14-mm entry into the rectus muscle sheath. A large Kelly clamp is then introduced into this space directly beneath the anterior rectus sheath and gently dissects an initial space inferiorly to begin to develop the retropubic space. The first trocar is a 12-mm balloon port, which is integrated with the AutoSuture (OMS-PDBS2, United States Surgical, Tyco Healthcare Group, Norwalk, Connecticut) dissecting balloon. The 0° laparoscope is introduced

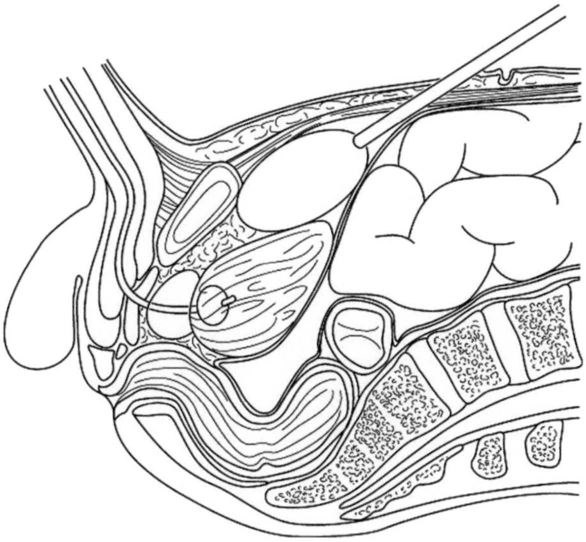

Fig. 12.2 Extraperitoneal access. The AutoSuture (OMS_PDBS2, United States Surgical, Tyco Healthcare Group, Norwalk, CT, USA) dissecting balloon is used to develop the preperitoneal space under direct vision with the 0° laparoscope

through the port and the balloon is inflated under direct vision to develop the preperitoneal space (Fig. 12.2). The dissecting balloon is deflated and removed, the balloon of the trocar is inflated then the lens is replaced and secured to the robotic arm. Pneumoretroperitoneum is established with insufflation pressure of 15 mmHg. At this point, the anterior aspect of the bladder, the pubic arch, and the external iliac vessels are visualized. The bed is placed in shallow Trendelenburg (10–15°).

A frequent complication of the retropubic dissection is disruption of the epigastric vessels and their branches to the anterior abdominal wall. We have had cases of delayed bleeding from these branches. It is important to carefully inspect the length of both epigastric vessels for avulsed tributaries. Even if they are not injured, the epigastric vessels frequently are left freely hanging in the surgical field and great care must be taken not to damage them (Fig. 12.3).

12.3.3.2 Trocar Placement

We use three working ports, in addition to the 12-mm infraumbilical camera port (Fig. 12.3). An 11-mm right paramedian port is placed approximately three finger breadths lateral to the median line and 5 cm inferior to the camera port, lateral to the rectus muscle. A blunt grasper

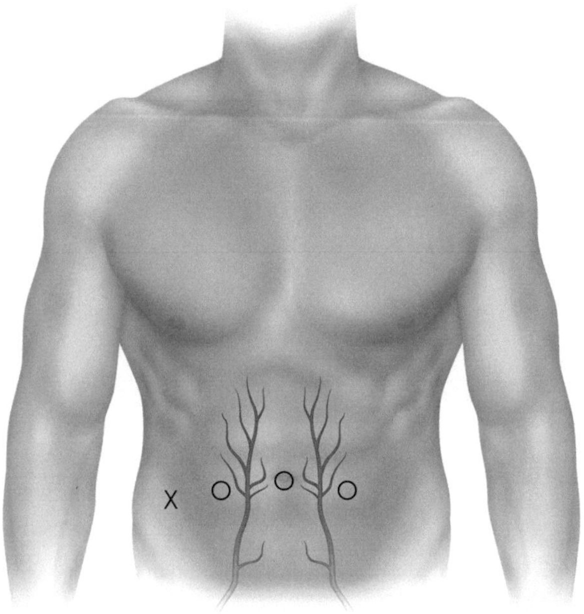

Fig. 12.3 Trocar positioning. Three working ports and one camera port are arranged as showed. O (infraumbilical): Camera Port (12 mm, Blunt Tip Trocar; United States Surgical), O (right paramedian): 11 mm working port, O (left paramedian): 11 mm working port. X: 5 mm working ports. Note that the inferior epigastric vessels are in close proximity to these ports. Care must be taken to avoid injury to these vessels during trocar insertion or while changing instruments

is placed through this port and used to complete the space between the spermatic cord and the epigastric vessels bilaterally. Then 5-mm ports are placed in the right lower quadrant, approximately 5 cm medial and superior to the anterior superior iliac spine and then on the left between the paramedian location and left lower quadrant. The inferior epigastric vessels run in close vicinity to the port placement sites and care must be taken to avoid injuring the vessels during port placement.

It is often cumbersome to develop the retropubic space. Because having an intact peritoneum allows the CO_2 gas to act as the retractor to expose the bladder and prostate for the surgery, it is worth the effort. If the peritoneum is violated, the peritoneal cavity will fill with CO_2, which will equilibrate with the retropubic space. Visualization will be hampered as the retropubic space is minimized and the use of suction or venting will preferentially collapse the extraperitoneal cavity. The greatest risk to breaching the peritoneum lies in the placement of the right lower quadrant trocar. If the peritoneum is inadvertently entered during trocar placement, then insufflation of the extraperitoneal cavity will be lost as pressure equalizes between the peritoneum and the space of Retzius.

Should the peritoneum be opened, mechanical retraction of the bladder can re-establish the working space. As noted above, an additional 5-mm trocar is placed in the region of the left lateral rectus border. The Civco arm can be used to hold a grasper, which is positioned to retract the bladder cephalad (see Fig. 12.1b).

We do not use a laparoscopic cautery device at any point during the eLRP. All dissections are performed with a 5-mm curved harmonic scalpel ACE (Ethicon Inc., Somerville, NJ) or with the laparoscopic scissors. Using graspers in the left lateral rectus port and the harmonic scalpel, the right-handed surgeon completes any additional development of the preperitoneal space. The assistant controls the suction/irrigation to assist with retraction via the right lateral quadrant port.

12.3.3.3 Pelvic Lymph Node Dissection

In our practice all patients with clinical T2 or higher cancer, PSA level greater than or equal to ten, or Gleason sum greater than or equal to seven, have a staging modified pelvic node dissection. The technique is identical to that performed in the open RRP, using the same landmarks. The lymph node packets are dissected from the region between the external iliac vein from the iliac bifurcation to the inguinal ligament, the obturator nerve, and the lateral pelvic sidewall. The lymphovascular tissue is ligated with Hem-o-Lok clips (Weck, USA). An accessory obturator vein is often visualized during the dissection and may be either preserved or divided between hemostatic clips.

We encountered an unexpectedly high incidence of pelvic lymphoceles in the beginning of the transition from a trans-peritoneal LRP as described by Vallencien and Guilloneau to the extraperitoneal approach.[17] Because any incomplete ligation of the lymphatics will result in drainage into the peritoneal cavity where it is absorbed, it had not been clinically significant in the first 250 cases performed by a transperitoneal approach. After several cases in which the patients treated with eLRP developed symptomatic lymphoceles requiring intervention, we modified our lymphatic dissection technique. Exquisite care is taken to ligate all lymphatic vessels, and the Hem-o-Lok clips are used in place of the metal clips previously employed. There have been no cases of symptomatic lymphoceles in the past 600+ cases with this approach.

The successful treatment of three of our patients with the symptomatic lymphoceles was transperitoneal laparoscopic marsupialization of the lymphocele into the peritoneal cavity.

12.3.3.4 Incision of the Endopelvic Fascia

The superficial dorsal vein is found in the midline, between the puboprostatic ligaments. This is divided using the harmonic scalpel. The endopelvic fascia then is dissected on either side of the prostate, first by sweeping the soft tissue aside with the blunt grasper, and then the laparoscopic scissors are used bilaterally to incise the fascia along the margins of the prostate. The prostate is retracted contralaterally to provide countertraction and facilitate incision from the lateral puboprostatic ligaments superiorly around the lateral lobes of the prostate to expose the apex of the prostate. The lateral puboprostatic ligaments are divided as necessary and the lateral attachments of the levator muscle are peeled off the prostate.

Accessory pudendal arteries may be visualized at this point. Recent reports suggest that up to 30% of patients will have an accessory pudendal artery. In a series of 377 LRP patients by Secin et al., 83% of these were spared and there was no difference noted in the incidence of positive margins.[18, 19] It has been suggested by many authors that preservation of the accessory pudendal arteries results in improved functional outcomes with respect to postoperative potency. Therefore, if the accessory pudendal arteries are identified, they are preserved if possible.[20, 21]

The assistant and the surgeon coordinate to retract the prostate while the surgeon suture ligates the deep dorsal venous complex (DVC) distal to the apex using a 0-Vicryl suture on a CT-1 needle using a right-handed forehand stitch from right to left. This step will limit back bleeding later in the procedure. Optimal placement of the suture is achieved by directing the needle time laterally through the inferior border of the plexus of Santorini between the DVC and the urethra (Fig. 12.4).

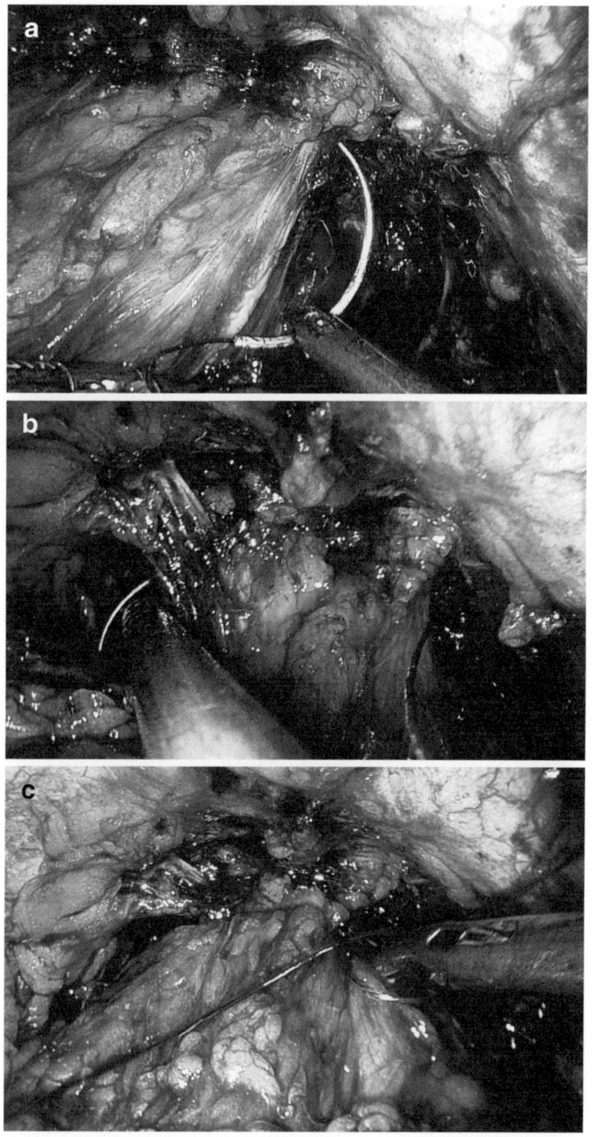

Fig. 12.4 Ligation of the dorsal venous complex. (**a**)The prostate is retracted to assist with suture ligation of the DVC distal to the prostate apex with a 0-Vicryl suture on a CT-1 needle using a right-handed forehand stitch. (**b**) This stitch is optimally placed by driving it diagonally through the tissue from right to left towards the contralateral iliac crest to encompass the entire DVC. (**c**) The completed suture ligation of the DVC minimizes back bleeding later in the procedure

12.3.3.5 Dissection of the Anterior Bladder Neck and Prostatic Pedicle Ligation, and Antegrade Neurovascular Bundle Preservation

The junction between the prostate and the bladder neck is identified by manipulating the Foley catheter balloon gently and by palpating the difference between the deflated bladder and the solid glandular tissue of the prostate. This is generally found approximately 2–3 cm proximal to the DVC suture. The harmonic scalpel is used to divide the venous tissue horizontally across the bladder neck. When the bladder is entered, the Foley catheter is removed and a metallic urethral sound is inserted. Retraction of the sound lifts the prostate anteriorly and facilitates the dissection of the lateral and posterior bladder neck. The sound is stabilized by the Civco arm, thereby freeing the assistant and surgeon's hands (see Fig. 12.1b).

12.3.3.6 Dissection of the Posterior Bladder Neck and Seminal Vesicles

As the bladder is entered, the ureteral orifices are identified laterally and the dissection is carefully continued across bladder mucosa crossing over the dorsal aspect of the prostate so as to preserve the orifices. An enlarged median lobe may also be identified at this point. In this case, the bladder neck is preserved by taking the dissection as close to the prostatic base as possible. This will minimize the degree of bladder neck reconstruction which will be required during the vesico-urethral anastomosis. As the incision between the posterior bladder and the prostate is developed, the posterior lip of the bladder neck is retracted cephalad.

As the posterior bladder is divided with the harmonic scalpel, the vasa deferentia are now identified and are dissected and divided harmonically close to the junction with the seminal vesicles. Following division of each vas deferens, they are held with a locking grasper and retracted anteriorly, to reveal the seminal vesicles, which are then dissected circumferentially to their junction with the prostate. The vascular supply to the seminal vesicles primarily enters laterally at the distal tip of the seminal vesicles in the seminal vesicle artery and multiple small vesicular vessels and can be taken with the harmonic scalpel, but rarely will require hemostatic clips. With the seminal vesicles and vasa retracted anteriorly, Denonvilliers' fascia is opened 1–2 mm posterior to the base of the prostate (Fig. 12.5). Blunt dissection in the midline between the prostate and the anterior rectum will help to develop the posterolateral vascular pedicles.

12.3.3.7 Hydrodissection of the Prostatic Capsule, Sparing of the NVB and Posterior Dissection of the Prostate

Once freed, the seminal vesicles and the vasa can be used to retract the prostate anteriorly to the contralateral side of the lateral pedicle and neurovascular bundle (NVB). The pedicle is taken harmonically distal to the NVB. Care must be taken at this point as the NVB lies in close proximity to the lateral pedicles of the prostate. When the pedicles are clearly defined, they are ligated with a clip and divided (Fig. 12.6).

An 18-gauge laparoscopic cyst aspiration needle is introduced through the lateral working ports and inserted on the anterolateral capsule of the prostate. Then 20–30 cc of 1:10,000 epinephrine solution diluted in buffered Ringers Lactate is injected to hydrodissect the interfascial plane of dissection laterally along the prostate[22] (Fig. 12.7). The harmonic scalpel or cold

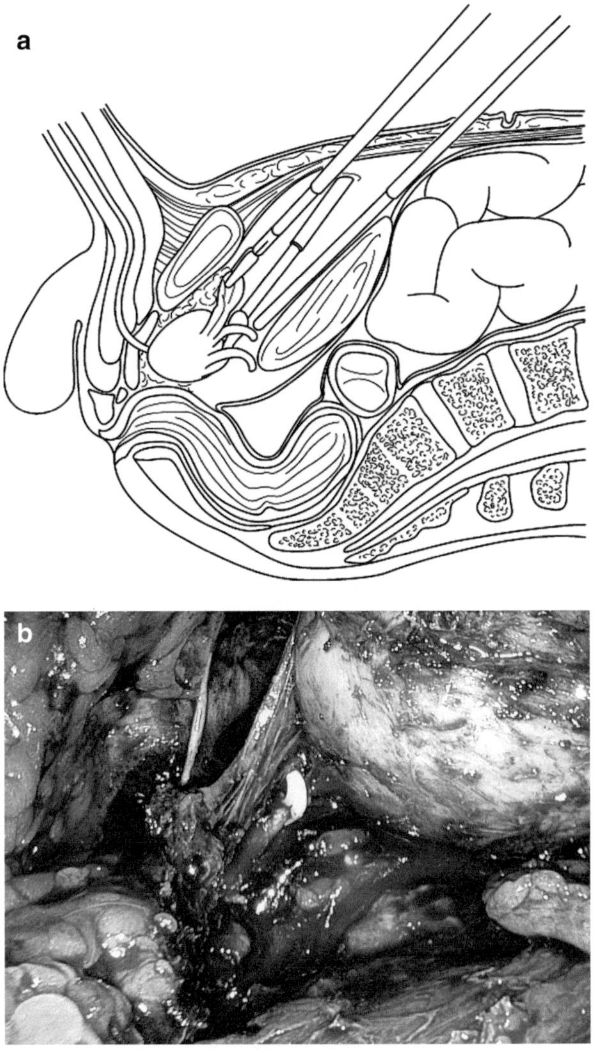

Fig. 12.5 Antegrade dissection. The prostate is retracted anteriorly by grasping the freed seminal vesicles and vasa (**a**) to assist in the antegrade posterior dissection in the plane between the prostate and the rectum (**b**)

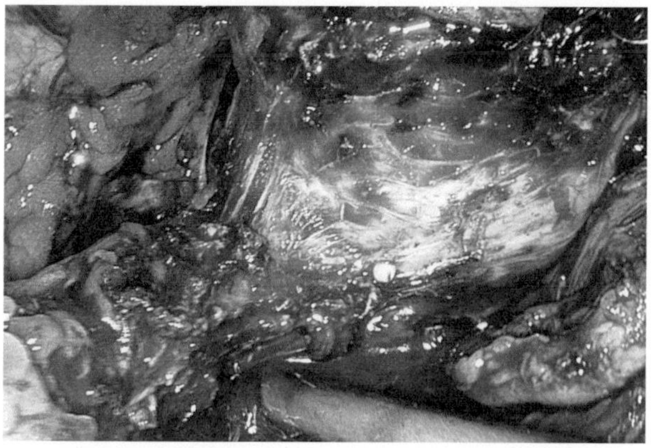

Fig. 12.6 Development of the pedicle. Using the Harmonic Scalpel, the vascular pedicles are identified. In the case where large vascular pedicles are isolated, they are ligated with a clip and divided

scissors are employed to divide the veil of Aphrodite tissue and allow the NVB to drop posteriorly towards the rectum to facilitate safe nerve-sparing during the posterior dissection of the prostate. The NVB is therefore released in an antegrade dissection along the posterior surface of the prostate using the endoshears after the pedicle has been controlled, to minimize thermal injury to the NVB. Importantly, we do not employ electrocautery at any point during the procedure. Instead, we extensively use the harmonic scalpel during key points of the dissection, which has been shown to cause less thermal damage to surrounding tissues and cause less charring while successfully coagulating and dividing tissues.[23]

In the non-nerve-sparing technique, generally undertaken when the patient has extensive disease on one or both sides of the prostate, we proceed with antegrade posterior dissection without hydrodissection and harmonically dissect the NVB and lateral edge of the prostate from the perirectal fat. The dissection is extended to the posterior aspect of the prostate apex.

During posterior dissection of the prostate, the anterior retraction of the prostate is initially accomplished with ratcheted graspers on divided vasa deferentia and dissected seminal vesicles. As the dissection progresses caudally, a tenaculum is often useful to provide countertraction as the prostate is held to the anterior-lateral side to that which the surgeon is operating. The assistant uses the suction tip to gently retract the ipsilateral NVB in the nerve-sparing technique or perirectal fat with overlying posterior leaflet of Denonvillier's fascia in the non-nerve-sparing technique, away from the prostate to maintain the tissues that are being divided on taut stretch and to keep the field of view clear. The goal of this maneuver is to provide adequate visualization of the planes of dissection to maximize oncologic control while minimizing the handling and traction on the cavernous nerve fibers to preserve function.

12.3.3.8 Apical Dissection, Division of the Dorsal Venous Complex and Urethra

When the prostate is fully freed posteriorly and laterally, and remains only tethered by the urethra at the apex, it is retracted cephalad and posterior using either

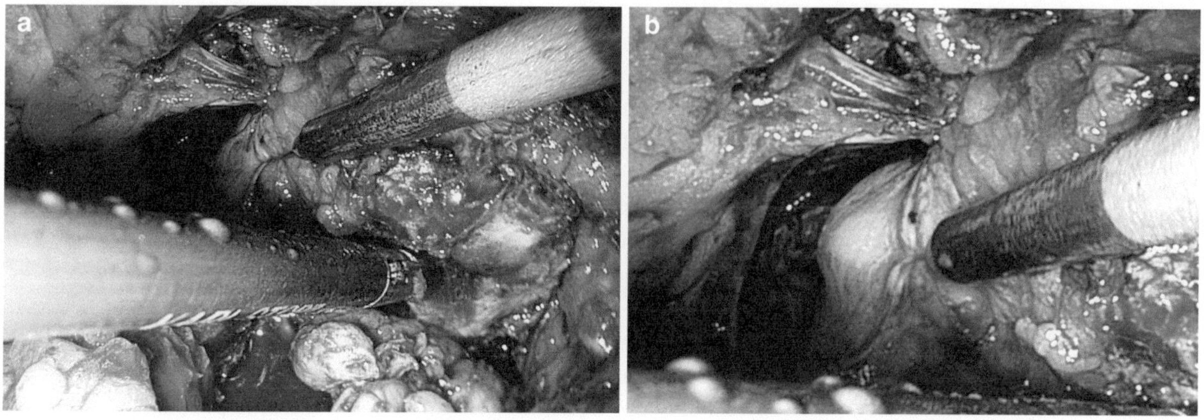

Fig. 12.7 Hydrodissection of the interfascial plane. An 18-gauge laparoscopic cyst aspiration needles is used to inject Tumescent solution (1:10,000 epinephrine solution diluted in buffered Ringers Lactate) into the interfascial plane (**a**) to assist division of the veil of Aphrodite tissue, permitting the NVB to drop posteriorly, away from the plane of dissection (**b**)

a laparoscopic grasper or the tenaculum. A metal Roth sound is useful to manipulate the urethra and can either be held by the Civco arm or by an assistant. The DVC is divided over the urethra first with the harmonic scalpel to reveal the anterior urethral wall. Meticulous hemostasis is necessary at this point. Compression of the urethra against the pubic symphysis anteriorly with the tip of the sound assists with hemostasis.

Then the scissors are used to transect the prostatic apex from the anterior urethra, following the concavity of the apex and paying careful attention to the potentially varied apical topography, such as a posterior lip, which may protrude caudally, posterior to the urethra. The goal of this dissection is to avoid a positive apical margin by preserving the apical prostatic capsule and to preserve maximal urethral length for the vesicourethral anastomosis. The metal urethral sound assists in delineating the extent of the urethra at this point of the dissection. To maximize visualization of the apex, the prostate can be retracted cephalad and toward the patient's contralateral side with the laparoscopic grasper or the tenaculum and rotated with the laparoscopic grasper on its urethral axis.

The caudad NVB lies in close proximity to the posterior prostato-urethral junction, therefore it is necessary to avoid use of cautery during the apical dissection to minimize thermal injury in the nerve-sparing technique. Taut retraction of the prostate to the alternate side of the NVB facilitates the posterior dissection. The posterior urethral wall and the rectourethralis muscles are then divided. The recto-prostatic dissection is completed safely at this point, avoiding entry into the rectum by continuing the division anterior to the perirectal fat up to the prostato-urethral junction. The assistant provides tension with the suction tip above the perirectal fat and below the rectourethralis muscle to facilitate this maneuver while the surgeon rotates the prostate alternately to the left and right while completing the posterior apical dissection.

Once the specimen is fully freed, the camera is switched to the right perirectus port and an endocatch bag (Autosuture, etc.) is advanced into the retroperitoneum via the midline port. The freed prostate is deposited into the endoscopic bag, which is closed and then set aside in the lateral cephalad margins of the space of Retzius while the vesico-urethral anastomosis is completed. The string on the bag is secured outside of the median port with a snap. Then the camera and lens are replaced in the infraumbilical port and reattached to the robotic arm. The dissection bed is irrigated with sterile normal saline and is inspected to assure hemostasis.

12.3.3.9 Vesicourethral Anastomosis

We perform an interrupted vesicourethral anastomosis with a series of six to eight 2-0 polyglactin sutures circumferentially. Prior to starting the anastomosis, the bladder neck is first examined and the ureteral orifices are identified and their position noted. Considerations for a water-tight anastomosis include ensuring mucosal reapproximation during the suturing of the bladder neck and urethra by directing the suture needle to incorporate sufficient extravesical or extraurethral tissue for strength. The bladder neck mucosa is slightly everted by the placement of the anastomosis sutures. Two posterior and two lateral sutures are placed and tied (Fig. 12.8). The two anterior sutures are placed, but not tied until visual confirmation that the 20 French Foley catheter is successfully placed in the bladder. Any narrowing of a patulous bladder neck is then accomplished with an anterior tennis racket bladder neck reconstruction (see Fig. 12.7c).

As with any hollow-viscous anastomosis, the sutures must be tension free. This is another area where lessons were learned from the switch from tLRP to eLRP. The retraction of the bladder which is facilitated by the approach puts greater tension on the anastomosis than with a trans-peritoneal approach. We had an increase in urethra-vesicle anastomotic urine leaks in the initial months after transition from tLRP to eLRP. By decreasing the CO_2 pressure and decreasing the degree of Trendelenburg during the tying of the anastomotic sutures, the anastomosis goes down tightly and urine leaks again became rare. The tying of sutures does require some modification with the eLRP. A three-throw surgeons knot is used for the first step of the knot. This holds well and prevents any slippage that could lead to a loose anastomosis.

Urethral suture placement is assisted with the Van Buren urethral sound. The first two sutures placed are posterior at 5 and 7 o'clock. The suture needle tip is placed against the sound in the urethral lumen and the sound is drawn into the urethra to guide the needle back 5–8 mm in the urethral stump. Then the needle is rotated into the urethral tissue to secure a good bite of tissue. The suture is then placed from outside the bladder to the inside of the bladder, taking great care to

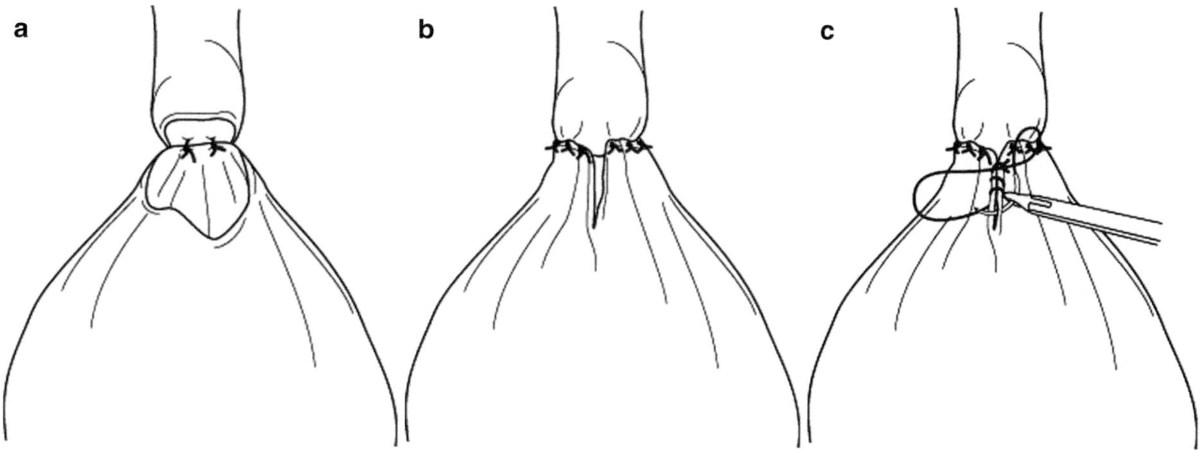

Fig. 12.8 Vesico-urethral anastomosis. (**a**) Two posterior sutures are placed at 5 and 7 o'clock. (**b**) Then interrupted sutures are continued laterally to complete the vesicourethral anastomosis with insertion of the Foley catheter into the bladder prior to tying down the two anterior sutures. (**c**) If the bladder neck requires narrowing, this is accomplished with a running anterior racquet closure

avoid injuring the ureters. The initial two knots are tied on the inside of the anastomosis (see Fig. 12.7a).

Interrupted sutures are then placed at approximately 3 mm intervals circumferentially around the urethra, using the urethral sound to assist with direction of the urethral stitches. Generally, sutures are placed at 3 and 9 o'clock from outside the bladder in, then inside the urethra out. These knots are therefore tied outside the bladder.

Two anterior sutures are placed from outside the urethra in, then inside the anterior bladder out. Prior to tying of the final two sutures anteriorly, the metal urethral sound is removed and the final 20 French silastic Foley catheter is inserted through the bladder neck with the assistance of a stylet. Then the anterior anastomosis is completed with tying the final two sutures (see Fig. 12.7b).

In the event of disparity between the size of the bladder neck and the urethra, we perform an anterior tennis racket reconstruction at the time of the anterior anastomosis. This is accomplished with a 2-0 Vicryl running suture in a right-handed forehand manner retrograde from the vesicourethral anastomosis to the apex of the reconstruction (see Fig. 12.7c). A Lapra-Ty (Ethicon) is secured to the distal end of the suture following placement of the first needle pass. The bladder tissue is then elevated anteriorly prior to each suture placement to avoid incorporating the Foley catheter in the suture. At the conclusion of the reconstruction, the suture is gently tightened, and then the proximal end is secured with second Lapra-Ty clip.

Rarely, a running suture is employed to close the anastomosis. This is particularly useful for cases when there is a great deal of tension on the anastomosis, or if the pelvis is so narrow or the bladder so thick that all visualization is lost with the tying of any knot. Following placement of the two interrupted posterior sutures at the 5 and 7 o'clock positions, two 2-0 Monocryl sutures, which are cut to approximately 10 cm in length, are secured beside the posterior sutures and are run to the anterior aspect of the anastomosis. The right-sided running suture is completed, followed by the left side, and then both sutures are independently tied. At this point, an anterior bladder neck reconstruction can be performed as is done with the interrupted anastomosis technique.

After the completion of the anastomosis and bladder neck reconstruction, if necessary, the Foley catheter balloon is filled with 8 cc of sterile water after ensuring that it has not been inadvertently included in the anastomosis. Then the integrity of the anastomosis is tested by instilling 120 cc of sterile normal saline into the bladder. If there is no leak evident, the Foley catheter balloon is gently manipulated against the closure. If any fluid escapes through the anastomosis, additional interrupted sutures are placed in the region of the leak, with careful attention to avoid incorporation of the ureteral orifices, the NVB, or the Foley catheter.

The bladder is then gently irrigated by hand to remove any blood clot, which could later obstruct the catheter. The surgical field is once again inspected for hemostasis and any additional irrigation is completed.

12.3.3.10 Drain Placement and Delivery of Specimen

An 18 French Blake drain (Johnson & Johnson) is inserted with the externalized end leading through the right pararectus port and grasped with a laparoscopic grasper inserted through the right lower quadrant port. Under direct vision, the port is then removed from the skin and the drain is pulled through this 5-mm port site and secured with a 0 silk suture. The drain is positioned intracorporeally close but not directly touching the anastomosis. Following completion of the operation and closure of the remaining port sites, closed suction is initiated.

The remaining trocars are each removed under vision with the laparoscope, with attention to the anterior abdominal wall to identify any injury to the epigastric vessels to assure no postoperative bleeding.

Then specimen in the endoscopic bag is then removed through the infraumbilical incision. The fascial incision is extended as necessary to allow for the delivery of the specimen.

12.3.3.11 Closure and Dressing

The anterior rectus incision of the infraumbilical port is closed in a running manner following removal of the specimen to prevent development of umbilical hernia. Then 20 cc of 2% lidocaine with epinephrine are injected into the port sites and in the region of the JP drain and the incisions are closed with 3-0 monocryl in a subcuticular manner and secured with sterile tape bandages.

12.3.4 Postoperative Management

Following recovery from anesthesia, the patient is encouraged to ambulate the evening following surgery. While in bed, the compression stockings and pneumatic compression boots are utilized. The patient is monitored carefully in the postoperative period for hemodynamic stability, adequate urine output via the Foley catheter, appropriate drain output, and good control of postoperative pain.

All patients receive two additional doses of perioperative antibiotics (generally cefazolin), and prophylaxis against gastro-intestinal reflux in the first 24 h following surgery. The patient starts a liquid diet the morning after surgery. One of the advantages of the extraperitoneal approach to this procedure is a generally minimal postoperative ileus. If the drain output is less than 10 cc/h during the day on postoperative day #1, the drain is removed in the mid-afternoon and the patient is generally to home late in the afternoon or the early evening, assuming adequate pain control and toleration of oral regimen.

While home, the patient is cautioned against sitting upright on firm surfaces for the first week to avoid placing pressure on the anastomosis and causing additional edema. He is instructed to sit in a reclined position until the catheter is removed.

The patient returns on postoperative day 7 for catheter removal and void trial. Oral ciprofloxacin is administered starting the day of catheter removal for a total of three consecutive days. This regimen sterilizes the bladder after removal of the catheter and prevents cystitis or pyelonephritis.

12.4 Discussion: Extraperitoneal Versus Transperitoneal Approaches

The transperitoneal approach to the LRP, introduced by the early work of Gaston and Piechaud (unpublished series) has been adopted most widely and is currently considered the gold standard of the minimally invasive approach to laparoscopic or robotic assisted prostatectomy.

The extraperitoneal approach and development of a preperitoneal space for laparoscopy was developed for the laparoscopic inguinal hernia repair.[24] The extraperitoneal approach to the LRP was first described in 1997 as an alternative approach to avoid intraperitoneal injuries, adhesive disease, and complications associated with bladder mobilization inherent in the standard transperitoneal LRP.[25] Access to this preperitoneal space is now utilized in many minimally invasive urological procedures such as pelvic lymph node dissection, varicocelectomy, and bladder neck suspension[24, 26]

Now the extraperitoneal approach with development of the preperitoneal space is accepted as a standardized approach to the minimally invasive treatment of prostate cancer. In comparison to the traditional transperitoneal LRP, some groups have found that the extraperitoneal approach is associated with shorter operative times (169.6 vs. 224.2 min, $P<0.001$), earlier return to a regular diet (1.6 vs. 2.6 days, $P=0.002$), and decreased narcotic requirement.[27] This may be due to the avoidance of a chemical peritonitis caused by entry of blood or urine into the peritoneal cavity which occurs to varying degrees during the transperitoneal approach, as well as the avoidance of manipulation of the bowel, the lack of necessity to lyse intraperitoneal adhesions or to mobilize the bladder. Early or prolonged anastomotic leak occurs in 2–17.2% of patients, and the intraperitoneal urine resulting from these leaks in the TP-LRP has been associated with prolonged ileus in 2.8–8.6% of patients.[4, 28-30] Longer time to return of continence in the TP-LRP in comparison to the EP-LRP has been reported and may be secondary to the greater degree of manipulation of the bladder inherent in the mobilization of during the transperitoneal technique.[31, 32]

Most groups have reported no significant differences between the two approaches. Specifically, the EP-LRP has been shown to have similar mean operative times, hemoglobin decreases or transfusion rates, complication rate, median catheter time, surgical margin positivity, or postoperative continence rates[28, 32-34]

In the extraperitoneal approach, the operative field is slightly smaller; however, the peritoneum forms a barrier, negating the necessity of manipulating or retracting the bowels, minimizing intraperitoneal injury, facilitating the LRP in patients with prior intraperitoneal surgery or inflammatory disease such as Crohn's disease or Ulcerative Colitis.

Limits of the extraperitoneal approach include the reduced working space, and the potential for increased tension on the vesico-urethral anastomosis as the bladder is not fully mobilized and remains fixed at the urachus. EP-LRP has also been related to slightly, although not statistically significantly, greater anastomotic leak rate (12% vs. 6%, $P=0.22$),[28] which may be related to the increased tension across the anastomosis in this procedure or, alternatively, to increased identification of the extravasation recognition because there is no confounding peritoneal fluid.

12.5 Results

Multiple recent comparisons between RRP and LRP have demonstrated equivalent oncologic and functional outcomes.[7, 29, 35-38] Positive margin rates are similar between the eLRP and tLRP,[28] and also in comparison to the open RRP.[7]

Although the learning curve is steep, and initial operative times of 5–6 h are common, after 20–30 patients, most surgeons reports durations of 3–4 h.[13, 28] The minimal invasive nature of LRP is associated with relative advantages in terms of decreased pain postoperatively,[39] however; a statistically significant improvement in postoperative pain has not been reported universally. This is largely thought to be due to the fact that following open RRP using a muscle-splitting infraumbilical incision, postoperative pain is relatively minimal. In our experience, following eLRP, the patient's pain is managed with low-dose IV morphine immediately postoperatively. On post-operative day 1, as patients resume a liquid diet, pain is managed with low dose oral narcotics (Percocet or Oxycodone) which is generally required for 1–3 days, after which most patients require only Acetaminophen or nothing at all.

In general, laparoscopic radical surgery of the prostate is associated with relatively lower blood loss in comparison to the open procedure as the majority of blood loss that occurs is secondary to loss from the venous sinuses, and the tamponade effect created by pneumoperitoneum or pneumoretroperitoneum reduces blood loss. Most series by experienced laparoscopists report blood loss of less than several hundred milliliters. In our experience, there was no significant difference in the decrease in hemoglobin between the transperitoneal and extraperitoneal approach (mean decrease 3.0 g/dL).[28]

12.6 Complications of the Extraperitoneal Laparoscopic Radical Prostatectomy

Recent large series of LRP cohorts suggest that complication rates may be lower than RRP when the LRP is performed by a surgeon with extensive laparoscopic experience.[29] The laparoscopic surgeon must be well versed in the physiologic effects associated with insufflation and general laparoscopic principles, which are beyond the scope of this chapter. The complications discussed here are those inherent to the radical resection of the prostate, with specific attention to the etiology, recognition, and management in the context of extraperitoneal laparoscopic approach.

Hemodynamic parameters are relatively similar between intraperitoneal insufflation and extraperitoneal insufflation. Comparison between the two methods has shown that with extraperitoneal insufflation, there is a slower increase in central filling pressures and end-tidal CO_2.[40] Intraperitoneal insufflation is also associated with significantly greater increases in CVP and MAP.[41] This is thought to be due to the relative distance of the space of Retzius from the intrathoracic cavity and that the additional soft tissues of the peritoneal cavity act as a buffer to the transmission of the pressures from the extraperitoneal space to the intrathoracic cavity. Theoretically, this may be of some benefit in those patients with limited cardiopulmonary reserve. Extraperitoneal insufflation is also associated with more pronounced carbon dioxide absorption in cases of prolonged insufflation (>8 h); however, with appropriate changes in minute ventilation by the anesthesia team, this does not produce any clinically significant changes in the acid–base status of the patient.[41]

12.7 Perioperative Complications and Management

12.7.1 Neurological Complications

Neurological injury can occur during LRP related to patient positioning or secondary to direct damage to nerves or traction injuries incurred during dissection. We noted three cases of genitofemoral nerve irritation in our series of eLRP in comparison to RRP.[6] Injury or transection of the obturator nerve is a known complication of LRP, occurring specifically during pelvic lymphadenectomy or instrument exchange through the lateral port sites.[42] During laparoscopic pelvic lymph node dissection in LRP, the obturator nerve must be identified prior to clip placement on the inferior aspect of the lymph node packet. If a clip is placed on the nerve, it can simply be removed at the time of identification, although the patient may develop transient symptoms secondary to the crush injury. Transection of the nerve can be managed with reapproximation of the nerve sheath using 7-0 polypropylene sutures in an interrupted manner.[42]

12.7.2 Bleeding and Vascular Injuries

Injury to the Inferior epigastric vessels, iliac vein, and dorsal venous complex are the most commonly cited vascular injuries associated with the LRP, occurring in 0–6% of cases.[27, 30, 43] In eLRP, injury to the inferior epigastric vessels occurs rarely (0.8%), whereas the most common site of intraoperative hemorrhage is in the dorsal venous complex and during division of small vessels adjacent to the neurovascular bundles.[44] We find control of these vessels can be adequately achieved with both early ligation of the DVC and use of the harmonic scalpel.

Postoperative hemorrhage or hematoma is noted in approximately 1% of eLRP.[28, 44] Hematoma occurs generally in the setting of an unrecognized injury to the epigastric muscles following trocar removal or from injury to the DVC. Delayed identification of a retrovesical hematoma may occur given that it is not drained by the drain overlying the anterior aspect of the anastomosis. In addition to the common sequelae of postoperative bleeding such as tachycardia and other hemodynamic changes associated with anemia, these patients may present with bilateral flank pain and renal failure secondary to obstruction of the ureters by extrinsic compression posteriorly on the anastomosis and ureteral orifices by the hematoma. In these cases, operative evacuation of the hematoma may become necessary, as percutaneous access is complicated and may not be sufficient.

12.7.3 Bowel and Rectal Injuries

In general, rectal and bowel injuries are uncommon in LRP (0.7–2.4%),[45, 46] and if identified at the time of surgery, can be repaired laparoscopically. Failure to recognize these injuries intraoperatively can result in significant morbidity and mortality. Bowel injuries commonly occur in LRP during trocar placement, instrument exchange, or tissue dissection. Additionally, thermal injury caused by electrocautery devices, the harmonic scalpel, or arcing of monopolar current to adjacent organs can cause delayed bowel injury and perforation, accounting for more than half of all laparoscopic bowel injuries.[47] Thermal injury to surrounding tissues is best prevented by maintaining instruments away from surrounding structures, and being attentive to position of nearby instruments that might conduct heat. Additionally, thermal energy can be transmitted to hollow viscus and cause injury by diffusion along tissue planes. Intraoperative repair by a two-layer closure can be performed laparoscopically. In the eLRP literature, injury to the small and large bowels by trocar placement has not been reported as it is avoided by the exclusion of the operative field from the peritoneal cavity.

Rectal injury has been reported in approximately 0.5–1.3% of eLRP in comparison to 0.5–9% in the LRP literature,[44, 46] most commonly during the posterior dissection of the apex, when the rectourethralis muscle is transected. Rectal injuries may also occur during sharp incision of Denonvillier's fascia after seminal vesical dissection. Finally, injury to the lateral border of the rectum has been reported when performing wide dissection of the neurovascular bundles in extensive disease. As with bowel injuries, perforation may result from sharp incision or by thermal injury, and the most important prognostic factor in rectal injuries is immediate intraoperative identification of the injury and closure of the defect in two layers (mucosal and serosal). Diagnosis of the injury and integrity of the repair can both be assessed by filling the pelvis with irrigant, and then insufflating the rectum with air and assessing for bubbles, which confirm a persistent injury.

In situations where rectal injury leads to gross fecal spillage, previous radiation, chronic steroid use, or where the urethrovesical anastomosis is under tension, we recommend consideration of diversion. Development of a rectourethral fistula is a recognized complication of rectal injury or inadequate repair of a rectal tear in LRP. Most of these injuries can be managed conservatively by urethral catheterization and/or diversion.[48] There appears no relative advantage between the eLRP and tLRP with respect to the rate of rectal as the posterior dissection is performed in both procedures in the same manner. Rectal injury is best prevented in LRP achieved either via the extraperitoneal or transperitoneal approach by meticulous dissection and careful use of thermal energy.

Injuries to the bowel not identified intraoperatively may present as ileus, nausea, vomiting, peritonitis, fever, and leukocytosis; however, a large study of laparoscopic access injuries by Chandler et al. found that the most common initial presenting symptom of bowel injury was persistent pain at a single trocar site without significant erythema or purulent discharge.[49]

Ileus occurs in 1–9% of patients following LRP, and is generally managed conservatively with nasogastric suction and management of anastomotic leaks in the cases where the cause of the ileus is a chemical peritonitis caused by urine leak in the transperitoneal approach. In cases of postoperative ileus, it is imperative to rule out small bowel hernia through a trocar site or unidentified bowel injury as the etiology. We found a 2.5% incidence of ileus with the transperitoneal approach in comparison to 0% in our extraperitoneal group, which is similar to the findings of the series of 1800 extraperitoneal LRP reported by Liatsikos.[28, 44]

12.7.4 Ureteral Injury

Ureteral complications are reported in 0–1% of patients undergoing eLRP, and are often related to thermal or electrical injury, or by suture placement near or through the ureteral orifices during the urethrovescular anastomosis.[44] The eLRP approach avoids potential injury to the ureters reported in the transperitoneal Montsouris technique during the posterior dissection of the vesiculodeferential junction, or during the dissection of the lateral vesical peritoneum.[36] Ureteral injury is ideally recognized intraoperatively and can be repaired laparoscopically either primarily over a ureteral stent or via ureteroneocystostomy.[29, 50] In cases where the ureteral orifices are identified in close proximity to the bladder neck, we recommend ureteral cannulation using 5 Fr pediatric feeding tubes, then completion of the posterior and lateral versiculourethral anastomosis. This allows confirmation that the ureteral orifices have not been injured by the posterior and lateral sutures by movement of the tubes within the orifices. In cases where ureteral injury recognition is delayed, it is generally managed with temporary percutaneous nephrostomy tube placement and anastomotic revision.

12.7.5 Bladder Injury

Injury to the bladder occurs rarely following eLRP, and largely occurs during the dissection of the posterior bladder neck and retrovesical space to achieve dissection of the seminal vesicles. Thermal injury to the bladder can also occur. These injuries can be identified and repaired intraoperatively with a single layer closure. Bladder injuries have specifically been reported in dissection of the extraperitoneal space in patients who have undergone previous extraperitoneal hernioplasty with mesh placement.[16]

12.7.6 Lymphocele

Lymphocele is a reported complication, which occurs following pelvic lymph node dissection and transection of lymphatic vessels. Significant lymphoceles may cause pelvic pain, voiding difficulty following catheter removal, and leg edema and discomfort. Furthermore, lymphoceles may become infected and be associated with fever and development of leukocytosis. In comparison to open series, where lymphocele rates are reported to occur in 4.7–61% of cases[51, 52] in the laparoscopic literature, lymphocele rates appear to be lower at 0–14%.[51, 53, 54] The transperitoneal approach allows lymphatic fluid to flow more readily out of the pelvis and to be absorbed by the peritoneum, whereas the extraperitoneal approach allows more rapid diagnosis of the lymphocele as it is restricted to the space of Retzius, where it may become symptomatic more rapidly. Management of the lymphocele in the eLRP population involves antibiotics and percutaneous drainage, sclerotherapy, and laparoscopic transperitoneal fenestration depending on the size and severity of symptoms.[54] We do not routinely perform peritoneal fenestration following eLRP with PLND; however, some authors advocate universally fenestrating the peritoneum, reporting a decrease in the incidence in symptomatic and asymptomatic lymphocele following this procedure.[54] Fenestration is performed by incising the peritoneum between the spermatic cord and the obturator fossa. When performing this procedure, it is important to take care to avoid ureteral injury.

12.7.7 Anastomotic Leak/Complications

The most common complication of LRP is the anastomotic leak, reported in 6–12% of the patients.[28, 36] It may occur as an early or late complication. This occurs more commonly than in RRP. Identification of the anastomotic leak is facilitated in the extraperitoneal procedure as increased drain output in the early postoperative period occurs exclusively of increased drainage secondary to peritoneal fluid output. The vast majority of anastomotic leaks are managed conservatively, with prolonged catheterization and drainage via the drain placed operatively, or by percutaneous drainage, if urinoma is noted after drain removal. As noted above, in the tranperitoneal approach, the urinary ascites can lead to significant intraperitoneal irritation causing a reflex ileus. This chemical peritonitis is avoided in the extraperitoneal approach.

The best method to prevent anastomotic leakage is to ensure a tension-free watertight anastomosis, with intravesical positioning of the bladder catheter under direct vision. Following completion of the anastomosis, the anastomosis can be tested for a leak by filling the bladder and tugging on the catheter to assess any irrigant leaks between the sutures. In the event where leak is identified intraoperatively, we place additional interrupted sutures to reinforce the anastomosis until there is no evidence of leak.

Management of anastomotic leak recognized in the postoperative period is by prolonged urethral catheterization and percutaneous drainage if necessary to drain the urinoma. In Guillonneau's series,[17] 57 of 567 patients experienced an anastomotic leak, and all but one were able to be managed conservatively with replacement of the urethral catheter. One patient required operative intervention. Some authors propose that if that urine output through the urethral catheter is less than the output of the drain for greater than 48 h, then reintervention and revision of the anastomosis is indicated via a laparoscopic approach.[44]

In our series, we report an anastomotic leak rate of 6% in the transperitoneal group and 12% of the extraperitoneal group ($P > 0.05$), all of which were managed conservatively.[28] Additionally we noted that drain management was easier in these patients with removal on average approximately 0.4 days earlier than in the group with a transperitoneal approach.

Acute urinary retention postoperatively is associated with early catheter removal, and occurs in 0.4–0.7% of patients whose catheters are removed in 3–5 days postoperatively.[44] We remove the urethral catheter on day 8–10.

Anastomotic stricture is a well-recognized late complication of LRP and is reported in 0.5–2% of patients. Risk factors for anastomotic stricture or bladder neck contracture include prior transurethral resection of the prostate, excessive intraoperative blood loss, and urinary extravasation. Some authors propose that there may be an association between bladder neck contracture and the running suture technique for the urethrovesical anastomosis.[55] However, a comparative study between a running suture and an interrupted sutured anastomosis showed that while the running suture reduced operative time and tension on the anastomosis, there was no significant difference in terms of leak, stricture, or continence rates.[56] We generally employ the interrupted suture technique, but in complicated cases where the extraperitoneal space is limited by a small pelvis or instrument mobility is limited by obesity, we will employ the running suture technique.

12.7.8 Thromboembolic Complications

Deep vein thrombosis and pulmonary embolus are rare but serious complications of pelvic surgery in general and well recognized following radical prostatectomy. A multi-institutional review of 5,951 patients demonstrated that symptomatic DVT and PE occurred in 0.5% patients within 90 days of surgery.[57] A multivariate analysis did not find that neoadjuvant therapy, body mass index, surgical experience or approach (extraperitoneal or transperitoneal laparoscopic or robotic), pathologic stage, perioperative transfusion, or heparin administration were significant predictors of thromboembolic complications. Therefore the authors conclude that the data do not support the administration of prophylactic heparin in all patients undergoing LRP. In our patient population, patients preoperatively have compressive stockings and pneumatic compression boots applied but do not prophylactically heparinize patients.

12.7.9 Open Conversion and Reoperation

Laparoscopic radical prostatectomy is one of the most technically demanding operations performed by urologists, and rates of complications clearly decline with surgeon experience.[43] Conversion to open surgery is reported in 0–6% of cases.[58] The most challenging portions of the case prompting conversion are the apical and posterior dissection, followed by dissection of the bladder neck. Additionally, one third of conversions in a multi-institutional study assessing conversion from LRP to open surgery occurred secondary to the need for open repair of injury to adjacent organs.[59]

12.7.10 Urinary and Sexual Function

From a patient's perspective, perhaps the two most concerning complications of radical surgery on the prostate are urinary incontinence and erectile dysfunction. Using laparoscopic technology, the magnification and improved visualization is thought to improve the accuracy of the apical dissection and sparing of the neurovascular bundles when clinically appropriate, theoretically improving functional outcomes. The data of many of the comparative studies that have been published is challenging to draw firm conclusions from, given the widely variable methods of data collections (e.g. telephone interviews, retrospective reviews of the medical record, surgeon assessment, and surveys) and lack of precise definitions of incontinence or impotence. However, it appears that rates of potency and continence are comparable between the open and laparoscopic (either transperitoneal or extraperitoneal approach) techniques.[36, 58, 60] In general, at high-volume centers, continence (defined as using less than one or no pads per day) rates of 40 to greater than 90% and potency (defined as the presence of spontaneous erections or erections sufficient for intercourse) rates of 23–>80% have been reported.[6, 61]

We recently published our experience comparing outcomes in patients who underwent either RRP or LRP in 2003–2004[6] using the following definitions:

- *Continence*: No leakage and no pad use.
- *Potency*: Erections firm enough for intercourse, with or without oral medications.

All patients were evaluated preoperatively and followed at monthly intervals postoperatively for 1 year. We found that at 12 months, 48% of patients in the RRP group and 59% of patients in the LRP group had total control of urinary function ($P=0.3$) and that 88% of patients after RRP and 83% of patients after LRP did not require any pads ($P=0.6$). Twenty-three percent of men after RRP and 32% of men after LRP experienced erections sufficient for intercourse ($P=0.22$). This study also identified the natural history of return to function following radical surgery of the prostate and the fact that function returns gradually following this surgery. Given the effect that radical prostatectomy has on personal bodily functions which have such emotional significance for patients, it is important to adequately educate patients preoperatively such that they will have realistic expectations for the time course and likelihood of return to preoperative function.

Between transperitoneal and extraperitoneal approaches to the LRP, there is no significant difference between these functional outcomes.[27, 31, 61] Interpretation of this data is further complicated by the multifactorial nature of continence and potency (Chapin et al., unpublished data, 2009), which is significantly influenced by preoperative function, medical comorbidities, and social habits (tobacco, drug, alcohol use). Overall, the basic surgical principles of meticulous dissection, gentle handling of tissues, ensuring optimal visualization, and avoiding electrocautery during dissection of the neurovascular bundles are essential for minimizing damage to these structures and maximizing postoperative function in either RRP, eLRP, or tLRP.

12.8 Summary

Over a relatively short period of time, the laparoscopic approach to the radical prostatectomy has become well accepted in the urological community for the surgical management of organ confined or locally advanced prostate cancer.

Extraperitoneal laparoscopic radical prostatectomy is a safe and effective technique for management of T2 or T3 prostate cancer. It is a technically challenging procedure with a steep learning curve; however, with experience, urologists can achieve oncologic and functional results comparable to the RRP or transperitoneal laparoscopic approach with similar and acceptable rates of complications.

References

1. Lau WY, Leow CK, Li AK. History of endoscopic and laparoscopic surgery. *World J Surg*. 1997;21(4):444-453.
2. Schuessler WW, Schulam PG, Clayman RV, Kavoussi LR. Laparoscopic radical prostatectomy: initial short-term experience. *Urology*. 1997;50(6):854-857.
3. Guillonneau B, Vallancien G. Laparoscopic radical prostatectomy: the montsouris technique. *J Urol*. 2000;163(6):1643-1649.
4. Dahl DM, L'esperance JO, Trainer AF, et al. Laparoscopic radical prostatectomy: initial 70 cases at a U.S. university medical center. *Urology*. 2002;60(5):859-863.
5. Guillonneau B, Abbou CC, Doublet JD, et al. Proposal for a "European scoring system for laparoscopic operations in urology". *Eur Urol*. 2001;40(1):2-6. discussion 7.
6. Dahl DM, Barry MJ, McGovern FJ, Chang Y, Walker-Corkery E, McDougal WS. A prospective study of symptom distress and return to baseline function after open versus laparoscopic radical prostatectomy. *J Urol*. 2009;182(3):956-965.
7. Dahl DM, He W, Lazarus R, McDougal WS, Wu CL. Pathologic outcome of laparoscopic and open radical prostatectomy. *Urology*. 2006;68(6):1253-1256.
8. Brown JA, Rodin DM, Lee B, Dahl DM. Laparoscopic radical prostatectomy and body mass index: an assessment of 151 sequential cases. *J Urol*. 2005;173(2):442-445.
9. Rodriguez AR, Kapoor R, Pow-Sang JM. Laparoscopic extraperitoneal radical prostatectomy in complex surgical cases. *J Urol*. 2007;177(5):1765-1770.
10. Fahy BG, Barnas GM, Flowers JL, Nagle SE, Njoku MJ. The effects of increased abdominal pressure on lung and chest wall mechanics during laparoscopic surgery. *Anesth Analg*. 1995;81(4):744-750.
11. Fahy BG, Barnas GM, Nagle SE, Flowers JL, Njoku MJ, Agarwal M. Effects of Trendelenburg and reverse Trendelenburg postures on lung and chest wall mechanics. *J Clin Anesth*. 1996;8(3):236-244.
12. Rassweiler J, Hruza M, Frede T, Teber D. Laparoscopic extraperitoneal ascending nerve-sparing radical prostatectomy: an effective and safe technique for apical tumors. *J Endourol*. 2009;22(9):13. discussion 2021.
13. Stolzenburg JU, Kallidonis P, Minh D, et al. Endoscopic extraperitoneal radical prostatectomy: evolution of the technique and experience with 2400 cases. *J Endourol*. 2009; 23(9):1467-1472.
14. Cook H, Afzal N, Cornaby AJ. Laparoscopic hernia repairs may make subsequent radical retropubic prostatectomy more hazardous. *BJU Int*. 2003;91(7):729.
15. Dulucq JL, Wintringer P, Mahajna A. Totally extraperitoneal (TEP) hernia repair after radical prostatectomy or previous lower abdominal surgery: is it safe? a prospective study. *Surg Endosc*. 2006;20(3):473-476.

16. Brown JA, Dahl DM. Transperitoneal laparoscopic radical prostatectomy in patients after laparoscopic prosthetic mesh inguinal herniorrhaphy. *Urology*. 2004;63(2):380-382.
17. Guillonneau B, Rozet F, Cathelineau X, et al. Perioperative complications of laparoscopic radical prostatectomy: the montsouris 3-year experience. *J Urol*. 2002;167(1):51-56.
18. Matin SF. Recognition and preservation of accessory pudendal arteries during laparoscopic radical prostatectomy. *Urology*. 2006;67(5):1012-1015.
19. Secin FP, Karanikolas N, Kuroiwa K, Vickers A, Touijer K, Guillonneau B. Positive surgical margins and accessory pudendal artery preservation during laparoscopic radical prostatectomy. *Eur Urol*. 2005;48(5):786-792. discussion 793.
20. Rogers CG, Trock BP, Walsh PC. Preservation of accessory pudendal arteries during radical retropubic prostatectomy: surgical technique and results. *Urology*. 2004;64(1):148-151.
21. Dubbelman YD, Dohle GR, Schroder FH. Sexual function before and after radical retropubic prostatectomy: a systematic review of prognostic indicators for a successful outcome. *Eur Urol*. 2006;50(4):711-718. discussion 718–20.
22. May J, McGovern F. Hemostatic hydrodissection: a new technique to promote nerve-sparing during radical retropubic prostatectomy. *Curr Urol Rep*. 2005;6(1):1.
23. Hayashi A, Takamori S, Matsuo T, Tayama K, Mitsuoka M, Shirouzu K. Experimental and clinical evaluation of the harmonic scalpel in thoracic surgery. *Kurume Med J*. 1999; 46(1):25-29.
24. Sayad P, Ferzli G. The extraperitoneal approach and its utility. *Surg Endosc*. 1999;13(11):1168-1169.
25. Raboy A, Ferzli G, Albert P. Initial experience with extraperitoneal endoscopic radical retropubic prostatectomy. *Urology*. 1997;50(6):849-853.
26. Raboy A, Albert P, Ferzli G. Early experience with extraperitoneal endoscopic radical retropubic prostatectomy. *Surg Endosc*. 1998;12(10):1264-1267.
27. Hoznek A, Antiphon P, Borkowski T, et al. Assessment of surgical technique and perioperative morbidity associated with extraperitoneal versus transperitoneal laparoscopic radical prostatectomy. *Urology*. 2003;61(3):617-622.
28. Brown JA, Rodin D, Lee B, Dahl DM. Transperitoneal versus extraperitoneal approach to laparoscopic radical prostatectomy: an assessment of 156 cases. *Urology*. 2005;65(2): 320-324.
29. Rassweiler J, Hruza M, Teber D, Su LM. Laparoscopic and robotic assisted radical prostatectomy – critical analysis of the results. *Eur Urol*. 2006;49(4):612-624.
30. Rassweiler J, Sentker L, Seemann O, Hatzinger M, Rumpelt HJ. Laparoscopic radical prostatectomy with the heilbronn technique: an analysis of the first 180 cases. *J Urol*. 2001;166(6):2101-2108.
31. Eden CG, King D, Kooiman GG, Adams TH, Sullivan ME, Vass JA. Transperitoneal or extraperitoneal laparoscopic radical prostatectomy: does the approach matter? *J Urol*. 2004;172(6 Pt 1):2218-2223.
32. Porpiglia F, Terrone C, Tarabuzzi R, et al. Transperitoneal versus extraperitoneal laparoscopic radical prostatectomy: experience of a single center. *Urology*. 2006;68(2):376-380.
33. Stolzenburg JU, Rabenalt R, Do M, et al. Complications of endoscopic extraperitoneal radical prostatectomy (EERPE): prevention and management. *World J Urol*. 2006;24(6): 668-675.
34. Stolzenburg JU, Rabenalt R, Do M, Kallidonis P, Liatsikos EN. Endoscopic extraperitoneal radical prostatectomy: the university of leipzig experience of 2000 cases. *J Endourol*. 2008;22(10):2319-2325.
35. Rassweiler J, Schulze M, Teber D, et al. Laparoscopic radical prostatectomy with the heilbronn technique: oncological results in the first 500 patients. *J Urol*. 2005;173(3): 761-764.
36. Guillonneau B, Cathelineau X, Doublet JD, Baumert H, Vallancien G. Laparoscopic radical prostatectomy: assessment after 550 procedures. *Crit Rev Oncol Hematol*. 2002;43(2):123-133.
37. Drouin SJ, Vaessen C, Hupertan V, et al. Comparison of mid-term carcinologic control obtained after open, laparoscopic, and robot-assisted radical prostatectomy for localized prostate cancer. *World J Urol*. 2009;27(5): 599-605.
38. Paul A, Ploussard G, Nicolaiew N, et al. Oncologic outcome after extraperitoneal laparoscopic radical prostatectomy: midterm follow-up of 1115 procedures. *Eur Urol*. 2010;50(4):267-272. 2009 Sep 17.
39. Bhayani SB, Pavlovich CP, Hsu TS, Sullivan W, Su LM. Prospective comparison of short-term convalescence: laparoscopic radical prostatectomy versus open radical retropubic prostatectomy. *Urology*. 2003;61(3):612-616.
40. Bannenberg JJ, Rademaker BM, Froeling FM, Meijer DW. Hemodynamics during laparoscopic extra- and intraperitoneal insufflation. An experimental study. *Surg Endosc*. 1997;11(9):911-914.
41. Meininger D, Byhahn C, Wolfram M, Mierdl S, Kessler P, Westphal K. Prolonged intraperitoneal versus extraperitoneal insufflation of carbon dioxide in patients undergoing totally endoscopic robot-assisted radical prostatectomy. *Surg Endosc*. 2004;18(5):829-833.
42. Hu JC, Nelson RA, Wilson TG, et al. Perioperative complications of laparoscopic and robotic assisted laparoscopic radical prostatectomy. *J Urol*. 2006;175(2):541-546. discussion 546.
43. Rassweiler J, Stolzenburg J, Sulser T, et al. Laparoscopic radical prostatectomy – the experience of the german laparoscopic working group. *Eur Urol*. 2006;49(1):113-119.
44. Liatsikos E, Rabenalt R, Burchardt M, et al. Prevention and management of perioperative complications in laparoscopic and endoscopic radical prostatectomy. *World J Urol*. 2008;26(6):571-580.
45. Katz R, Borkowski T, Hoznek A, Salomon L, de la Taille A, Abbou CC. Operative management of rectal injuries during laparoscopic radical prostatectomy. *Urology*. 2003;62(2): 310-313.
46. Guillonneau B, Gupta R, El Fettouh H, Cathelineau X, Baumert H, Vallancien G. Laparoscopic [correction of laproscopic] management of rectal injury during laparoscopic [correction of laproscopic] radical prostatectomy. *J Urol*. 2003;169(5):1694-1696.
47. Bishoff JT, Allaf ME, Kirkels W, Moore RG, Kavoussi LR, Schroder F. Laparoscopic bowel injury: incidence and clinical presentation. *J Urol*. 1999;161(3):887-890.
48. Blumberg JM, Lesser T, Tran VQ, Aboseif SR, Bellman GC, Abbas MA. Management of rectal injuries sustained during laparoscopic radical prostatectomy. *Urology*. 2009;73(1): 163-166.

49. Chandler JG, Corson SL, Way LW. Three spectra of laparoscopic entry access injuries. *J Am Coll Surg*. 2001;192(4):478-490. discussion 490–1.
50. Modi P, Goel R, Dodiya S. Laparoscopic ureteroneocystostomy for distal ureteral injuries. *Urology*. 2005;66(4): 751-753.
51. Solberg A, Angelsen A, Bergan U, Haugen OA, Viset T, Klepp O. Frequency of lymphoceles after open and laparoscopic pelvic lymph node dissection in patients with prostate cancer. *Scand J Urol Nephrol*. 2003;37(3):218-221.
52. Ojeda L, Sharifi R, Lee M, Mouli K, Guinan P. Lymphocele formation after extraperitoneal pelvic lymphadenectomy: possible predisposing factors. *J Urol*. 1986;136(3):616-618.
53. Herrell SD, Trachtenberg J, Theodorescu D. Staging pelvic lymphadenectomy for localized carcinoma of the prostate: a comparison of 3 surgical techniques. *J Urol*. 1997;157(4): 1337-1339.
54. Stolzenburg JU, Wasserscheid J, Rabenalt R, et al. Reduction in incidence of lymphocele following extraperitoneal radical prostatectomy and pelvic lymph node dissection by bilateral peritoneal fenestration. *World J Urol*. 2008;26(6):581-586.
55. Remzi M, Klingler HC, Tinzl MV, et al. Morbidity of laparoscopic extraperitoneal versus transperitoneal radical prostatectomy verus open retropubic radical prostatectomy. *Eur Urol*. 2005;48(1):83-89. discussion 89.
56. Teber D, Erdogru T, Cresswell J, Gozen AS, Frede T, Rassweiler JJ. Analysis of three different vesicourethral anastomotic techniques in laparoscopic radical prostatectomy. *World J Urol*. 2008;26(6):617-622.
57. Secin FP, Touijer K, Mulhall J, Guillonneau B. Anatomy and preservation of accessory pudendal arteries in laparoscopic radical prostatectomy. *Eur Urol*. 2007;51(5):1229-1235.
58. Gargollo Patricio C, Dahl Douglas M. Complications of laparoscopic radical prostatectomy. In: Loughlin KR, ed. *Complications of Urologic Surgery and Practice: Diagnosis, Prevention, and Management*. 2nd ed. New York: Informa Healthcare USA, Inc; 2007:349. 52 Vanderbilt Avenue, New York, NY 10017.
59. Bhayani SB, Pavlovich CP, Strup SE, et al. Laparoscopic radical prostatectomy: a multi-institutional study of conversion to open surgery. *Urology*. 2004;63(1):99-102.
60. Rassweiler J, Schulze M, Teber D, Seemann O, Frede T. Laparoscopic radical prostatectomy: functional and oncological outcomes. *Curr Opin Urol*. 2004;14(2):75-82.
61. Rassweiler J. Open vs. laparoscopic radical prostatectomy ... and laparoscopy is better! *Eur Urol*. 2006; 50(1):26-28.

Robot-Assisted Extraperitoneal Laparoscopic Prostatectomy

13

Thomas T. Hoang, Satya B. Allaparthi, and Ingolf A. Tuerk

Abstract Extraperitoneal surgery for the prostate has been the gold standard for open surgeons. The technique can be applied by minimally invasive surgeons if the principles of extraperitoneal space formation are followed. We have endeavored to provide the reader with a stepwise team approach to achieve robotic extraperitoneal laparoscopic prostatectomy in a safe and reproducible manner.

Keywords Extraperitoneal • Laparoscopy • Prostate cancer • Prostatectomy • Robotics

Key Points

- It is more difficult to learn and familiarity with the transperitoneal approach is very beneficial
- Excellent approach for patients with prior transabdominal surgery (colon and small bowel resection) because of the avoidance of significant intraperitoneal adhesions
- Reduced risk of injury of intraperitoneal organs (bowel), while increased risk of lymphocele formation
- Very mild Trendelenburg position required due to the retraction of the bowel by the intact peritoneum, therefore significantly reduced risk of morbidity and side effects of prolonged steep Trendelenburg
- Less irritation of the peritoneal cavity and therefore faster recovery of patients particularly with respect to bowel function (les ileus)
- In case of complications (urine leak, bleeding, rectum injury), separation of urine, blood, and stool from the peritoneum with avoidance of peritonitis and less overall morbidity

13.1 Introduction

Since the first laparoscopic nephrectomy was performed in 1991, laparoscopic urology has grown by leaps and bounds.[1] This technology was applied to pelvic lymphadenectomy for staging prostate cancer in the early 1990s.[2] Transperitoneal as well as extraperitoneal approaches were described. Soon the radical

I.A. Tuerk (✉)
Department of Urology, St. Elizabeth's Medical Center, 736 Cambridge St, Boston, MA 02136, USA
e-mail: ingolf.tuerk@semc.org

J.V. Joseph and H.R.H. Patel (eds.), *Retroperitoneal Robotic and Laparoscopic Surgery*,
DOI: 10.1007/978-0-85729-485-2_13, © Springer-Verlag London Limited 2011

prostatectomy was performed entirely laparoscopically and this procedure has been established in some institutions as a first-line therapy for organ-confined prostate cancer.[3] Most of the early technique was strictly transperitoneal but eventually an extraperitoneal technique was developed.[4] The oncologic and functional outcomes have been compared to the gold standard of open radical retropubic prostatectomy and relatively few differences are actually seen.[5] Next, robot-assisted laparoscopic surgery was introduced and applied to the radical prostatectomy.[6] The initial approach was described as transperitoneally but also an extraperitoneal approach has been described which combines all the advantages of robotic laparoscopic surgery but stays away from the peritoneal cavity.[7] The specific advantages include avoidance of the peritoneal cavity, resulting in fewer incidences of postoperative ileus and bowel injury. A patient with multiple abdominal surgeries who most likely has severe adhesions can be operated on safely as this technique avoids those obstacles.[8] Also, the peritoneal cavity acts like a self-retaining bowel retractor so the patient does not have to be in steep Trendelenburg as in the transperitoneal procedure. Certain patients with poor pulmonary reserve certainly benefit from not having to be in steep Trendelenburg. The extraperitoneal technique mirrors the open technique in that the procedure takes place in the exact same area as the open surgery. Most urologists are very comfortable operating in this area if they have performed numerous open radical retropubic prostatectomies. Another advantage is in the event of a urine leak from the anastomosis, the urine is contained in the extraperitoneal space. Urine has long been known to be irritating to the bowel and can cause a moderate to severe peritonitis if prolonged contact is made. A urine leak can be managed with a Foley catheter just as one manages an extraperitoneal bladder rupture in the trauma setting.[9]

13.2 Indications/Contraindications

The primary indication to undergo a robot-assisted extraperitoneal laparoscopic prostatectomy is organ confined (stage cT1 or cT2) prostate cancer. The size of the patient also does play a factor although some of the literature disputes this notion. We have experienced that a larger patient with a BMI > 35 will be a more difficult case if the extraperitoneal approach is used. The size of the prostate also plays a factor and may further prolong the case and add to the blood loss. A narrow pelvis does not preclude an extraperitoneal approach. The patient must be in good enough health to undergo surgery under general anesthesia. A cardiac evaluation is imperative if the patient reports a history of cardiac disease. A benefit of the extraperitoneal approach as opposed to the transperitoneal approach is the amount of Trendelenburg used. An extraperitoneal approach uses minimal Trendelenburg while the transperitoneal approach uses steep Trendelenburg which could compromise a patient with poor pulmonary function and other significant comorbidity. Absolute contraindications include uncorrected coagulopathy, metastatic prostatic cancer, poor performance status, and recent myocardial infarction or stroke. Relative contraindications include severe obesity and previous radiation therapy to the prostate. Previous laparoscopic inguinal herniorrhaphy with mesh will not allow for an extraperitoneal access and a transperitoneal route is preferred. However, in patients with extensive surgery via laparotomy an extraperitoneal approach has the significant benefit of avoiding the expected massive intraperitoneal adhesions. Also in a patient with high-risk prostate cancer requiring an extended pelvic lymph nodes dissection (PLND) (up to the aorta) the transperitoneal approach is favorable over the extraperitoneal approach.

13.3 Preoperative Preparation

Upon initial evaluation the patient is given a comprehensive packet detailing all the steps leading up to, during, and after the surgery. It has been shown that pelvic floor exercises after prostatectomies assist in patients recovering continence.[10] We have extrapolated this data to start the Kegel exercises before the surgery. At the initial visit the patient is specifically instructed to perform Kegel exercises immediately to help promote faster return of continence after the surgery. The patient is thoroughly worked up and if the patient has significant comorbidities, a cardiac workup is initiated prior to surgery. The patient obtains standard preoperative lab work including a complete blood count, a chemistry panel, and coagulation studies. The patient should have a light diet starting noon the day before surgery and 8-h fasting before surgery is required. No bowel or rectal preparation is mandatory but a fleet enema or a laxative suppository may be recommended for patients who suffer from constipation or in the postradiotherapy salvage prostatectomy setting. A single dose of a first-generation cephalosporin is administrated preoperatively in order to prevent wound infection, especially at the umbilical site. No antibiotics are indicated postoperatively. No antibiotics are either routinely indicated before or after Foley catheter removal unless the patient is at risk of distant infections (heart valves, prostheses, etc.). In case a cystogram is planned before Foley removal, antibiotic coverage is mandatory. Prevention of deep venous thrombosis remains an essential element of preoperative care in patients at high risk of thrombo-embolic events, such as tobacco exposure, prolonged hospital stay, re-operation, or patients with large volume glands. Patients are given 3,500 IU of low-molecular-weight heparin subcutaneously 2 h before the operation. Patients continue with this daily dose until they are discharged from the hospital. Pneumatic compression stockings are regularly used during the surgery and postoperatively until the patient resumes ambulation.

13.4 Operative Room Set Up

13.4.1 The Patient

The patient is positioned in the dorsal supine position. Thoracic wrap with elastic adhesive tape is used to secure the patient to the table and avoid backward slide with Trendelenburg positioning. Hard shoulder supports are not appropriate because of the risk of postoperative shoulder pain due to prolonged pressure on the acromio-clavicular joints. Arms are placed along the body side to avoid the risk of injury to the brachial plexus. Hands are protected with mittens to avoid any inadvertent injury to the fingers while flexing and unflexing the table. Legs are split (an operating room table with split leg function is preferred although Allen stirrups have also been used) and positioned in flexion-abduction on foam supports after pneumatic compressive stockings have been placed. Particular attention should be paid to the calves due to the reported risk of compartment syndrome during long procedures when the leg is placed in the lithotomy position. Combined with a prolonged surgical time, this position may cause an acute compartment syndrome. Therefore, spread bars should be used instead of stirrups.

The anesthesia team provides general endotracheal anesthesia and an orogastric tube is placed to decompress the gastric contents. After usual skin preparation, the abdomen is disinfected from the costal margins to the perianal region and the patient is draped. Legs are covered individually to allow easy access to the perineum. An 18-french Foley catheter is inserted, the balloon filled with 10 cc of water, and the bladder drained.

13.4.2 Surgical Team

The da Vinci S® (Intuitive Surgicals, California, USA) robot is set up before the entry of the patient in the operating room. The system is turned on and performs a self-testing procedure during which it recognizes its own spatial position and various components. The camera is black-and-white balanced and calibrated. The surgical cart is then draped with sterile plastic sheaths. All these procedures take approximately 20 min and can be performed by a trained nurse. We prefer the use of the Da Vinci S robot with its four arms that are all utilized during the procedure thereby reducing the need of additional surgical assistance. We do place the fourth arm on the patient's right side which will alternate with the right-hand scissors and has the advantage that during the use of the fourth arm (usually Pro-grasp) that we have two grasping instruments available for better instrument assistance. While the surgeon operates at the console, the first assist stands on the patients left side utilizing the suction device and assists through the left-side assistant port in addition to the responsibility of exchanging the instruments of the left robotic arm and the scrub nurse is located on the right side of the patient exchanging the instruments of the right robotic arm as well as the fourth arm.

13.5 Operative Steps

13.5.1 Space Creation and Port Placement

The procedure starts with a 10-mm incision in the infraumbilical crease. A same size incision is performed on the anterior rectus fascia and the rectus muscle fibers vertically separated by blunt dissection with Kelly forceps until the anterior aspect of the umbilico-prevesical fascia is exposed. Finger dissection between the rectus muscle anteriorly and the umbilico-prevesical fascia posteriorly gives access to the retropubic space. Care must be taken to stay close to the rectus muscle while performing this maneuver, thereby avoiding inferior epigastric vessel injuries. This creates the extraperitoneal space and an Auto Suture® (Covidien, Mansfield, MA) balloon trocar is placed and inflated under direct vision with a 0° laparoscope. After the pubis is exposed adequately from the balloon dissection, the trocar is removed and a 5-mm suction assistant port is placed on the left, superior and lateral to the umbilical incision. Using manual assistance through the umbilical incision, the tip of the trocar is guided into the extraperitoneal space. An Auto Suture balloon trocar is placed into the infraumbilical incision while inflating the balloon for fixation and a CO_2 pneumoperitoneum is obtained with a 15 mmHg pressure maximum. The patient is then placed in a very mild Trendelenburg position. The 0° laparoscope is placed into the trocar and under direct vision the extraperitoneal space is further extended laterally while mobilizing the peritoneum from the lateral abdominal wall with the scope itself to accommodate the placement of the lateral ports. Then the robotic and assistant trocars are placed in the typical standard fan-shaped distribution.

Two 8-mm robotic trocars are placed infraumbilically 8–9 cm laterally away from the camera port. A right-sided fourth arm 8-mm robotic trocar is placed just medial to the anterior superior iliac spine. A left-sided 12-mm assistant port is placed as lateral as possible just above the anterior superior iliac spine. The robot is then positioned between the split legs of the patient and each arm is docked to its respective port in a way that avoids any compression or excessive traction of the patient's skin during the operative movements (Fig. 13.1).

Bipolar forceps are placed in the robotic left arm, monopolar shears are placed in the right arm, and the Pro-Grasp forceps are used for the fourth arm (right side of the patient). The assistant at the bedside uses the 5-mm port for suction and irrigation and the 12-mm port to introduce/remove needles and to also help retract. The whole procedure will be performed with a 0° lens; no 30° downward or upward optic is required (Fig. 13.2).

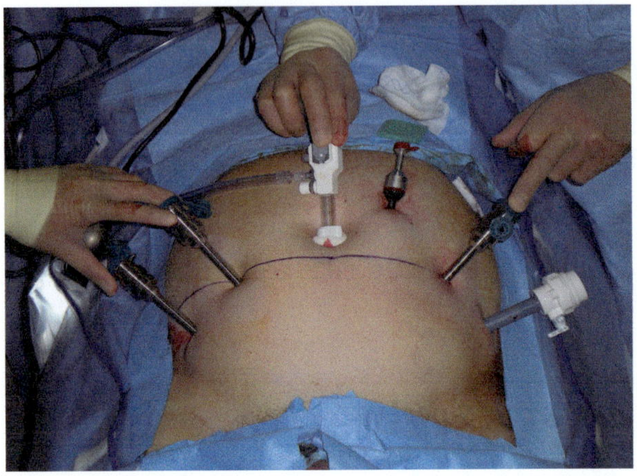

Fig. 13.1 Location and arrangement of the trocars for extraperitoneal robotic radical prostatectomy

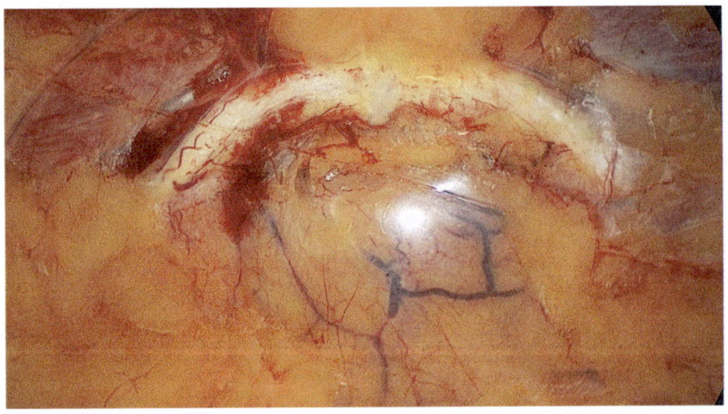

Fig. 13.2 Inside view during inflation of extraperitoneal balloon

13.5.2 Template and Technique of the Extraperitoneal PLND

If clinically indicated, a unilateral or bilateral pelvic lymph node dissection is done at this point. The external iliac artery forms the lateral border of dissection. Dissection is carried down to Cooper's ligament. The superior limit of dissection is defined by the bifurcation of external and internal iliac vessels. The posteromedial limit of dissection is formed by the internal iliac vessels and the anteromedial limit is represented by the medial umbilical ligament (obliterated umbilical artery).

It should be reinforced that a complete extended PLND within the template as described elsewhere is only feasible with a transperitoneal approach. In order to perform an accurate PLND, certain landmarks have to be visualized (Fig. 13.3).

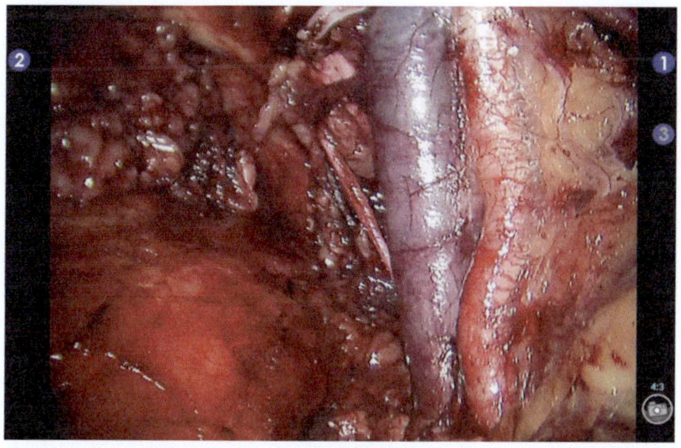

Fig. 13.3 Iliac external vessels and obturator nerve after extraperitoneal lymph node dissection

Utilizing bipolar forceps (left hand) and monopolar shears (right hand) the pubic bone is identified and following the arc of the pubic bone the dissection is continued laterally until the encounter of the iliac vessels. The bladder also is mobilized and separated from the iliac vessels along the medial umbilical ligament. Another important landmark is the identification of the vas deferens (VD) crossing over the iliac vessels since it represents the extent of the peritoneum and helps to avoid incising the peritoneum.

On the right side, the best exposure for a PLND will be achieved with the Pro-grasp retracting the peritoneal sack cephalad and a grasper from the first assist (left side) retracting the medial umbilical ligament to the left side. After initial dissection of the iliac vessels, the Pro-grasp also can be used to retract the external iliac vein. On the left side, the Pro-grasp will retract the bladder in the area of the medial umbilical ligament toward the right and the suction device will retract the vas deferens with peritoneum and or the iliac vessels. With appropriate mobilization of the peritoneum and the ideal retraction, the lymph node dissection can be carried out removing all tissue from the extern iliac artery and extern iliac vein all the way to the bifurcation of the common iliac vessels, including the obturator fossa and along the intern iliac vessels. To minimize the risk of lymphocele formation, the use of Weck clips prior to the transection of major lymph vessels is recommended. In addition, it is my routine to create at the end of the procedure large windows into the peritoneum to facilitate lymph drainage into the peritoneal cavity to further reduce the risk of lymphocele formation.

13.5.3 Exposing the Endopelvic Fascia

The fat of the retropubic space must be swept laterally to expose clearly the internal obturator muscles, the endopelvic fascia, and the puboprostatic ligaments. Control of tiny vessels within the fat is necessary. This dissection exposes the superficial dorsal vein that is easily identified emerging through the puboprostatic ligaments; it must be coagulated in this area with bipolar forceps and then transected. Once the superficial dorsal vein is transected, the fat covering the endopelvic fascia can be easily swept off.

The entire endopelvic fascia is then identified, covering the prostate. It is incised laterally on its line of reflection, starting at the level of the base of the prostate and extending anteriorly toward the apex (Fig. 13.4). This plane should leave the levator ani fascia covering the homonym muscle laterally and the prostatic fascia covering the sidewall of the prostate. In the event of bleeding, attempt to fulgurate periprostatic veins is always unsuccessful and very frustrating. It is better either to tamponade the area of bleeding or to ignore it and continue with the dissection. Temporary increase of the intra-abdominal pressure up to 15 or 20 mmHg helps with tamponading any venous bleeding.

Toward the pubic bone, the endopelvic fascia is reinforced by fibers from the puboprostatic ligament and the levator ani fascia becomes more adherent to the prostatic fascia. Small vessels, which penetrate into the prostatic apex or anastomose to branches of the dorsal vein complex (DVC) as well as apical accessory pudendal arteries (APAs) can be identified at this level if the

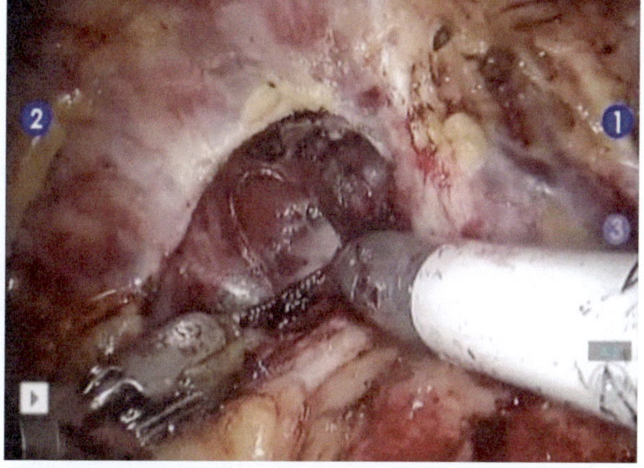

Fig. 13.4 Exposing endopelvic fascia

dissection is developed toward the apex. While the veins should be identified and fulgurated to allow complete access to the lateral aspect of the apex, the APAs should be preserved as they may contribute to both penile and urethral irrigation. These APAs rather than penetrating into the prostate, continue their course parallel to the DVC towards the anterior perineum. APAs can give off small branches to the prostatic apex that need to be fulgurated and transected.

13.5.4 Ligation of the Dorsal Vein Complex

Incision of the puboprostatic ligaments is done at a safe distance from the DVC, as close as possible to the prostatic fascia in order to maintain the integrity of the suspensor mechanism of the urethral sphincter. Any overdissection of the urethra may contribute to postoperative urinary incontinence. The section of the puboprostatic ligaments allows accurate visualization of the lateral aspect of the DVC, covered by the extension of the prostatic fascia. This fascia can be delicately incised to facilitate further dissection and cleanly expose the lateral aspects of the veins and their inferior limit.

In case of inadvertent bleeding from any of the veins forming the DVC, it is again useless to try to control them with any kind of fulguration and the intra-abdominal pressure can be transiently raised up to 15 or even 20 mmHg while the definitive ligature is placed.

The DVC is ligated with a 0-Vicryl suture on a # 1 CT needle. It is necessary to stretch the curve of the needle out so that it can cross the entire width of a particularly wide DVC. For a right-handed surgeon, the needle is grabbed backhand with the right needle-holder and passed from right to left under the DVC. The needle is situated such that the curve of the needle follows the curve of the symphysis, i.e., inverted U shape. A "figure of 8" suture is placed around the dorsal vein complex and the suture is tied but the dorsal vein complex is not transected at this point in time (Fig. 13.5).

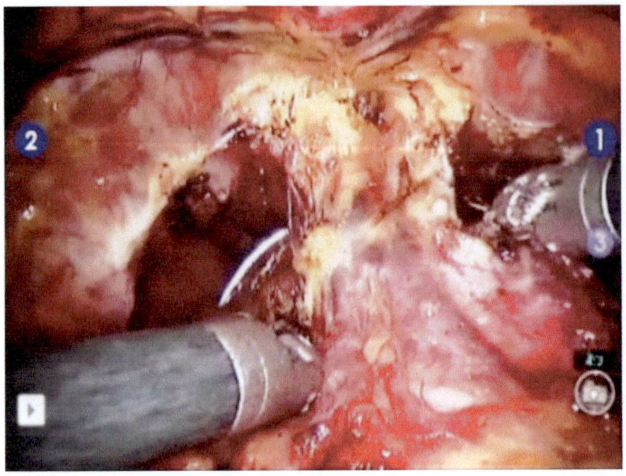

Fig. 13.5 Dorsal vein stitch

13.5.5 Bladder Neck Dissection

This step is often claimed to be difficult since the anatomical landmarks are not as well defined as in other phases of the surgery. Adequate identification and dissection of the prostato-vesical junction is crucial in order to minimize the risk of a positive surgical margin at the base of the gland and to preserve as much bladder neck as possible. The place where the bladder neck should be incised is exactly where the fat becomes adherent to the anterior bladder wall. To recognize this area, the anterior prevesical fat must be swept off superiorly causing a faint outline of the prostato-vesical plane. (This retraction of the preprostatic fat is possible because the superficial dorsal vein had been previously transected). The fat tends to be more adherent at the level of the bladder surface (adventitia) than to the endopelvic fascia covering the prostate. The opening of the prostato-vesical junction should be done at the level of this adherent fat. The prostatic fascia is then transversally incised at this landmark with careful coagulation as several veins run in this layer. This maneuver is accomplished by maintaining traction of the bladder cephalad with the fourth arm (Pro-grasp) while the other instrument incises (scissors) or coagulates (bipolar forceps) fibers and vessels. The assistant clears the operative field by aspirating blood and smoke. It is generally easy to develop the plane of dissection between the bladder and the prostate with sharp and blunt dissection. The mucosa of the anterior bladder neck is identified by a sudden change in the orientation of the muscular fibers that become longitudinal rather than circular or plexiform. It is possible to recognize the origin of the prostatic urethra as the mucosa of the anterior bladder neck continues under an "arch" created by the base of the prostate that corresponds to the level where the anterior bladder neck can be safely incised. The bladder neck is dissected, not only anteriorly but also laterally on each side. The bladder is checked again to be empty and the catheter balloon is deflated.

The anterior bladder neck is incised transversally and the tip of the Foley catheter is pulled upwards with the Pro-grasp utilizing the fourth arm in order to tent and lift up the prostate exposing the posterior bladder neck wall. The entire thickness of the posterior bladder neck wall is then incised. This is a step when the dissecting pace should be reduced as this is a highly vascularized area and discrete coagulation alternating the use of the tip of the scissors and the bipolar forceps is needed. The first assistant can improve the exposure by retracting the bladder with a grasper (introduced through the left-side assistant port) and gently pulling the bladder neck down with the suction device. To have an adequate access to this plane, the dissection should be extended laterally. Conceptually, the goal of the dissection of the posterior bladder neck is to free the bladder off the prostate (rather than the prostate off the bladder). It is important to direct the dissection straight posterior, following the posterior bladder wall (instead of the contour of the prostate). A common mistake is to confuse this plane with the surgical capsule and develop a plane dissection between the central and the peripheral zone of the prostate rather than between the prostate and the bladder. This wrong plane is very "attractive" because it is very easy to develop. If inadvertently opened, the dissection should be redirected more posteriorly to find the correct plane. In other words, if the plane is easily developed, it is probably the wrong one! The correct plane of dissection leads to the recognition of the longitudinal fascia of the detrusor muscle fibers inserting into the prostate base. Inexperienced surgeons might confuse these fibers with the rectal wall, but these fibers should be incised in order to gain access to the retrovesical space where the vas deferens (VD) and seminal vesicles (SV) are located.

13.5.6 Dissection of Vas Deferens and Seminal Vesicles

Once the longitudinal fascia of the detrusor is identified at the posterior bladder neck, it should be incised horizontally in the midline. The ampullary portion of the vas deferens is identified in the midline covered by the adventitia of the bladder, which should also be incised. At that point, one VD is grasped with the Pro-grasp (fourth arm) and retracted anteriorly. The

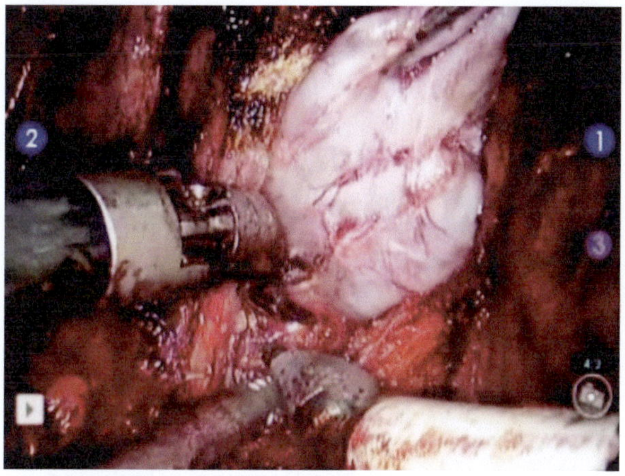

Fig. 13.6 Retraction of seminal vesicle

assistant uses a grasper to retract the bladder for exposure and uses the suction cannula as needed. The VD is dissected a few centimeters from the ampulla and coagulated with bipolar forceps or clipped and then transected. The deferential artery runs between the vas and the SV, therefore it will not be visible until the vas is sectioned. Division of the vas and deferential artery allows access to the seminal vesicle.

At this point, the Pro-grasp (fourth arm) grasps the prostatic end of the vas in order to expose and facilitate SV dissection while retracting the bladder posteriorly with the suction cannula to widen the working space. Seminal vesicles are gently dissected to avoid any injury to the inferior hypogastric plexus. Coagulation of the seminal vesicle vessels must be performed precisely on the surface of the seminal vesicle. During this dissection, the Pro-grasp will progressively grasp the seminal vesicle and retracts it anteriorly and contralaterally (Fig. 13.6).

It is important to mobilize the seminal vesicles completely before opening Denonvilliers' fascia and before starting the prostatic pedicle dissection to avoid injury of rectal fibers tented when the seminal vesicles are lifted upwards by the assistant.

13.5.7 Incision of the Denonvillier's Fascia and Rectum Mobilization

Incision of Denonvilliers' fascia during this step detaches the prostate from the rectum and delineates the medial aspect of the neurovascular bundles (NVBs).

After complete mobilization of both VD and both SV, the Pro-grasp pulls both VD anteriorly in order to expose Denonvillier's fascia and the rectum. Denonvillier's fascia is incised close to the base of the prostate and the rectum is mobilized of the posterior prostate with a combination of blunt and sharp dissection. The dissection is taken as far distal toward the apex as possible and also as far lateral as possible to facilitate the identification of the prostatic pedicles and the recognition of the neurovascular bundle (NVB).

13.5.8 Control of the Prostatic Pedicles and Dissection of the NVB

The prostatic pedicles are taken down with meticulous dissection and the use of Weck clips. This procedure is facilitated by anterior traction from the SV or the base of the prostate. Depending on how wide the surgeon is planning to perform the NVB dissection, control of the prostatic pedicles can be performed at variables distances from the gland. The amount of periprostatic tissue removed with the specimen will depend on the characteristics of the tumor, location, Gleason score, serum PSA, clinical stage, and imaging findings.

The pedicles are separated in smaller portions creating windows with the bipolar forceps in one direction and verified by the shears in the other direction (Fig. 13.7). The right arm shears are switched out for a robotic Weck clip applier and the clip (medium) is placed around the isolated pedicle tissue and transected (Fig. 13.8). This process is used repeatedly until the whole prostatic pedicle is controlled and transected. Smaller perforating arteries or veins are controlled with small titanium clips (introduced with the right robotic arm) thereby avoiding the use of electrocautery around the neurovascular bundles (Fig. 13.9).

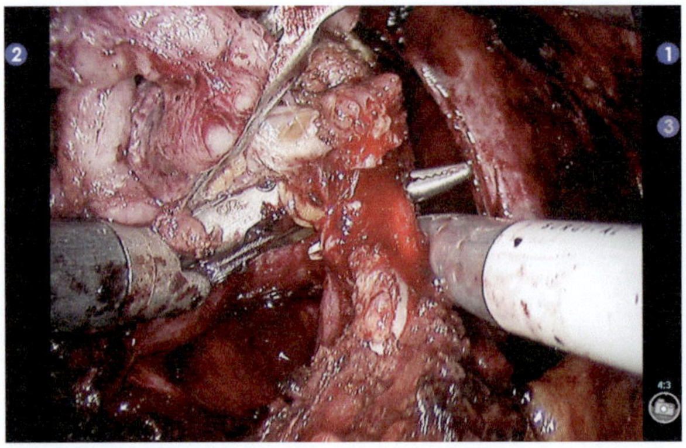

Fig. 13.7 Separation of the right prostate pedicle

To achieve an optimal preservation of the neurovascular bundles, it is necessary to consider three landmarks: Denonvillier's fascia posteromedially, the prostatic fascia posterolaterally, and the prostatic pedicle in between them. The proper incision of Denonvilliers' fascia during the earlier step detaches the prostate from the rectum and delineates the medial aspect of the neuro-vascular bundle. The prostate should be pulled medially to expose the lateral aspect of the prostate upholstered by the prostatic fascia. Incision on the prostatic fascia from the base toward the apex demarcates the lateral limit of the NVB (Fig. 13.10).

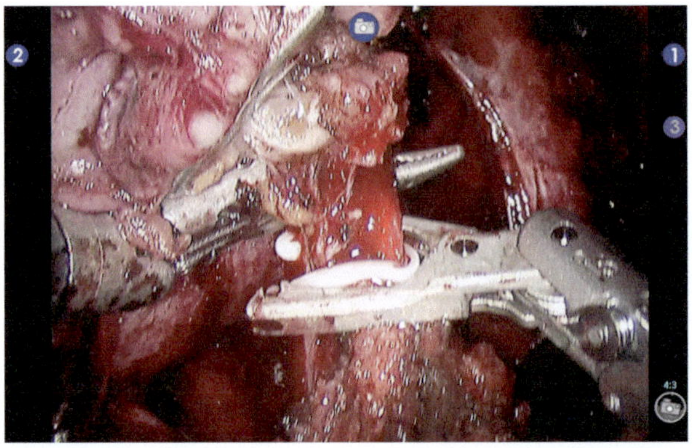

Fig. 13.8 Applying robotic-delivered Weck clip for pedicle control

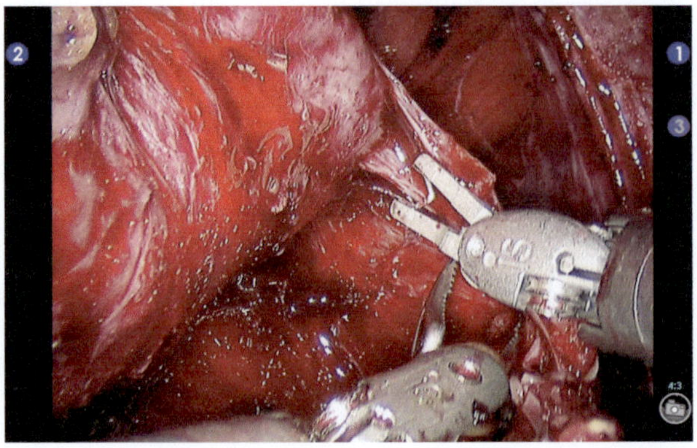

Fig. 13.9 Utilizing robotic-delivered small titanium clips for perforating vessels between neurovascular bundle (NVB) and prostate

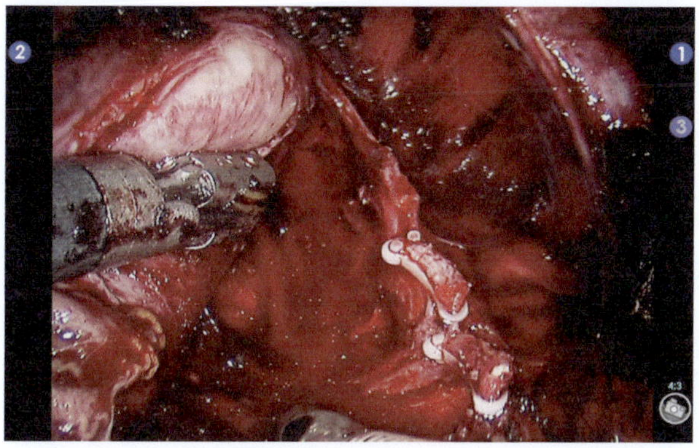

Fig. 13.10 Completed right side nerve sparing

Having established the medial and lateral limits of the NVB by incising Denonvilliers' fascia and the prostatic fascia, respectively, the next step is to "connect" or "bridge" these two landmarks following the contour of the prostatic capsule. The last components of the prostatic pedicle require transection in order to gain access to the posterolateral aspect of the gland and develop a plane between the prostatic capsule and the prostatic fascia. In this process, the NVB will be swept laterally. Using the "cut and peel" technique, the neurovascular bundle is swept posterolaterally. Posteriorly, the prostate is left covered by the prostatic fascia that is in continuity with Denonvilliers' fascia.

This intrafascial dissection allows gentle and progressive detachment of the bundle from the prostate. Again, as surgeons we should be aware of the possibilities of a capsular tear that may lead to a positive surgical margin. In any doubt, it is always preferable to dissect wider rather than compromising the oncological efficacy of the procedure.

The shape and volume of the prostate will usually dictate how far the surgeon can progress with the dissection of the NVB. It is often necessary to free the apex of the prostate anteriorly and transect Santorini's plexus before actually dissecting the distal extent of the NVB. This maneuver gives mobility to the gland facilitating the final freeing of the NVB and subsequent sectioning of the urethra.

13.5.9 Apical Dissection of the Prostate

At this point in the operation, the prostate is anchored by four structures: the DVC, the urethra, the distal attachment of Denonvillier's fascia to the rectourethralis muscle, and the distal extension of both NVB.

The incision of the DVC should be done tangential to the prostate to avoid a positive surgical margin at the apex, particularly posterior to the urethra. The DVC is divided until an avascular plane of dissection between the DVC and the urethra is developed. This plane exposes the anterior and lateral urethral wall but should not be developed too widely in an effort to avoid any injury to the sphincter mechanism (Fig. 13.11).

Should excessive bleeding from the DVC occur, never aspirate through the suction cannula while the DVC is bleeding, this will make bleeding worse!

1. Increase the pneumoperitoneum to a maximum of 20 mmHg
2. Complete the sectioning of the DVC all the way down to the urethra
3. Suture the bleeding laparoscopically with 2/0 Vicryl on an SH needle

At the apex, the neuro-vascular bundles are divergent from the prostate, but they must be followed until their entrance into the pelvic floor, below and lateral to the urethra to avoid any injury. Once the NVBs have been dissected off the apex, the urethra will be incised and transected with cold scissors. During this step, excessive traction on the prostate should be avoided so as not to stretch the urethra and the sphincter complex. The transection of the posterior urethra will be facilitated keeping the catheter tip visualized in the urethra stump. After the complete transection of the urethra, the distal attachments of Denonvillier's fascia (rectourethralis muscle) are incised. It is individualized at the apex and dissected off the posterior aspect of the

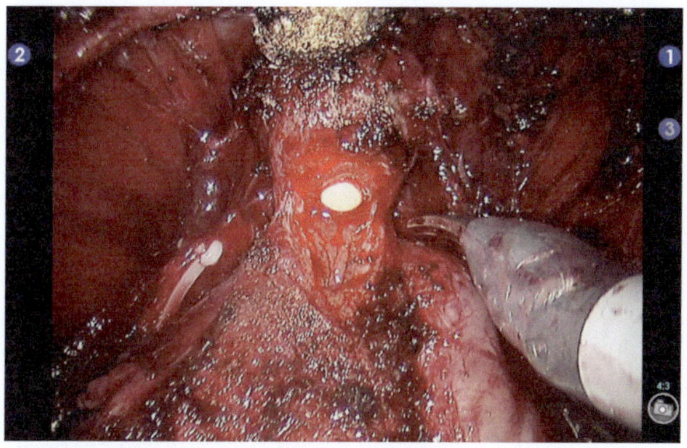

Fig. 13.11 Apex and urethra dissection

urethra. The surgeon should pay attention not to go all the way across with the shears to avoid any injury of the NVB on the opposite side.

Once free, the specimen is placed into a 10-mm laparoscopic bag and placed in an extraperitoneal pocket on the right side (proximal to the trocar of the fourth arm).

13.5.10 Urethrovesical Anastomosis (Running Suture)

We never evert the bladder mucosa. Even when the opening in the bladder neck is large, we do not narrow it before starting the anastomotic suture. In cases of a large bladder neck, an anterior tennis racquet – rather than posterior – is performed at the end of the anastomosis, once the posterior and lateral approximations are done.

A running urethrovesical anastomosis is performed using a modified van Velthoven technique.[11] One dyed and one undyed 3–0 Monocryl suture (approx. 6 in. long) with RB-1 needle are used each with a Lapra-Ty clip placed at the end of the sutures over a knot. The first suture is started at the 5 o'clock position on the bladder neck as well as urethra and run clockwise to the 12 o'clock position. Then the other suture is started at the 5 o'clock position and run counterclockwise to the 12 o'clock position. The posterior lip of the bladder neck is left (1–2 cm) apart from the posterior urethra as the first two throws on the urethra and the first three throws on the bladder are completed. When this is achieved, gentle traction is exerted on each thread simultaneously or alternately; the system of loops acts as a "winch" to bring the bladder in contact with the urethra without excessive traction. After performing a transition stitch of the undyed suture from the urethra to the bladder, the ends of the running sutures are tied to one another at 12:00 o'clock.

The Foley catheter is placed towards the end of the anastomosis and 10 cc of sterile water is used to inflate the balloon. The anastomosis is tested with 120 cc of normal saline injected gently through the Foley. If there is no leak, then no pelvic drain is placed. If a moderate leak is noticed then it may be prudent to place a bulb suction drain down in the pelvis but not directly on the anastomosis and bring it out through one of the lateral trocar sites.

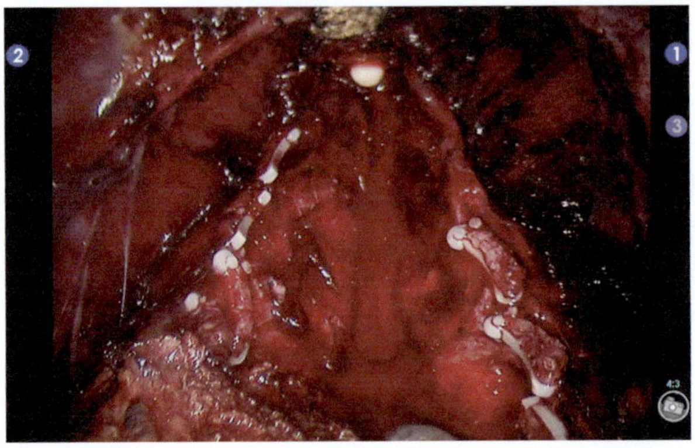

Fig. 13.12 Completed prostatectomy with bilateral preservation of the NVBs

13.5.11 Specimen Removal and Completion of the Operation

After completion of the anastomosis, meticulous attention is paid to the inspection of the operating field for bleeding. The area of the preserved NVBs is inspected and usually I place Surgicel between NVB, bladder, and rectum to support hemostasis since the NVBs tend to "ooze" after cold dissection (Fig. 13.12).

The tie to the Endo-bag is then brought through the trocar site and placed directly on the bag. The robot is then undocked and the rest of the case is concluded with conventional laparoscopy. The endocatch tie is then transferred under direct vision to the umbilical port. All trocars are removed under direct vision making to ensure there is no bleeding on the anterior abdominal wall. The umbilical skin incision is lengthened inferiorly to allow for removal of the specimen. The fascia is divided and the specimen removed. The fascia is closed with a running suture using 0-Vicryl, UR-6 needle and the skin incisions are closed with a skin adhesive.

13.6 Postoperative Care

The patient is admitted to the Post Anesthesia Care Unit and later to the floor with the Foley catheter to gravity drainage and secured to the leg. Postoperative labs are drawn in the recovery room as well as on the morning after surgery including a complete blood count and chemistry panel. The patient is put on a clear liquid diet and advanced to a regular diet as tolerated the evening of the surgery day (dinner). The patient is encouraged to ambulate as soon as possible. Subcutaneous heparin and sequential lower extremity compression devices are used until the patient is discharged. Pain is usually controlled with an oral narcotic and ketorolac is given if the patient's creatinine is below 1.2 g/dl. The patient is observed overnight and is usually discharged the next morning if clinically indicated (less than 24 h).

13.6.1 Postoperative Instructions

Patients usually start passing gases on postoperative day 1–2 and have their first bowel movement on postoperative day 2–4. We tend to support the bowel activity by administrating a Glycerin suppository on postoperative day 1 and encourage the patient to take stool softeners while at home in addition to ambulation.

Foley catheter is removed 7 days after surgery without a cystogram and Kegel exercises are started the day after catheter removal.[10]

Patients who underwent a nerve sparing procedure are offered the regular intake of Tadalafil[12] immediately after catheter removal and are allowed to resume sexual activity as soon as possible.[13]

13.7 Complications and Management

13.7.1 Intraoperative Complications

13.7.1.1 Bleeding from the DVC

The size and anatomic shape of the DVC varies from one patient to another. A wide DVC in patients with a narrow and deep pelvis is most challenging. Although laparoscopy allows a clear vision of the apex and the pneumoperitoneum provides a tamponade effect, bleeding from the DVC can be significant and may impact on the remainder of the operation as it affects visibility. A meticulous apical dissection defining the principal elements around the DVC is essential to preventing unnecessary hemorrhage.

First, all the apical adipose tissue should be dissected off the pubic symphysis superiorly and off the prostate posteriorly and laterally. This brings into view the superficial dorsal vein, which is easily controlled and gives access to the pubovesical ligaments. The latter should be taken down close to their bony attachment. This maneuver widens the access to the DVC and allows the opening of the periprostatic fascia covering the DVC laterally. By doing so, the limit between the DVC is clearly exposed facilitating the placement of the ligating suture accurately engulfing the whole complex.

At times when the ligating suture is loose, placed too proximal or cut during the transection of the DVC, bleeding can be controlled by either increasing the pneumoperitoneum pressure up to 20 mmHg or by clamping the DVC with a grasper. This allows a tamponade effect while the surgeon can calmly prepare a second ligating suture. Precipitation during the placement of the suture may cause more harm. Once tied, the DVC stitch can eventually be anchored to the periosteum of the pubic symphysis to ensure its compression.

13.7.1.2 Bladder Injury

The bladder is more likely to be damaged at three different moments of the transperitoneal laparoscopic radical prostatectomy.[14]

First, during the posterior dissection of the seminal vesicles: dissection in fatty tissue should alert the surgeon of a plane either too close to bladder or to the rectum.

Second, during the development of retropubic space, especially when the dissection is carried out in the incorrect plane and the avascular plane is not adequately identified. Any excessive bleeding should alert the surgeon of a dissection taken too close to the bladder. Filling the bladder with 120–180 ml of saline may help to delineate the contours and identify any leakage.

Third, during the dissection of the posterior bladder neck, the area at risk is the trigone and retro trigonal bladder wall. When identified, the surgeon should verify the integrity of the ureters and ureteral orifices and repair the bladder with one layer of polygalactin suture.

13.7.1.3 Rectal Injury

There are two mechanisms in which the rectum can be injured. The first one is through a rectal tear, which most commonly occurs during the dissection of the posterior surface of the prostatic apex. It should be recognized intraoperatively, otherwise, will lead to a pelvic abscess and peritonitis. The risk of rectal tear increases when there is a substantial amount of periprostatic inflammatory reaction, prior prostate surgery or radiation, large volume gland with a narrow pelvis and/or during a non-nerve sparing procedure. Intrarectal digital manipulation or insertion of a rectal bougie or balloon may be of help to stay away from the rectal wall during the dissection of the posterior surface of the prostate. Their use is also recommended for tear identification purposes. While opinions on early postoperative care (antibiotics, low fiber diet, anal dilatation) are similar, management of the rectal injury itself remains debatable in regards to interposition of healthy tissue between the rectal repair and the urethrovesical anastomosis, and the need for a diverting colostomy. In the absence of gross fecal soiling, it is advised to repair the defect with a two-layer primary closure after debridement of any devitalized tissue. While interposition of an omental flap or pararectal fat flap provides extra safety, it is routinely not necessary. However, in face of a large, devitalized rectal laceration or gross soiling, a temporary diverting colostomy is advisable.[15,16]

The second kind of rectal injury is secondary to ischemia of the anterior rectal wall following vigorous dissection or excessive cauterization of vessels on the rectum surface. This devascularization injury may not be recognized intraoperatively and is frequently manifested by a delayed rectourethral fistula after the Foley catheter is removed. The first therapeutic option is to reinsert the Foley catheter until the fistula heals spontaneously. If this conservative approach fails, elective surgical approach of the rectourethral fistula should be considered.[17]

13.7.1.4 Ureteral Injury

It may occur either during the PLND or by an inadvertent thermal injury. Urine will not be seen coming out of a sectioned ureter as anyone might expect. Even if ureteral sectioning goes unnoticed, uro-peritoneum may not be an immediate event, especially if the ureter was fulgurated before being sectioned. When the injury is not identified intraoperatively, a persistent urine leakage or uro-peritoneum with a watertight anastomosis suggests the diagnosis. Ureteral reimplantation is the treatment of choice. To prevent this, it is essential to identify the vas deferens and its relationship with the peritoneum, in order to avoid going into the peritoneal cavity and getting lost in the wrong plane. The best way to avoid this is to mobilize the whole peritoneal sac cephalad from the iliac vessels, which will usually take the ureter with the peritoneum.

Another kind of ureteral complication is the occlusion of the ureteral orifice(s) caused by incorporating the ureteral orifices in the urethrovesical anastomotic sutures. If this is identified postoperatively, which can present with pain and, anuria, the anastomosis should be redone laparoscopically/robotically.

13.7.1.5 Inferior Epigastric Vessels Injury

The inferior epigastric vessels are at risk of injury during port placement. Bleeding around the trocar either internally or externally suggests a vessel injury. Transillumination to locate the epigastric vessels is not reliable; however, in thin patients the lateral umbilical ligament is an important landmark to help locate the inferior epigastric vessels. Placement of the port lateral to the rectus abdominalis muscle is safer. Venous injury can be managed successfully by tamponade, whereas arterial injury requires surgical hemostasis using a suture, a Reverdin, or a Carter-Thomason needle. As a fundamental rule of laparoscopic surgery, all the trocars should be removed under direct vision with a decreased abdominal pressure.

13.7.2 Postoperative Complications

13.7.2.1 Urethrovesical Anastomotic Leak

An increased and prolonged urine output from the pelvic drain suggests the diagnosis. In the majority of cases, the posterior aspect of the anastomosis is compromised particularly considering the higher tension with the extraperitoneal approach. This is managed conservatively by prolonging the bladder and pelvic drainage. If the leak persists despite conservative management, a ureteral injury or an eversion of the ureteral orifice outside of the anastomosis needs to be ruled out.

To prevent a severe leak, whatever the suture techniques – running or interrupted – it is essential to pay attention to the posterior aspect of the anastomosis, particularly on the left side. The anterior portion of the anastomosis is rarely a source of prolonged postoperative leaks.

13.7.2.2 Small Bowel Injury

The risk of small bowel injury is low given the extraperitoneal approach. The injury can occur either early in the operation by direct puncture or by thermal injury during dissection. A missed bowel injury will manifest itself postoperatively initially by ileus, mild abdominal pain particularly around the umbilicus, and normal or even decreased white blood cell count. Clinical signs of infection are subtle until sepsis suddenly takes place. Prompt computed tomography (CT) scan imaging with oral contrast may lead to the diagnosis, but in any doubt laparoscopic re-exploration should be considered.[17]

Rather than abscess formation (rectal injury), peritonitis usually occurs with the clinical picture described previously at the early stage. The treatment requires an exploratory laparotomy with inspection of the small bowel from the ligament of Treitz to the ileocecal junction and inspection of the large bowel as well.

13.7.2.3 Nerve Compression and Compartment Syndrome

Ulnar and brachial neuropraxia have been reported following LRP and resulted in a transient paresis. This type of complication is related to patient positioning. We place our patients in a low lithotomy position with both arms alongside the body. The shoulders, elbows, and wrists are adequately padded, and the patient is secured to the operating table with surgical tape. It is also important to remind the surgeon and assistant not to inadvertently lean on the patient's arm.

Obturator nerve neuropraxia can be associated with PLND. It is manifested by different degrees of postoperative throbbing, unrelenting leg pain, and weakness. Abducting capacity of the leg is markedly diminished and more frequently takes place on the left side due to the greater difficulty of the LND on this side for right-handed surgeons.

We prefer the low lithotomy position because it allows easy access to the rectum if needed. However, care should be taken to have a wide angle of flexion at the hip and knee levels. Over-tightness of the calves by the sequential compressive devices and stirrups should be avoided. Increased calf pressure for long periods of time may lead to a compartment syndrome: an emergency that should always be ruled out. Distal pulses should always be assessed pre- and postoperatively as well as distal capillary refill at the nail beds for it usually precedes cessation of arterial flow. Myoglobinuria, electrolyte disturbances, disorders of acid–base balance, and serum CK values over 2,000 U/l after surgery may be considered a warning sign in ventilated and sedated patients, in whom early clinical symptoms of the compartment syndrome such as pain and paresthesias cannot be ascertained.

In the presence of postoperative leg pain think first of acute compartment syndrome, particularly if symptoms are bilateral, outside the abductor muscle territory and in a patient in whom LND had not been performed. The treatment is emergent fasciotomy of the muscular groups involved.

13.7.2.4 Lymphocele

Another potential complication that could happen is a lymphocele after extended pelvic lymph node dissection. The incidence in the literature ranges from 2% to 5%.[13-15] However, the extraperitoneal approach seems to have a slightly higher incidence due to the separation from the peritoneal cavity. Meticulous closure of major lymph vessels with clips will reduce the formation of lymph fluid collections. Also a bilateral fenestration of the peritoneum at the end of the procedure will allow for drainage of the lymph fluid into the peritoneal cavity and will reduce the risk of lymphocele formation. If the lymph collection becomes large enough it can cause pain, ipsilateral leg edema, voiding symptoms due to bladder compression, hydronephrosis, or even deep vein thrombosis. Patients will present with vague or localized lower abdominal pain, voiding symptoms, leg pain, leg swelling, or ipsilateral flank pain from ureteral obstruction. Lymphoceles may become infected and patients may present with persistent fevers and chills. If a lymphocele is suspected then a CT scan should be ordered to determine the extent and size of the lymphocele. The preferred treatment would be a laparoscopic peritoneal fenestration but percutaneous drainage with or without sclerotherapy is an alternative treatment option.[16]

13.8 Advantages and Pitfalls

There are numerous advantages in using the extraperitoneal technique for robot-assisted laparoscopic prostatectomy. Most of them have been mentioned previously but here are the main points. By avoiding the peritoneal cavity, there is a significantly less chance of postoperative ileus and an even lesser chance of a bowel injury.[17] If the patient has had prior abdominal surgeries, he most likely will have intestinal adhesions depending on how many surgeries and the type of surgeries. These adhesions can be a major problem during a transperitoneal approach but can be avoided all together with an extraperitoneal approach. Another advantage is in the event of a urine leak postoperatively from the anastomosis, the urine is contained in the extraperitoneal space. Urine has long been known to be an irritant to the peritoneal contents so a minor peritonitis can be avoided during an extraperitoneal approach. The same is true for postoperative bleeding also, which has a better chance to be contained and therefore conservatively handled compared to the transperitoneal approach. The extraperitoneal approach mirrors the standard open radical retropubic prostatectomy procedure in almost every facet. The fact that most urologists are very comfortable in this area of the body can be an advantage if one attempts to learn the robot-assisted extraperitoneal laparoscopic prostatectomy technique. Yet another advantage of the extraperitoneal approach lies in the fact that the peritoneum acts as a self-retaining retractor for the entire bowel contents. Therefore, a very minimal amount of Trendelenburg is used which significantly reduced risks associated with prolonged steep Trendelenburg position.[18]

The disadvantages of the extraperitoneal approach are very few. Some authors have advocated that the transperitoneal approach should be learned first because it is the quickest way to become proficient with the robot and get over the learning curve. The extraperitoneal access is known to be somewhat more difficult to develop, and certainly lacks familiar landmarks during the dissection compared to the transperitoneal approach. One postulated disadvantage of the extraperitoneal approach is the limited working space as well as a more unstable pneumoperitoneum. An extended pelvic lymph node dissection all the way to the aorta is certainly not possible during the extraperitoneal approach. Another disadvantage is certain obese individuals have a body habitus that is not conducive to the extraperitoneal approach. The patient has a very short umbilicus to pubis area. Upon placing the trocars and robotic arms, the angle between the instrument and the pubic bone is so steep that reaching the apex of the prostate is extremely difficult and a thorough and well-performed surgery is not possible. Therefore, in patient with a BMI > 30, a transperitoneal approach is favorable by bringing all the trocar sites superiorly slightly to allow more working space.

References

1. Clayman RV, Kavoussi LR, Soper NJ, et al. Laparoscopic nephrectomy. *N Engl J Med*. 1991;324:1370-1371.
2. Ferzli G, Trapasso J, Raboy A, Albert P. Extraperitoneal endoscopic pelvic lymph node dissection. *J Laparoendosc Surg*. 1992;2:39-44.
3. Schuessler WW, Schulam PG, Clayman RV, Kavoussi LR. Laparoscopic radical prostatectomy: initial short-term experience. *Urology*. 1997;50:854-857.
4. Stolzenburg JU, Do M, Pfeiffer H, et al. The endoscopic extraperitoneal radical prostatectomy (EERPE): technique and initial experience. *World J Urol*. 2002;20:48-55.
5. Rassweiler J, Schulze M, Teber D, Seemann O, Frede T. Laparoscopic radical prostatectomy: functional and oncological outcomes. *Curr Opin Urol*. 2004;14:75.
6. Wolfram M, Bräutigam R, Engl T, et al. Robot-assisted laparoscopic radical prostatectomy: the Frankfurt technique. *World J Urol*. 2003;21:128-132.
7. Gettman MT, Hoznek A, Salomon L, et al. Laparoscopic radical prostatectomy: description of the extraperitoneal approach using the da Vinci robotic system. *J Urol*. 2003; 170:416-419.
8. Stolzenburg JU, Rabenalt R, Do M, et al. Endoscopic extraperitoneal radical prostatectomy: the University of Leipzig technique of 2000 cases. *J Endourol*. 2008;22: 2319-2325.
9. Joseph JV, Rosenbaum R, Madeb R, Erturk E, Patel HR. Robotic extraperitoneal radical prostatectomy: an alternative approach. *J Urol*. 2006;175:945-950.
10. Filocamo MT, Li Marzi V, Del Popolo G, et al. Effectiveness of early pelvic floor rehabilitation treatment for post-prostatectomy incontinence. *Eur Urol*. 2005;48:734-738.
11. Ball AJ, Bordeau KP, Davis JW, et al. Modified running vesicourethral anastomosis after robotically assisted laparoscopic radical prostatectomy: use of solitary Lapra-Ty to secure posterior approximation. *Urology*. 2005;66: 16-18.
12. Montorsi F, Nathan HP, McCullough A, et al. Tadalafil in the treatment of erectile dysfunction following bilateral nerve sparing radical retropubic prostatectomy: a randomized, double-blind, placebo controlled trial. *J Urol*. 2004;173:664.
13. Madeb R, Golijanin D, Knopf J, et al. Patient-reported validated functional outcome after extraperitoneal

robot-assisted nerve-sparing radical prostatectomy. *JSLS*. 2007;11:315-320.
14. Hoznek A, Antiphon P, Borkowski T, et al. Assessment of surgical technique and perioperative morbidity associated with extraperitoneal versus transperitoneal laparoscopic radical prostatectomy. *Urology*. 2003;61:617-622.
15. Stolzenburg JU, Rabenalt R, Do M, et al. Complications of endoscopic extraperitoneal radical prostatectomy (EERPE): prevention and management. *World J Urol*. 2006;24:668-675.
16. Guillonneau B, Gupta R, El Fettouh H, et al. Laparoscopic management of rectal injury during radical prostatectomy. *J Urol*. 2003;169:1694-1696.
17. Bishoff JT, Allaf ME, Kirkels W, et al. Laparoscopic bowel injury: incidence and clinical presentation. *J Urol*. 1999; 161:887-890.
18. Madi R, Daignault S, Wood DP. Extraperitoneal v intraperitoneal robotic prostatectomy: analysis of operative outcomes. *J Endourol*. 2007;21:1553-1557.

Laparoendoscopic Single-Site Retroperitoneal Surgery

14

Michael A. White and Jihad H. Kaouk

Abstract Initial reports of single-port laparoscopic surgery, now known as laparoendoscopic single-site surgery (LESS), are gaining momentum. LESS has become more sophisticated in part due to flexible tip laparoscopes and advancements in operating instruments. These newer instruments have improved the surgeon's range of motion and the ability to "triangulate" instruments despite in-line placement. Feasibility reports have focused almost exclusively on transperitoneal single-port surgery through the umbilicus, with little data to support LESS through a retroperitoneal approach.

The retroperitoneum is familiar to the urologist and the retroperitoneal approach can be superior to the transperitoneal technique in unique clinical presentations especially in those who have undergone previous intraabdominal surgery. We present our LESS retroperitoneal surgical technique and discuss our outcomes.

Keywords LESS • Retroperitoneal • Single port • Single-port laparoscopic retroperitioneal surgery • Single-site surgery

Key Points

- Single-port laparoscopic surgery is known as laparoendoscopic single-site surgery (LESS), but other names exist such as SILS (single-incision laparoscopic surgery).
- Improvements in the tools used for LESS allow for better "triangulation" during surgery which eases the technical demands on the surgeon.
- Robot-assisted LESS is now beginning an evolution, potentially simplifying still further the ease of performing LESS.
- Transperitoneal LESS is simple to perform compared to retroperitoneal LESS.
- Retroperitoneal LESS will be easier to undertake using advanced reticulating instruments or robotic assistance.

14.1 Introduction

LESS represents the latest evolution in minimally invasive urologic surgery and has a prime focus on esthetics and a reduction in postoperative morbidity. Advancements in laparoscopic instrumentation, improved optics, and robotics have allowed many different complex urological procedures to be performed through a single incision. LESS requires a solid background in standard laparoscopic surgery to minimize technical challenges posed by inserting all instruments in parallel without triangulation.

J.H. Kaouk (✉)
Director, Robotic and Laparoscopic Surgery,
Department of Urology, Cleveland Clinic Foundation,
9500 Euclid Ave, Q-10,
Cleveland, OH 44195, USA
e-mail: kaoukj@ccf.org

J.V. Joseph and H.R.H. Patel (eds.), *Retroperitoneal Robotic and Laparoscopic Surgery*,
DOI: 10.1007/978-0-85729-485-2_14, © Springer-Verlag London Limited 2011

14.2 Background

One of the early reports on LESS was in 2007 by Rane et al. who performed a simple nephrectomy through a retroperitoneal incision in the flank using a single port and a pyelolithotomy performed through a transumbilical single port.[1] Their results were presented as an abstract and the functional outcomes were not reported. During the same year Raman et al. used a variation of single-incision surgery with a multitrocar configuration inserted through a single skin incision to complete transumbilical nephrectomy on three patients. Two were completed through a single incision while one required an additional port for liver retraction.[2] The mean operative time was 133 min with an estimated blood loss of 30 ml. The specimens were extracted through 2–4.5 cm incisions.

In 2007 Kaouk et al. reported a series of LESS cases encompassing cryotherapy, kidney biopsy, and sacrocolpopexy in seven patients.[3] There were no complications and functional outcomes were good. Gill et al. further expanded the complexity of renal LESS by performing laparoscopic donor nephrectomy on four patients through a transumbilical incision. They named this procedure embryonic-natural orifice translumenal endoscopic surgery (E-NOTES) in reference to the embryonic origin of the umbilicus.[4]

Since these initial reports, clinical experience has grown to greater than 200 cases performed worldwide and has included a single institution's experience with more than 100 consecutive cases.[5] LESS has included: simple and radical nephrectomy, pyeloplasty, ileal ureter, ureteroneocystostomy and psoas hitch, radical prostatectomy, radical cystoprostatectomy with extended pelvic lymph node dissection, ureterolithotomy, partial nephrectomy, transvesical simple and radical prostatectomy, adrenalectomy, varicocelectomy, orchiectomy, orchidopexy, and augmentation enterocystoplasty.[6-17]

14.3 Ports

Several multichannel single-port devices are commercially available. Each of these ports has a set of advantages and disadvantages (Table 14.1).

14.4 Instrumentation

In addition to specially designed ports, instrumentation is critical to successful LESS. The necessary equipment consists of standard laparoscopic, bent, or flexible instrumentation. Flexible graspers, needle holders, and scissors are available (RealHand; Novare Surgical Systems, Cupertino, CA, USA and Autonomy Lapro-Angle; Cambridge Endo, Framingham, MA, USA). Since operative space is limited, a 5-mm endoscope is essential and is available in either the rigid 30° or the flexible variety (Olympus Surgical, Orangeburg, NY, USA).

Although equipment technology continues to expand and the scope and volume of LESS cases is on the rise, significant limitations to LESS exist requiring significant technical skill from an experienced laparoscopic team. The primary limitation to LESS is reduced ability to triangulate, resulting in instrument clashing. Retraction of tissues is another limitation. In traditional laparoscopy, retraction can be performed effectively since ports are placed distant from each other, but in LESS this is difficult due to the instruments lying parallel. A possible solution is the use of percutaneous sutures that can be placed at suitable points to allow adequate tissue retraction and help avoid the need for an additional port placement.

An additional limitation relates to the body habitus of the patient. In traditional laparoscopy, ports can be configured and shifted according to body habitus, a luxury that is not possible in LESS.

14.5 Robotic LESS

The impact of the limitations encountered during LESS is most recognizable during intracorporeal suturing. To combat these limitations the da Vinci Surgical System (Intuitive Surgical, Sunnyvale, CA, USA) has been used for LESS. Some advantages of using robotic technology are articulation of instruments, three-dimensional visualization, motion scaling, and tremor filtration. Robotic LESS procedures have been documented in the literature with encouraging outcomes.[18-21]

Table 14.1 Available single-port access devices

Port	Manufacturer	Lumens	Fixation	Valve
R-Port	Advanced surgical concepts, Dublin, Ireland	One 12 mm Two 5 mm	Inner/outer ring with plastic sleeve	Gel elastomer
Triport	Advanced surgical concepts, Bray, Co Wicklow, Ireland	One 12 mm Two 5 mm	Inner/outer ring with plastic sleeve	Insufflation line
Gelport	Applied medical, Rancho Santa Margarita, CA, USA	Gelface plate with central opening	Inner/outer ring with plastic sleeve	No insufflation site
Gelpoint	Applied medical, Rancho Santa Margarita, CA, USA	Gelface plate with insufflation port on side no openings	Inner/outer ring with plastic sleeve	Peripheral insufflation line
SILS	Covidien, Mansfield, MA, USA	One 12 mm Two 5 mm	Malleable conforms to incision	Insufflation line

14.6 Retroperitoneal Versus Transperitoneal Laparoscopy

The retroperitoneoscopic nephrectomy (RPN) may be useful in patients with previous intraabdominal surgery. Since the RPN approach involves reduced bowel manipulation, it may also promote earlier return of bowel function and reduced hospital stay. Several investigators have studied these approaches, both prospectively and retrospectively, and while not all the outcomes are the same, it appears that RPN and TPN have no significant difference in operative times, estimated blood loss, hospital stay, pre- and postoperative complications, and analgesic requirements.[22-26] Two studies have reported an earlier return to oral intake in the RPN cohort.[27,28] Obese patients seem to benefit from RPN and there have been demonstrated shorter operative times and shorter hospital stay compared to the nonobese.[29]

There are several limitations associated with the retroperitoneoscopic approach. Surgical working space is limited and may be challenging, especially during the robotic approach to allow for placement of bulky robotic arms. Additionally, anatomical surgical landmarks may be difficult to identify. An additional limitation is related to postoperative pain after retroperitoneal surgery. Nadler et al. reported higher subjective pain scores months to years after patients have undergone RPN, they theorize that this is due to proximal disruption of the somatic and cutaneous nerves innervating the abdominal musculature and skin.[24]

14.7 LESS Retroperitoneal Surgery

The retroperitoneal approach may be appealing during LESS procedures since bowel may be held away from the surgical field by the intact peritoneum thereby minimizing the need for additional retraction. In addition, LESS is appealing during retroperitoneal surgery since the surgery is performed entirely through a single incision at the tip of the twelfth rib thus eliminating a potentially painful posterior laparoscopic port.

14.7.1 Indications

The feasibility of LESS retroperitoneal surgery has been reported recently and applied during lap cryoablation, cyst decortication, and partial nephrectomy.[30] The retroperitoneal approach may be appealing for obese patients and those with significant abdominal surgery.

14.7.2 Contraindications

LESS retroperitoneal surgery is contraindicated in patients that have undergone prior retroperitoneal surgery and in patients with large or locally advanced tumors. Additionally, general laparoscopic contraindications apply, and patients with significant cardiopulmonary comorbidity, uncorrected coagulopathy, and abdominal sepsis are excluded.

14.7.3 Preoperative Preparation

Detailed informed patient consent is obtained. Bowel preparation involves two bottles of magnesium citrate self-administered in the afternoon prior to surgery. Intravenous broad-spectrum antibiotics and sequential compression stockings bilaterally are routine.

14.7.4 Operative Steps

14.7.4.1 Positioning

The patient is placed in the full flank position (90°) with the kidney rest elevated and the operative table flexed. This maximizes the space between the iliac crest and the lowermost rib. Arm boards are used to support the upper extremities in a neutral position. All bony prominences are padded and the patient is secured to the table with adhesive tape. The surgeon and assistant stand facing the patient's back.

14.7.4.2 Retroperitoneal Access and Port Placement

Retroperitoneal access is achieved with an open (Hasson) technique. A 1.5-cm transverse skin incision is made at or just below the tip of the 12th rib. The flank muscle fibers are separated with two S-retractors to visualize the anterior thoracolumbar fascia, which is incised to enter the retroperitoneal space with the tip of the index finger. Digital dissection is performed along the anterior surface of the psoas muscle and fascia, posterior to Gerota's fascia (to create a space for the balloon dilator) (Fig. 14.1). A PDB balloon dilator (US Surgical, Norwalk, CT) is inserted into the retroperitoneum and approximately 600 ml of air is instilled in the balloon to create the retroperitoneal space (Fig. 14.2). This maneuver ensures that the peritoneal reflection is mobilized medially. In this manner, the *en bloc* kidney and surrounding Gerota's fascia are mobilized medially, thus exposing the posterior aspect of the renal hilum and the adjacent vessels.

The balloon is subsequently deflated and the single port of choice is utilized according to surgeon preference (Fig. 14.3). A pneumo-retroperitoneal pressure of 15 mmHg is achieved by instilling carbon dioxide through the insufflation channel of the port.

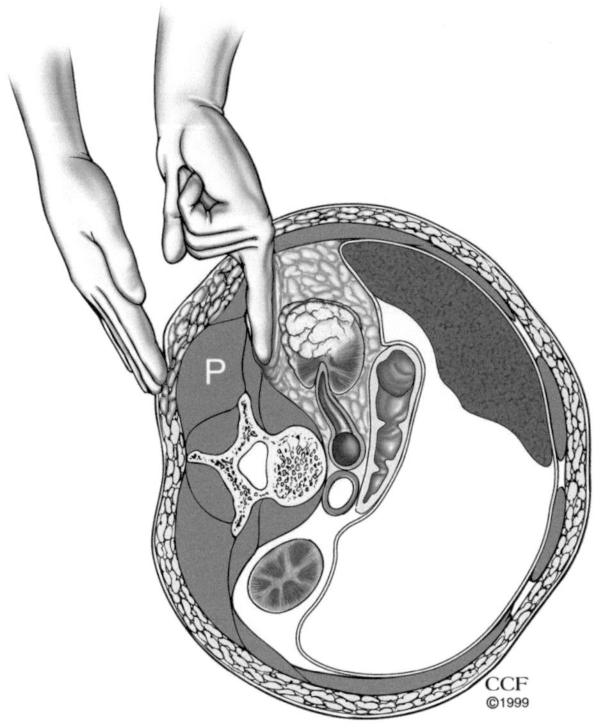

Fig. 14.1 Depiction of development of the retroperitoneal space. The surgeon's finger is inserted at the tip of the 12th rib to develop an initial space through which the balloon dilator will be positioned (PSOAS) (Reprinted with permission, Cleveland Clinic Center for Medical Art & Photography © 1999–2010. All Rights Reserved)

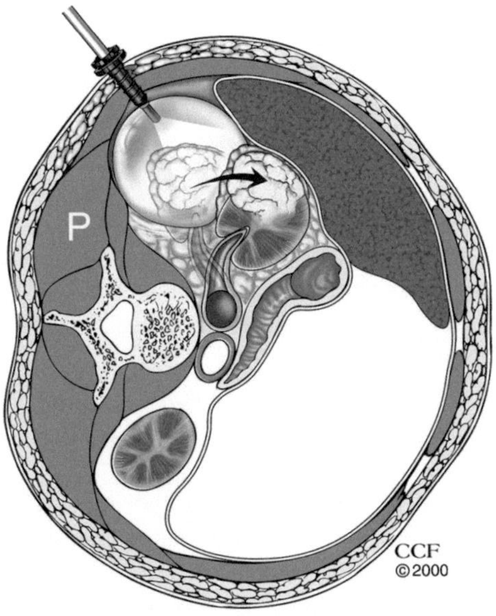

Fig. 14.2 Depiction of development of the retroperitoneal space. The retroperitoneal balloon dilator positioned behind the kidney and anterior to the psoas muscle to create the surgical space (Reprinted with permission, Cleveland Clinic Center for Medical Art & Photography © 1999–2010. All Rights Reserved)

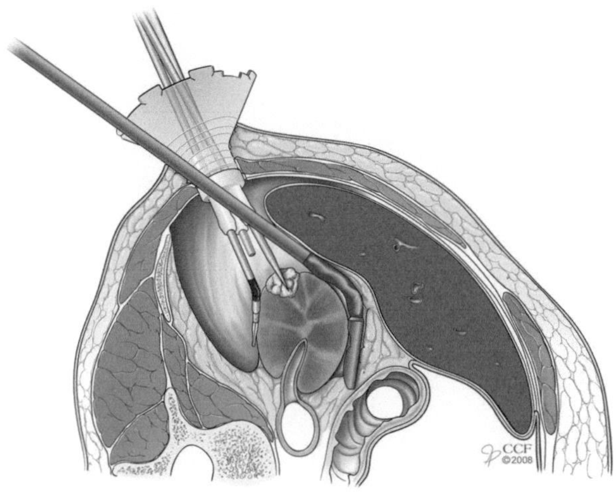

Fig. 14.3 Illustration of the single port and instruments in place during cryoablation (Reprinted with permission, Cleveland Clinic Center for Medical Art & Photography © 1999–2010. All Rights Reserved)

A 5-mm, 0° laparoscope with a flexible tip (Olympus Surgical, Orangeburg, NY) is helpful to avoid clashing of instruments, and assist in identifying the salient landmarks. Given the limited internal space of the retroperitoneum, the use of articulating instruments may minimize the clashing of instruments and maximize the external range of motion.

14.7.4.3 Cryoablation

After creating a retroperitoneal working space the kidney is completely mobilized within Gerota's fascia, exposing the entire renal surface, including the tumor. The perirenal fat overlying the tumor is removed for histopathological examination. Such mobilization of the kidney has two advantages: complete ultrasound examination of entire kidney surface is feasible, and the tumor can be properly aligned for cryoprobe puncture. A 10-mm flexible laparoscopic ultrasound probe is inserted through the fascial defect adjacent to the multichannel port (BK Medical, Denmark).

Under ultrasound guidance, intraoperative biopsy is performed using an 18-gauge Tru-Cut needle (Cardinal Health, Dublin, OH) inserted percutaneously or directly through the multichannel port and sent for permanent section analysis. The tip of the cyroprobe should be advanced up to, or just beyond, the inner margin of the tumor. An appropriately sized cryoprobe (Endocare, Irvine, CA) is placed into the tumor through the operative port. Additional cryoprobes can be introduced percutaneously, as needed. A double freeze–thaw cycle is performed under real-time endoscopic ultrasound monitoring and laparoscopic visualization. Obliteration of vascularity and blood flow within the anechoic ice ball is confirmed by color Doppler. Laparoscopic visualization confirms that the entire exophytic surface of the tumor is covered with the ice ball, including approximately 1 cm of healthy margin (Fig. 14.4).

On removal of the cryoprobes, hemostasis is achieved with a hemostatic agent such as FloSeal (Baxter, Deerfield, IL) and continuous pressure with a Surgicel bolster. The bolster is removed after approximately 10 min, and the probe entrance site is coagulated with the argon beam coagulator as needed. The insufflation pressure is decreased to 0 mmHg, and the operative field is inspected for hemostasis.

14.7.4.4 Partial Nephrectomy

Partial nephrectomy is a relatively complex laparoscopic procedure and should be attempted after experience has already been achieved with other LESS procedures. Patient selection in the above is the utmost importance.

The ureter with surrounding fibro-fatty tissue is mobilized off the anterior surface of the psoas and then laterally retracted. The anterior surface of the psoas is cleared of loose areolar tissue in a cephalad direction to create space for the vascular clamp posterior to the renal hilum. Fibro-fatty tissue in the renal hilum is carefully dissected using a laparoscopic hook dissector to expose the renal artery and vein. Gerota's fascia is entered and the kidney defatted. Under real-time ultrasonographic guidance, the proposed line of tumor excision is circumferentially scored around the tumor with the tip of a monopolar J-hook electrocautery. The oncological adequacy of this scored margin is reconfirmed ultrasonographically prior to initiating tumor resection.

LESS partial nephrectomy has been reported with or without hilar clamping.[20]

The harmonic scalpel (Ethicon Endo-Surgery, Cincinnati, OH) is used to excise the tumor without

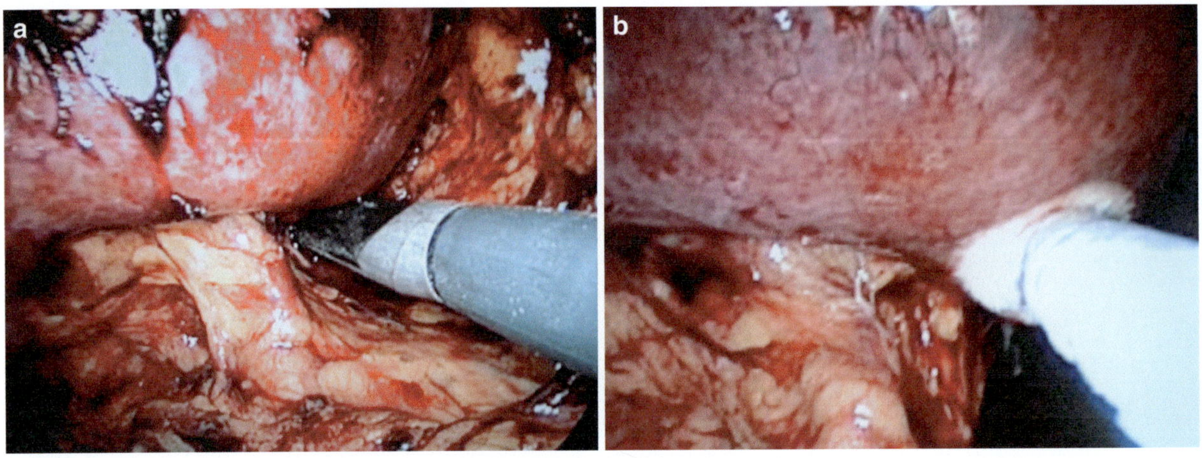

Fig. 14.4 Intraoperative image during left-sided retroperitoneal LESS cryoablation. (**a**) Note the deflectable ultrasound probe scanning the tumor after defatting the kidney. (**b**) Cryoablation probe inserted into the tumor and ice covering the exophytic portion of the renal mass

inducing renal ischemia. The renal hilum is identified and isolated in all cases should vascular control be needed. Hemostasis is achieved using the harmonic scalpel. The entire operative bed is thoroughly coagulated with argon beam. A mixture of hemostatic agents and Surgicel are applied to the defect. The insufflation pressure is decreased to 0 mmHg to assess the adequacy of the hemostasis. The retroperitoneal space is thoroughly irrigated and suctioned free of blood and solution. The specimen is entrapped and extracted through the fascial defect. A Jackson–Pratt drain is introduced through the wound, and the fascia is closed around the drain using one of the previously placed fascial sutures.

14.7.4.5 Renal Cyst Decortication

For patients undergoing cyst decortication, initial access mimics that of partial nephrectomy and cryotherapy. With parapelvic cysts or large cysts in close proximity to the collecting system, cystoscopy is performed and a ureteral catheter placed through which retrograde injection of methylene blue can be performed as needed to identify the collecting system. Subsequently, the patient is positioned and access obtained to the retroperitoneum, as stated previously. After release of the peritoneum, the cyst is identified and incised sharply with endoscopic shears. The roof of the cyst is sent for pathologic evaluation. The base of the cyst is coagulated with the argon beam, and hemostasis is checked as stated previously. Subsequently, the port is removed, and the fascia and skin are closed.

14.8 Postoperative Management

Postoperative management for LESS retroperitoneal surgery does not differ from its straight laparoscopic counterpart. Patients undergoing cryotherapy and cyst decortication are mobilized on the evening of surgery. Two Dulcolax suppositories are administered on the morning of postoperative day 1. In the majority of our cases, the patient is discharged on the evening of postoperative day 1, after resumption of oral fluid intake. Given the developmental nature of cryoablation, follow-up is rigorous to ensure oncological adequacy. Our protocol comprises biochemical and radiological evaluation. The aim of this follow-up is to document continuous shrinkage of the cryoablated tumor without any evidence of tumor growth, lack of shrinkage, or suspicious nodular enhancement. We obtain a computed tomography (CT) scan on postoperative day 1 to obtain a baseline image. Follow-up CT scans are performed at 1, 3, and 6 months and every 6 months thereafter for 2 years followed by yearly CT scanning. Chest X-ray is performed at yearly intervals. Complete blood count and metabolic panel, including serum creatinine, are performed.

Patients undergoing partial nephrectomy are advised strict bed rest for 24 h, followed by gradual mobilization. The ureteral and Foley catheters are removed on the morning of postoperative day 2 as the patient begins ambulation. Following discharge from the hospital, the patient is advised restricted activity for 2 weeks. A MAG-3 radionuclide scan is performed at 1 month to evaluate renal function and assess pelvicaliceal system integrity. In patients with pathologically confirmed renal cancer, a follow-up CT scan and a chest X-ray are obtained at 6 months. Subsequent oncological surveillance is as per the individual pathological tumor stage.

14.9 Outcomes of LESS Retroperitoneal Surgery

14.9.1 Initial Experience

At our institution eight patients underwent LESS retroperitoneal surgery. Cryoablation was performed for five patients and partial nephrectomy for a single patient secondary to radiographic evidence of an enhancing renal mass. An additional patient underwent metastectomy for isolated recurrence of renal cell carcinoma while the remaining patient underwent renal cyst decortication for unrelenting pain.

The LESS retroperitoneal group was then compared retrospectively to a matched, contemporary cohort of patients who had undergone similar procedures using a traditional retroperitoneal laparoscopic approach. No intra- or postoperative complications were noted. The mean hospitalization was 1.4 days. The mean visual analog pain scale score at discharge was 0.4 of 10 (range 0–2). Patients who underwent cryoablation reported lower visual analog pain scale scores ($P = .023$).[30]

14.10 Complications

In our analysis of complications in the initial patients undergoing LESS retroperitoneal partial nephrectomy, cryoablation, cyst decortication, and metastectomy, we did not have any complications. Yet we feel as though the complication rate should not differ from our data reported for similar procedures performed via a standard transperitoneal approach. This includes hemorrhagic complications in 3%, urine leak in 1.5%, and open conversion in 1%, with no perioperative mortality mirroring current open surgical outcomes.

14.11 Future Advancements in LESS Retroperitoneal Surgery

The future of LESS retroperitoneal surgery will most likely involve the introduction of robotic systems. We are still far from having a perfect system and are in the infancy of robotic single-site surgery. The robot that is currently available is bulky and not specific for what is necessary in single-site surgery. The limited range of motion is often frustrating and significant improvement is needed before this technique can diffuse into widespread practice. Advances in the field of robotics will hopefully overcome these limitations and provide improved triangulation, degrees of freedom, dexterity, and visualization, either through miniaturized robots, flexible robotics, or robot- controlled internal retraction platforms.[31]

14.12 Advantages and Pitfalls of the Technique

The primary advantage of retroperitoneal LESS is that it provides an alternative to the traditional laparoscopic retroperitoneal approach with three ports placed and the discomfort and scars which accompany. It appears that the visual analog pain scale scores are less for the LESS retroperitoneal surgery compared to the traditional laparoscopic retroperitoneal surgery.

The pitfalls of this procedure revolve around the need for advanced laparoscopic skills prior to attempting this procedure. We suggest gaining experience with transperitoneal LESS prior to embarking on the LESS retroperitoneal surgery.

Disclosure Funding was not received for this work from any organizations including National Institutes of Health, Wellcome Trust, Howard Hughes Medical Institute, and others.

References

1. Rane A, Rao P, Bonadio F, Rao P. Single port laparoscopic nephrectomy using a novel laparoscopic port (R-port) and evolution of single laparoscopic port procedure (SLIPP). *J Endourol*. 2007;21:A87.
2. Raman JD, Bensalah K, Bagrodia A, et al. Laboratory and clinical development of single keyhole umbilical nephrectomy. *Urology*. 2007;70:1039-1042.
3. Kaouk JH, Haber GP, Goel RK, et al. Single-port laparoscopic surgery in urology: initial experience. *Urology*. 2008;71:3-6.
4. Gill IS, Canes D, Aron M, et al. Single port transumbilical (E-NOTES) donor nephrectomy. *J Urol*. 2008;180:637-641.
5. White WM, Haber GP, Goel RK, et al. Single-port urological surgery: single-center experience with the first 100 cases. *Urology*. 2009;74:801-804.
6. Desai MM, Stein R, Rao P, et al. Embryonic natural orifice transumbilical endoscopic surgery for advanced reconstruction: initial experience. *Urology*. 2009;73(1):182-187.
7. Desai MM, Aron M, Canes D, et al. Single port transvesical simple prostatectomy: initial clinical report. *Urology*. 2008; 72(5):960-965.
8. Sotelo Noguera RJ, Astigueta JC, Carmona O, et al. Laparoscopic augmentation enterocystoplasty through a single trocar. *Urology*. 2009;73(6):1371-1374.
9. Aron M, Canes D, Desai MM, et al. Transumbilical single-port laparoscopic partial nephrectomy. *BJU Int*. 2009; 103(4):516-521.
10. Kaouk JH, Goel RK, Haber GP, et al. Single-port laparoscopic radical prostatectomy. *Urology*. 2008;72(6):1190-1193.
11. Ponsky LE, Cherullo EE, Sawyer M, et al. Single access site radical nephrectomy: initial clinical experience. *J Endourol*. 2008;22:663-666.
12. Stolzenburg JU, Kallidonis P, Hellawell G, et al. Technique of laparo-endoscopic single-site surgery radical nephrectomy. *Eur Urol*. 2009;56(4):644-650. Epub 2009 Jun 23.
13. Raman JD, Caddedu JA, Rao P, et al. Single incision laparoscopic surgery: initial urological experience and comparison with natural-orifice transluminal endoscopic surgery. *BJU Int*. 2008;101(12):1493-1496.
14. Rane A, Rao P, Rao P. Single port access nephrectomy and other laparoscopic urologic procedures using a novel laparoscopic port (R-Port). *Urology*. 2008;72(2):260-263.
15. Kaouk JH, Palmer JS. Single-port laparoscopic surgery: initial experience in children for varicocelectomy. *BJU Int*. 2008;102:97-99.
16. Kaouk JH, Goel RK. Single port laparoscopic pelvic surgery: a scar-less approach. Abstract presented at: Annual meeting of the society of gastrointestinal and endoscopic surgeons; April 9–12, 2008; Philadelphia, PA. Abstract 201.
17. Msezane LP, Mushtaq I, Gundeti MS. An update on experience with the single instrument port laparoscopic nephrectomy. *BJU Int*. 2009;103(10):1406-1409.
18. Kaouk JH, Goel RK, Haber GP, et al. Robotic single-port transumbilical surgery in humans: initial report. *BJU Int*. 2009;103(3):366-369.
19. Barret E, Sanchez-Salas R, Kasraeian A, et al. A transition to laparoendoscopic single-site surgery (LESS) radical prostatectomy: human cadaver experimental and initial clinical experience. *J Endourol*. 2009;23(1):135-140.
20. Kaouk JH, Goel RK. Single-port laparoscopic and robotic partial nephrectomy. *Eur Urol*. 2009;55(5):1163-1169.
21. Stein RJ, White WM, Goel RK, et al. Robotic laparoendoscopic single-site surgery using gelport as the access platform. *Eur Urol*. 2009;57(1):132-136. Epub 2009 Mar 31.
22. Nambirajan T, Jeschke S, Al-zahrani H, et al. Prospective, randomized controlled study: transperitoneal laparoscopic versus retroperitoneoscopic radical nephrectomy. *Urology*. 2004;64:919-924.
23. Desai MM, Strzempkowski B, Matin SF, et al. Prospective randomized comparison of transperitoneal versus retroperitoneal laparoscopic radical nephrectomy. *J Urol*. 2005; 173:38-41.
24. Nadler RB, Loeb S, Clemens JQ, Batler RA, Gonzalez CM, Vardi IY. A prospective study of laparoscopic radical nephrectomy for T1 tumors: is transperitoneal, retroperitoneal of hand assisted the best approach? *J Urol*. 2006;175: 1230-1234.
25. Berdjis N, Hakenberg OW, Leike S, et al. Comparison of transperitoneal versus retroperitoneal approach in laparoscopic radical nephrectomy for renal cell carcinoma: a single-center experience of 63 cases. *Urol Int*. 2006;77: 166-167.
26. Berglund RK, Gill IS, Babineau D, Desai M, Kaouk JH. A prospective comparison of transperitoneal and retroperitoneal laparoscopic nephrectomy in the extremely obese patient. *BJU Int*. 2007;99:871-874.
27. McDougall EM, Clayman RV. Laparoscopic nephrectomy for benign disease: comparison of the transperitoneal and retroperitoneal approaches. *J Endourol*. 1996;10:45-49.
28. Okegawa T, Noda H, Horie S, et al. Comparison of transperitoneal and retroperitoneal laparoscopic nephrectomy for renal cell carcinoma: a single-center experience of 100 cases. *Int J Urol*. 2008;15:957-960.
29. Colombo JR, Haber GP, Aron M, et al. Laparoscopic partial nephrectomy in obese patients. *Urology*. 2007;69:44-48.
30. White WM, Goel RK, Kaouk JH. Single-port laparoscopic retroperitoneal surgery: initial operative experience and comparative outcomes. *Urology*. 2009;73(9):1279-1282.
31. Canes D, Lehman AC, Farritor, et al. The future of NOTES instrumentation: flexible robotics and in vivo minirobots. *J Endourol*. 2009;23(5):787-792.

On the Horizon

15

Jean V. Joseph and Hitendra R. H. Patel

Abstract Laparoscopy and robotic surgery have provided much excitement in our operating theaters over the last two decades. Continued technological improvements have added a number of new tools to our surgical armamentarium promising to better the care we deliver to our patients. From open surgery, to multiport laparoscopic surgery, to needlescopic, and most recently to single-port surgery, the ultimate goal remains to lessen the insult associated with surgical intervention. Herein we address several technological innovations that will continue to change how we operate. The challenges associated with surgical innovation are also addressed.

Keywords Augmented reality • Future robots • Minimally invasive urology • Surgical innovation • Technology

Key Points

- Laparoscopy and robotic surgery continue to evolve.
- Current robots are in a growth phase.
- Technology that further augments the surgical reality are necessary, to allow surgeons to use all available information.
- Surgical innovation will continue to be disruptive, rendering techniques referred to as gold standard obsolete.
- Proper multidisciplinary collaboration is necessary to ensure safe evaluation of new technologies.

Minimally invasive urology continues to evolve at a staggering pace. Within a short time period we have gone from open to laparoscopic, and to robot-assisted procedures. Robots, which were recently being developed for military purposes, are now commonplace in our operating rooms. In less than a decade, we have witnessed the evolution of robotic systems, with newer generations promising and delivering greater agility, improving a surgeon's ability to perform complex surgical tasks. The success story of robotic technology in surgery has rather been a story of serendipity. Similarly, the adoption of the technology in urology has also been one of serendipity as the technology was developed for cardiac surgery. As we glimpse over the horizon, there are a number of technologies in development geared for surgical applications. Our prediction is that for one reason or another a handful of these will succeed, while serendipitous successful applications will continue to redefine our work.

J.V. Joseph (✉)
Head-Section of Urologic Laparoscopy and Robotic Surgery, Department of Urology Wilmot Cancer Center, Center for Robotic Surgery and Innovation, University of Rochester Medical Center, Rochester, NY, USA
e-mail: jean_joseph@urmc.rochester.edu

J.V. Joseph and H.R.H. Patel (eds.), *Retroperitoneal Robotic and Laparoscopic Surgery*,
DOI: 10.1007/978-0-85729-485-2_15,

Although we are in awe when we look at the improved visualization afforded by high-definition endoscopes, or when we look into the three-dimensional, high-definition view of the da Vinci robot, we can speculate that these technologies are in a growth phase. They have improved the view for the surgeons, but have yet to augment the surgical reality. The surgeon operates only based on visual cues targeting a predefined problem. Current robots improve surgical dexterity through motion scaling and tremor filtration. Coarse movements made at the surgical console are converted into fine delicate manipulations of the instruments positioned inside the patient. The range of motion provided by the available robotic system, along with the added precision and dexterity previously mentioned, go well beyond what can be provided by available videoendoscope systems, or the human hand. They facilitate dissection and suturing in anatomical areas that are not easily accessible. They have, however, in the process nullified the surgeon's sense of touch. The loss of proprioception has been perhaps the greatest source of criticism from opponents of robotic surgery. Haptic feedback is necessary to allow a surgeon to regain the sense of touch.

Robots of the future will allow a surgeon to make the most of all their senses, beyond the visual cues, to obtain relevant information from the surgical site, and go beyond giving the feel of open surgery. They will not only improve the view, but also provide the surgeon with intrinsic anatomical details. They will allow differentiation between tissues from one organ to another, differentiation of nerves from blood or lymphatic vessels, overall improving a surgeon's diagnostic capability.

Single-port surgery, whether with pure laparoscopic or robot-assisted, will likely become more widespread. Advanced laparoscopists are adopting this modality. There have been a number of reports of a variety of urologic procedures performed using single-port access.[1] A variety of trocars and instruments have been developed to facilitate this. One of the main difficulties of single-port surgery is the inability to triangulate at the target organ. Laparoscopic or robotic trocars are generally placed to facilitate triangulation. The surgery becomes counterintuitive, as the instrument on the surgeon's right hand is positioned on the left side, and vice versa inside the patient. A robotic single-port system, which is not yet approved by the Food and Drug Administration (FDA), is currently available for the da Vinci Si, promising to allow surgeon to overcome this difficulty. The developed cannulae are curved and crossed at the entry point, allowing triangulation at the target. The computer interface corrects the laterality such that the instruments on one side are controlled by the surgeon's hand on the same side (Fig. 15.1).

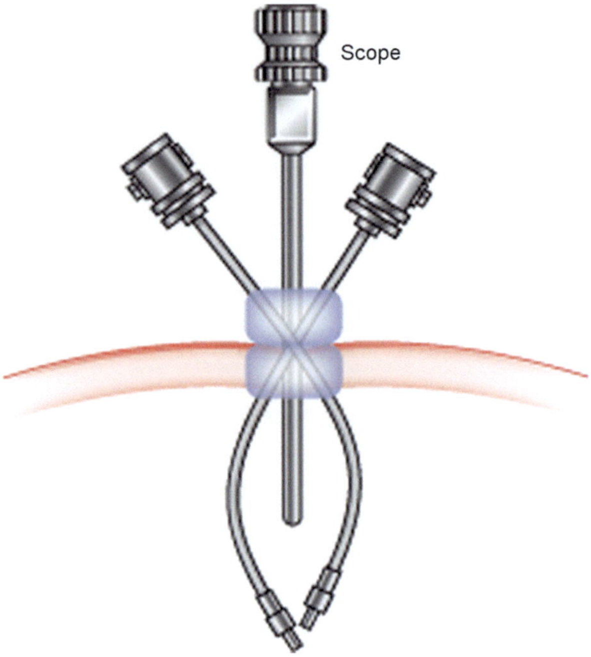

Fig. 15.1 Diagram of curved cannulae for single-port surgery

15.1 Augmenting the Surgical Reality

Current videoendoscopic and robotic systems allow the surgeon a superb, well-defined view of the surgical field. However, no detailed anatomy is provided regarding the structure or contour of a particular structure. The surgeon only has access to the information exposed at the surface, or what can be gathered directly from intraoperative visual cues. The future of surgery will be targeted toward rendering opaque organs transparent to the surgeon. Structures rendered invisible by overlying fat, important vital anatomy, margins of infiltrating tumor can be made visible through augmented reality.

The incorporation of tile protechnology in the latest robot generations has been a significant leap forward in augmenting the visual cues available to the surgeon. A live ultrasound image can be incorporated in the surgeon's screen showing details of the surgical field.

This tool has found its greatest application in nephron sparing surgery where it allows robotic surgeons to better delineate the extent of a tumor prior to its resection. The surgeon however relies on the bedside assistant to insert and navigate the ultrasound probe. Future technology may perhaps allow this to be an integral part of the surgeon's instrument, where maneuvering this device can be carried out just as a surgeon toggles to take control over the fourth arm of the robot.

Augmented reality systems have been commonplace in neurosurgery where "stereotactic surgery" is routinely performed. Preoperative imaging is used to target treatment for specific brain lesions with great accuracy. The rigid skull limits motion and facilitates reconstruction of the surgical anatomy in three dimensions. Abdominal surgery, on the other hand, requires abdominal insufflation, which alters anatomical location. In addition, diaphragmatic excursions, surgical manipulation, make any preoperative surgical mapping significantly unreliable. The organ is in constant motion. Live imaging systems taking into account these limiting factors are needed for abdominal surgery. Imaging modalities such as computed tomography (CT) scan and magnetic resonance imaging (MRI), which are routinely used for diagnostic purposes, are not readily available in the operating room. Due to its versatility and ease of use, ultrasound remains the most commonly used imaging modality, despite its limitations.

To overcome the current limitations of augmented reality in the abdominal cavity, body-GPS systems and surgical radars are being developed to assist in surgical navigation. Real-time serial imaging is necessary to allow effective tracking with dynamic reconstruction of the target organ, taking into account organ displacement and changes in anatomy as the surgery progresses. With surgical tracking, the surgeon can potentially sets the instruments to provide a warning, or to stop when the dissection is in excess, or strays from the preset target. The extent of a surgical resection can perhaps be set to the same accuracy, as the focal shock zone is set on a lithotripsy unit. Alternatively developments are underway using agents that selectively target a potential tumor, facilitating its identification, ensuring the dissection plane avoids violation of the tumor margins. These will ensure the true meaning of minimally invasive surgery where only the disease organ is extirpated. In nephron-sparing surgery, the surgeon can remove only the diseased tissues, leaving as much healthy kidney as possible unaltered.

Collateral damage can also be avoided in procedures such as prostatectomy, where identification of the cavernous nerves and sphincteric muscles can further assist in their preservation. Work is underway with agents that can be administered, which are selectively taken by nerve tissues to allow their visual identification. Information on the conductive properties of tissues can be obtained in real time to help the surgeon decides whether a neurovascular bundle is being encroached. Similarly tactile feeling and information on tissue vascularity can help a surgeon identify a tumor. Sensors can help differentiate between normal tissues versus abnormal ones. Ultimately tumor markers coupled with visible dye can help identify the location of the tumor and the presence of disease extension, requiring a wider excision and improving cure rates.

15.2 Beyond the Bulky Tools

Current day laparoscopic and robotic systems are bulky. Despite recent modifications of the available robotic systems, they remain large and bulky occupying significant space in an already crowded operating room. Microrobots have been designed to overcome some of these challenges. In collaboration with surgeons and engineers from the University of Nebraska, we have previously used microrobots in an animal model to perform a laparoscopic nephrectomy and prostatectomy.[2] These microrobots, when placed inside the abdominal cavity, provide an additional view, or an extra frame of reference, which potentially enhance the cues available to the surgeon (Fig. 15.2). Initial prototypes were cumbersome with a cord transmitting signals out of the abdominal cavity. Recent prototypes have been tetherless, adding to their versatility. In their current state, however, these microrobots are not ready for our surgical armamentarium. If equipped with sensors capable of providing information on tissue composition, consistency, temperature, oxygen status, and conductivity, they can add significant value justifying their use. Perhaps they can be equipped with instruments that can be deployed when needed to perform specific surgical tasks. While this may be seen as only theoretical presently, one must be reminded of wireless capsule endoscopy, which is currently in everyday use. In 2001 the FDA approved the Given Diagnostic Imaging System. The capsule is ingested and transmits

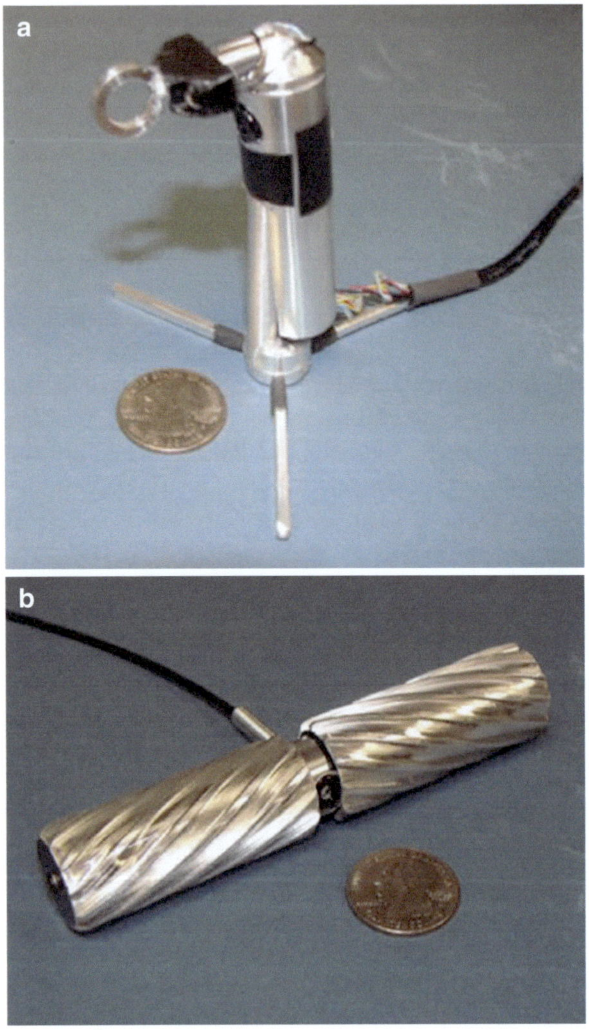

Fig. 15.2 (**a**) Pan-tilt and (**b**) crawler microrobot prototypes

views of the gastrointestinal tract as it passes from one segment to another, propelled by peristalsis. It is made of biocompatible material that can withstand the acidity of stomach fluid, and the destructive power of digestive enzymes. The capsule is smooth and easily swallowed, with patients reporting it being easier to swallow than aspirin. Images are sent to a recording device, until the capsule passes without any discomfort with a bowel movement.

Scaling down further, true microrobots barely noticeable to the human eye may eventually become available for clinical use. Microendoscopic trocar systems with instruments-oriented electronically using fluid have been developed. These devices measuring 0.6 mm in diameter can be oriented to specific locations targeting pathologies. Micrograspers and scissors, which can be controlled electronically, are available to perform specific tasks.[3]

Robots at the nanoscale or nanorobots may eventually see their way in routine urological care. Just as the aforementioned capsule makes its way in the alimentary tract, nanorobots may be placed in the bloodstream, designed to travel to different targets, performing diagnostic and therapeutic maneuvers. They can potentially be designed to deliver drugs or clean an obstructed blood vessel. Nanorobots will eventually allow us to work at the cellular or molecular level, ushering unprecedented forms of intervention. In the postgenome coding era, nubots or nucleic acid robots may eventually make their appearance in clinical care, allowing physicians to intervene by altering genetic-based abnormalities.

15.3 Pace of Surgical Innovation

Over the last decade we have seen a flurry of new technology in our operating rooms. The pace of surgical innovation has been unparalleled. New products emerge, while some not fully mature are put aside. Disruptive innovation can be used to categorize many of the products we currently use. This term is used to describe innovations that have led to improvement in ways that mainstream users did not expect.

Although experienced laparoscopic surgeons performed early cases of robotic surgery, the technology was embraced primarily by laparoscopy-naïve surgeons. The use of robotic surgery has been much simpler and easier to adopt. While training remains essential, the skills required for a laparoscopist to perform a partial nephrectomy on an intrarenal hilar lesion are far more than those required from a trained robotic surgeon. The feasibility of laparoscopy to perform complex procedures was demonstrated, but the complexity of the technique itself prevents it from disrupting mainstream open surgeons the way robotic surgery has done. Most laparoscopic and open surgeons had been content in performing or improving the procedures they routinely perform. Market forces or patient demand have been the main drivers of this disruption. As is seen in other industries, institutions with a strong reputation in open surgery were slow to explore laparoscopic applications. Similarly, those with laparoscopic expertise have often been unwilling to explore robotic surgery. In this information age, the traditional pace of innovation in medicine, slow and incremental, has been rapidly changing. While we all seek to improve our work, it remains our responsibility to best serve our patients, providing high level of evidence on any new or potentially disruptive innovation prior to its adoption.

Medical advances in cardiology have led to widespread use of stents in the management of coronary artery disease, significantly reducing the number of cardiac bypass graft surgeries performed, the original target operation for the da Vinci robot. While deliberate pursuit of technology will lead to newer and better tools, emerging technology often being developed for a completely unrelated discipline is likely to come forth fulfilling an unintended need. Collaboration between surgeons, inventors, industry, and government as for the da Vinci robot is necessary to take advantage of potentially beneficial technology.

15.4 Conclusions

Laparoscopy and robotic technology were first applied to several other disciplines. The growth of these minimally invasive approaches, particularly robotic surgery, has been most profound in urology. Computer-enhanced instrumentation will undoubtedly continue to help surgeons improve the care they deliver to their patients. In less than two decades, we have seen procedures hailed as "gold standard" practically used only when there are contraindications or a skilled minimally invasive surgeon is not available. The pace of surgical innovation will continue to be disruptive. The danger has been when innovators clinging on to their own innovations, gathering data on ways to further perfect their innovation, do not give a fair and objective appraisal of competing innovations. In the quest of minimal invasiveness, to improve patient care while avoiding harm, we should be poised to disrupt ourselves, or our own innovations, and critically assess promising technologies looming on the horizon.

References

1. Stein RJ, White WM, Goel RK, Irwin BH, Haber GP, Kaouk JH. Robotic Laparoendoscopic single-site surgery using gelport as the access platform. *Eur Urol.* 2010;57: 132-137.
2. Joseph JV, Oleynikov D, Rentschler M, Dumpert J, Patel HRH. Microrobot assisted laparoscopic surgery in a canine model. *J Urol.* 2008;180:2202-2205.
3. Schurr MO, Heyn SP, Menz W, Buess G. Endosystems-future perspectives for endoluminal surgery. *Minim Invasive Ther Allied Technol.* 1998;7:37-42.

Index

J.V. Joseph and H.R.H. Patel (eds.), *Retroperitoneal Robotic and Laparoscopic Surgery*,
DOI: 10.1007/978-0-85729-485-2, © Springer-Verlag London Limited 2011

MIX
Papier aus verantwortungsvollen Quellen
Paper from responsible sources
FSC® C105338

If you have any concerns about our products,
you can contact us on
ProductSafety@springernature.com

In case Publisher is established outside the EU,
the EU authorized representative is:
Springer Nature Customer Service Center GmbH
Europaplatz 3, 69115 Heidelberg, Germany

Printed by Libri Plureos GmbH
in Hamburg, Germany